HEALTHIER LIVING
HIGHLIGHTS

HEALTHIER LIVING HIGHLIGHTS

A College Text in Personal and Environmental Health

Justus J. Schifferes, PH. D.

Director, Health Education Council; Formerly: Medical Editor,
National Foundation for Infantile Paralysis; Associate in Hygiene,
Columbia College; Instructor in Health Education, Teachers
College, Columbia University

With the editorial assistance of

James M. Pryde

American River College

John Wiley & Sons. Inc.   New York   London   Sydney   Toronto

TO MY FAMILY
Cecile, Stephen, Sande

A Health Education Council Book

Books by Justus J. Schifferes include

Essentials of Healthier Living
Third Edition

Healthier Living
Third Edition

The illustration on the cover is a New York State Department of Commerce Photo. The frontispiece is by John H. Atkinson, Jr./DPI

Library of Congress Catalogue Card Number: 73-142141

ISBN 0-471-76070-6

Printed in the United States of America.

10 9 8 7 6 5 4 3 2 1

PREFACE

THIS SHORT NEW BOOK, *Healthier Living Highlights,* HAS BEEN PREPARED TO MEET a demand in some colleges for a less extensive (and less expensive) text for a basic course in health education.

This book is the seventh in the series of *Healthier Living* texts: the original edition, 1954; revised editions, 1965 and 1970; and three briefer versions (but not so brief as the present book), *Essentials of Healthier Living,* 1960, 1963, and 1967. *Healthier Living Highlights* retains editorial features that prompted adoption of the earlier versions in some 250 colleges and universities in the United States.

This new text should prove particularly useful in courses which labor under severe time pressure, that is, courses in which there is barely enough classroom time for instruction in the highlight topics of modern health education—drugs, mental health, sexual problems, nutrition, smoking, and environmental health (ecology).

To meet the needs of such courses, this book covers the main fields of college health education but does not include all topics presented in earlier editions. It is divided into five major parts, which may be considered the major concerns of present-day health education. These are (1) mental health, (2) personal health, (3) family living, (4) health hazards, and (5) environmental health. A more detailed view of each topic can be gleaned from the Table of Contents.

The basic premises on which this book is written are time-tested. To quote briefly from prefaces of earlier editions:

"This is a book on health, not disease. It stands on the premise that promotion of health, for which you may read happiness, is something different from and beyond the prevention of disease, though not completely divorced from it.

"I see the aim of modern health education as that of inspiring a course of human conduct illumined by an understanding of the structure and function of the human body. . . . But bodily function is modified and controlled by the human mind and emotions and it takes place within a social framework. I have given fuller consideration, therefore, to the social factors that play upon mind and body and thus account for bodily function or malfunction (disease)."

This book seeks to stimulate and motivate readers to wise health behavior, based on well-marshalled scientific facts and well-considered attitudes. Hence it does not preach. On many important but unresolved health issues, it frankly presents pro-and-con opinions, drawn from recent authoritative sources. It is left to the reader—the student—to come to intelligent, personal decisions in his health conduct.

No textbook can take the place of good teaching, but I hope that this book may make good teaching easier. The Summary Review Questions at the end of each chapter should help in this direction. So should the striking illustrations in the text and the "Glossary and Selective Dictionary of Common Medical Terms."

A text such as this must draw its facts from many sources. These have been duly credited in earlier editions, in instructor's manuals, in footnotes, and in the "Chapter References and Bibliography" at the end of the book. I also want to acknowledge the help of James Pryde in readying this text for collegiate use.

It is my hope that this text—with its carefully chosen subject matter, its scientific background, and its lucid style of presentation—may lead a substantial number of students along the way to healthier living.

Justus J. Schifferes, Ph.D.
Livingston, New Jersey
January 1971

CONTENTS

PART FIVE ENVIRONMENTAL HEALTH

HEALTHIER LIVING
HIGHLIGHTS

1

MENTAL HEALTH: MIND AND BODY

MANY DEFINITIONS OF "MENTAL HEALTH" have been attempted. A simple and sensible concept is that proposed by Freud: a person is mentally healthy to the extent that he can *love* and *work*. Conversely, he is mentally ill to the degree that he *cannot* love or work. This concept leaves a wide range for normal behavior. It also suggests that, just as perfect happiness comes to no one, even so no one is ever in perfect mental health all the time. Imperfection is the distinctive badge of the human race, and we are wise when we acknowledge this about ourselves.

The mentally healthy person has learned to live with the frustrations of human existence, but they do not disenchant him from continuing the struggle. He accepts the fact that human beings will make mistakes so long as they keep trying. He keeps his tolerance for frustration, disappointment, and grief at a high level. He also realizes that the ancient Socratic doctrine, "Know thyself," is at the heart of mental health but that it is a hard doctrine to apply.

If one really knows himself, he knows his own weaknesses, shortcomings, and failures. Yet the humility to accept these shortcomings is rare. Dr. Karl Menninger has put it this way: "That curious emotional defense which impels some people to believe themselves exempt from all failure, from all weakness, from the taboo of 'abnormality,' is perhaps the greatest enemy of healthy-mindedness."

We must not think of mental health as a sheer abstraction. It has a locale in the body and mind of each individual. But problems arise if we attempt to assign exact bodily locations to the multitudinous functions of the mind and emotions. The best we can say is that these functions occur in or are mediated by the human nervous systems, sometimes assisted by the endocrine system. We shall seek later in this chapter to provide a brief description of the human nervous systems and, beyond that, to offer some explanation of the physiology of thought and feeling.

Mental health is a 24-hour-a-day possession. It is present during sleep as well as waking. Indeed, one of the positive indications of lack of mental health is constantly disturbed sleep—sleeplessness or insomnia. In the mentally healthy man or woman there is a regular cycle of sleep and wakefulness. Throughout all of this the unconscious mind remains in operation. Since sleep and rest are critical factors in mental health, we shall also deal with these subjects later in this chapter.

Toward Conscious Control of Unconscious Forces

Human beings have the power to think and reason and to govern their actions, within limits, by the higher faculties of the mind. 'Schools' of philosophy have exalted man's reason implying that mankind could attain Utopia through the exercise of reason. But it has always been sensed, and twentieth-century research in psychiatry and psychology has clearly demonstrated, that human conduct is never completely reasonable. Motives for conduct are always a mixture of conscious thought and unconscious or preconscious impulses in undiscoverable proportions.

The unconscious motives in behavior are often described as emotional reactions.

The value of conscious thought and reasonable effort in directing our behavior, in opening new horizons, and in illuminating new goals for us should never be discounted or negated. But we must also recognize that deep in the psyche unconscious, emotional forces are constantly at work to modify, influence, and sometimes overwhelm our intellectual powers.

To know this in general, and to pinpoint it as far as possible for our own particular psyche, is to take a great step forward in achieving conscious control of our unconscious drives. The control will never be complete, but it will usually be adequate to get along in the world and sustain reasonable achievement. Serious failure of the conscious mind to control the unconscious forces by which it is besieged and bombarded can result in such life tragedies as mental illness, "purposive accidents," suicide, chronic alcoholism, narcotic addiction, antisocial and even criminal behavior.

The Unconscious Mind. To understand why people think, feel, speak, and act the way they do we must grasp the concept of the unconscious mind. To anticipate a fuller description in the following chapter, we shall give a very brief résumé at this point.

The unconscious mind is the repository of thoughts and feelings of which we are unaware. It files and remembers (but does not necessarily release to conscious memory) *all* our past experience. Indeed, it releases comparatively little, largely because we *want* to forget or repress unpleasant memories. We can assign a *theoretical* structure to the unconscious mind which helps to comprehend its operation.

The unconscious mind is assumed to consist of three parts: *id, ego,* and *superego.* The id may be said to represent the primitive drives and instincts of the human being. The ego represents the conscious self, which makes contact with reality and tries to keep the demands of the id in tune and touch with the real world. The superego is, crudely, the conscience, which also seeks to direct the ego.

The ego has a tough job. It must seek to satisfy the demands of the id, the superego, and external reality at the same time. To protect itself, the ego must adopt defenses; it must find compromise solutions which at least temporarily stabilize conflict in the unconscious mind and permit the individual to carry on. These compromises are often called mental mechanisms. The ego represents that part of the psyche which looks, acts, and builds toward individual satisfactions and socially commendable achievements in human life.

Interaction of Mind and Body

Physical health and mental health are certainly intertwined. For purposes of discussion we may separate mind (psyche) and body (soma), but in the everyday business of living they are indivisible. What we think and feel, consciously or unconsciously, is reflected in the cells of our bodies. Consider, for example, the shiver of fear and the blush of shame. Conversely, damage, deprivation, or disorder of the body affects the mind. Take, for instance, the delirium produced by high fever. Furthermore, our feelings and conduct can be drastically altered by drugs—for example, alcohol, narcotics, tranquilizers, and cerebral stimulants. These are fairly extreme examples. A more subtle interaction goes on all the time under the mediation, regulation, and control of the two important integrative systems of the body—the nervous system and the endocrine system.

The simple principles for maintaining a reasonably good state of physical health—adequate diet, sufficient rest and exercise, attention to warning signals of disease—apply also the quest for mental health. One cannot pursue mental health as if it were a butterfly to be caught in a net. Indeed constant concern over health is itself unhealthy. One attains and maintains mental health by indirection. The positive steps are outward. A person in a good state of mental health is identified by the fact that he enjoys good personal and social relationships with other people. He is not brooding about himself, nor introspectively exploring the state of his unconscious mind. He is living out, within the framework of the culture around him, something that may be called a satisfying and mature philosophy of life.

An excellent summary and overview of the problems of and opportunities for mental health was presented at the International Conference on Health and Health Education held in Philadelphia in July 1962 by Dr. Cyrille Koupernik, of the Children's Clinic of the Neuropsychiatric Faculty of Medicine in Paris. The essence of Dr. Koupernik's observations (originally in French and with some emendations and additions [in brackets] by this writer and translator) is as follows:

The whole idea of "mental hygiene" [or mental health as we prefer to call it in the United States] is relatively recent. It is more difficult to formulate both the methods and limitations of this area of preventive medicine than those of more traditional fields. Smallpox, tuberculosis, and poliomyelitis are ills which afflict mankind without regard to any of cultural, social, or ethical conceptions. But even on questions of diet, as a result of differences in climate around the globe, it is impossible to arrive at a unanimity of opinion. To expect any unanimity on the specific goals of mental health is doubly difficult. [The difficulty in setting standards or criteria to determine who is and who is not mentally healthy is highlighted in an 8-year study, published in 1962 under the title *Mental Health in the Metropolis* in which it is averred that only one out of every 5 adults aged 20–59 living in a particular section of midtown Manhattan can be considered as "essentially well" in terms of mental health.]

Nevertheless there is general agreement on these three points:

1. [Good] mental health permits the healthy development of the individual [his spirit and even soul, if you will; and respects individual differences between people and peoples].
2. At the same time a [good program of mental health] favors the integration of the individual in the group within which he is destined to live.

Since every individual will eventually leave the family group into which he is born, a third valid goal of mental health might well be to teach him gradually how to live in the world outside his immediate family, and to prepare him for the "world of tomorrow" in which he must inevitably live.

3. Finally, it must be recognized that our traditional concepts [in this relatively new discipline of mental hygiene] are applicable principally to Western societies and culture, which have certain [built-in] traditions which it is imprudent to expect to change [overnight]. Optimism about rapidly altering the current concepts of Western civilization are [to put it mildly] unjustified.

The goal of modern mental health has apparently been a [negative one]: not to return to the dogmatic and authoritarian concepts of the Victorian era. But we should not move toward the reverse excess and affirm that truth resides only in the concept of *laissez-faire*.

From the [psychoanalytically oriented teachings of the past half century—the teachings of Freud—viewed as a method of research rather than a method of therapy, and greatly revised since their original pronouncements]—we can accept certain principles as well established. These include:

¶ Most important, the demonstrated need of the infant and child for love and affection. It cannot be repeated too often that the child needs to love and be loved as its natural right, and that no other institution can replace the family for this indispensable end—certain political theories (Spartan and *kibbutzim*, for example) notwithstanding.

¶ Equal recognition of the fact that there are [normal] periods and points of discomfort and inquietude in the evolution of the infant toward maturity. We must accept the facts that infants usually begin to refuse proffered food at about the age of six months (this, however, appears to be a problem principally in the "well-developed" nations of the world); that they develop sleeping difficulties (possibly because their physiologically geared sleeping habits are not in phase with the socially dictated sleeping habits of the older members of their families); that a "negativism" and crisis of opposition to authority usually develops during the second or third year of life; that a [set of feelings] is often crystallized in a refusal to abide by social proprieties; that jealousy of an older child toward a younger brother or sister (an interloper in the family system) is almost inevitable; that children at about the age of three years become notably interested in their bodies, including their sex organs, and in the sexual life of adults.

It is not necessary, however, for parents to give preschool children exhaustive explanations of adult sex relations and the mysteries of procreation—for the intelligence of children at this age cannot comprehend the genuine and mature significance of this subject. However, the young child should not be so shielded from all knowledge of human anatomy and reproduction that he becomes an object of derision to his schoolmates (from whom he is all too likely to obtain distorted versions of sexual matters which may have unforeseen consequences on his later development toward a full heterosexual maturity in love relationships).

Writers, teachers, and parents must avoid creating a sense of anxiety about [sex matters] among their readers, students, and children. They must be equally blameless of inculcating others with a sense of guilt or forcing them into unnatural attitudes about these matters.

In dealing with the problems that agitate adolescents we should not forget that the educative process is a [two-way street], and that unless we listen attentively to their problems and complaints we are more likely to aggravate than to diminish the conflicts between older and younger generations.

Teamwork for Mental Health Is Vital. The concept of teamwork among professional disciplines and cooperation between peoples is vital to any scheme of mental health. The field of mental health and human relations is far from being the exclusive property of the physician or even of "technicians" trained in the methods of psychotherapy—orthodox Freudian, psychobiologic, or somewhere in between. It may even be argued that the physician, trained in objective observations of facts, is less well trained than members of some other professions,[1] notably the social caseworker and the clinical psychologist, in dealing with problems of general psychotherapy and human relations.

Professionals in the field of mental health must thoroughly appreciate what an illness means to its victim. The sick man feels sick, and his feelings must be respected. He must not be looked upon as a field of battle upon which one team (or school) of psychiatric creed will win a "victory" over rival schools.

The revolution in psychiatry and psychiatric treatment which began with Freud is not to be wiped out; but the Freudians (especially since the advent of a new psychopharmacology in the 1950's) can no longer assume the role of the only legitimate priests and prophets in the further development of the mental health of individuals, communities, and nations. The help of all professional groups, psychologists, physicians, social workers, teachers, nurses, parents, and others, and of the people themselves, is necessary if the high goals of mental health are ever to be achieved. With such cooperation mental hygiene is not a vain hope but rather a major weapon in the armament with which mankind can fight successfully against the mounting menace of its mental ills.

Some Principles of Mental Health

There is no "magic formula" for personal happiness or mental health. The positive tenets of mental health can be expressed in the same words as the age-old ethical teachings of all great religions. The Golden Rule—"Do unto others as you would have them do unto you"—is one of the greatest recipes for mental health, unless, of course, this great moral axiom is itself neuroti-

[1]A sign in the window of a busy bar in Washington, D.C., once read: "Quick service inside. Four 'psychiatrists' in constant attendance."

cally abused. The difficulty is not to put the principles of mental health into words but rather to put them into practice. This every individual must do for himself.

We offer the following simple principles for improving mental health and decreasing the burden of what Freud called "everyday unhappiness":

Have faith in something beyond yourself.
Show appreciation to and of other people.
Face your responsibilities.
Live one day at a time—in "daytight compartments."
Set your life in order.
Lead your own life.
Don't take your troubles and your negative feelings out on other people.
Strike a balance of work, play, love, and worship in the daily cycle of your activities.

Emotions

It would be naive to think that any human being can consistently and invariably follow the simple principles of mental health just set forth or any other valid statement of similar "good advice." Emotions, positive and negative, are constantly breaking in upon our conscious striving for a happy, well-adjusted life. A favorable balance can be struck; but we cannot deny the emotional stresses always operating in our unconscious minds.

"Emotion" is a difficult concept to pin down. In the most popular concept "to be in love" is an "emotion," to cry easily or to fly off the handle on the slightest provocation is to be "emotional." In more sophisticated connotations we use such phrases as "emotional reactions," "emotional stability," and "emotional maturity."

All this implies that emotions must be kept under control. This is true enough, but we must also recognize that the powerful, primitive, inner forces that we call emotions animate *all* human behavior—for better or worse. Emotions are feelings. We become consciously aware of them when they are heightened to a certain degree, but they are constantly resident in the unconscious mind. The operation of the emotions offers testimony

to the unity of body and mind in the human being.

This was observed by William James, the father of modern psychology, who formulated one of the early theories of emotion in the 1880's and who wrote:

If we fancy some strong emotion, and then try to abstract from our consciousness of it all the feelings of the characteristic bodily symptoms, we find we have nothing left behind. . . . What kind of emotion would fear be left if the feelings neither of quickened heartbeats nor of shallow breathing, neither of trembling lips nor of weakened limbs, neither of goose flesh nor of visceral stirrings, were present, it is quite impossible to think. . . . Every passion in turn tells the same story. A purely disembodied human emotion is a nonentity.

James's theory of emotions has been largely superseded, but his descriptions are still valid. Emotions do not live in thin air; they must have some bodily expression. Certain modern physiologists describe emotions as "visceral actions."

Another important investigator of human emotions was the great Harvard physiologist Walter B. Cannon. He observed that fear, rage, pain, and hunger are emotional reactions that human beings share with lower animals. He explained these reactions in part as a result of the mediation of the endocrine system, particularly the release of adrenalin under conditions of stress, excitement, or danger. He saw these bodily reactions as "purposeful reflexes" designed and developed to assist survival in critical emergencies. He accounted for the similarity in the expression of strong emotions on the part of man and animal on the grounds that there is "an ancient and primitive part of the brain which is the common possession of all vertebrates." Some of Cannon's conclusions have been challenged, but of the central thesis there is no doubt: emotions stimulate the mobilization of body forces for action. When action cannot be taken, harmful effects may result. Emotions may be "converted" into physical illness.

Emotions in general and emotional stress in particular obviously have innumerable effects upon human physiology. Efforts of scientists to study hormonal and other physiologic changes that occur under such types of emotional stress as depression and anger have been hampered by the difficulties of inducing these emotions in realistic experimental settings. Recent studies, however, have made use of hypnosis to study the effect of emotions without situational complications that might distort the findings. Under these conditions of study, some made by U. S. Public Health Service investigators, it has become possible to observe some of the more subtle effects of emotions upon human physiology. It has been demonstrated now, for example, that various types of emotional stress, such as depression, fear, and anger, are associated with an increase in free fatty acids in the blood stream. This finding bears importantly on further investigations both in the field of nutrition (Chapter 6) and heart disease (Chapter 11).

Sleep

Man spends approximately a third of his life in sleep. Yet for an activity so common and universal, we still know surprisingly little about its fundamental mechanisms. The most scientific explanations of the function of sleep hardly surpass Shakespeare's seventeenth-century description:

Sleep that knits up the ravell'd sleave of care,
The death of each day's life, sore labour's bath,
Balm of hurt minds, great nature's second course,
Chief nourisher in life's feast.

During sleep the sleeper becomes unconscious, unaware, and more or less unresponsive to the environment about him. However, this is a relative matter. Some sense and some parts of the body remain more alert and more in function than others. For example, a sleeper may sleep through a loud noise but awake at the lightest touch. Again, while the lungs and heart may work more slowly during sleep, the sweat glands and some parts of the brain and nervous system may become more active. This increased, even though temporary, activity of the nervous system is the explanation of dreams, sleepwalking

(somnambulism), and talking in one's sleep. Exactly why these events occur to a specific person on a given night cannot be explained, but the fact of their occurrence demonstrates that sleep and waking are both part of the same cycle of living. It is questionable whether the unconscious mind ever completely rests. Anxiety, certainly, is one of the great enemies of sleep.

Most of the measurable physiological functions of the body are diminished during sleep. The body temperature falls, indicating a general decline in metabolism and a decrease in the tone of muscles. Muscular relaxation is one of the key components of sleep. During sleep also the heart beats more slowly, blood pressure and pulse rate fall, breathing is slower, and secretion from nearly all glands diminishes.

But sleep is more than a time of rest and relaxation. It is also a time of recuperation and repair, of growth and regrowth. During the normal course of living, cells of the body wear out and must be replaced. This regeneration takes place more rapidly during sleep. It has been shown, for example, that the cells of the skin divide and make new cells about twice as fast during sleep.

The amount of sleep a person needs is therefore influenced by his rate of growth. Rapidly growing infants need more sleep than children; children more than adults. Again in old age, when the reparative processes of the body are less active, an increase in sleep may be required. Furthermore during the period of recovery from a debilitating illness or operation (convalescence) and in some stages of pregnancy, added increments of sleep or rest may be essential.

REM. Experiments undertaken in the 1950's and 1960's have added a great deal to our concepts of the sleeping state. The use of the electroencephelograph (EEG), which records "brain waves," was one of the best new tools for studying sleep. The new concept pointed out the fact that every sleeper's night is punctuated by regular periods of body change and dreaming accompanied by rapid-eye-movement (REM).

About two dozen sleep laboratories in the United States are now observing the REM characteristics and other bodily changes during sleep. In spite of their research efforts, the exact nature of the sleep phenomenon both in men and animals still eludes analysis.

We have only begun to learn what people mean when they say they slept "well" or "poorly." The differences can be partly determined by brain-wave patterns, heart rates, and temperature changes noted during sleep. The poor sleepers do not seem to follow the 24-hour rhythm of sleep and wakefulness. (This rhythm is sometimes called the "circadian" rhythm, from the Latin phrase *circa dies,* translated to mean "about one day.") The poor sleepers show an unusually small amount of REM sleep. By EEG monitoring of sleeping persons, who are fitted with tiny electrodes on their bodies (including the eyes), it has been possible to detect four stages of sleep. Stage IV is the sleep of the weary, the time when recuperative powers are at their best and sleep at its deepest. This stage comes normally within the first few hours of sleeping.

The treatment for sleep problems, both sleeplessness (insomnia) and oversleeping (narcolepsy), has been made more complicated by these recent discoveries about sleep. Alcohol, barbiturates, and tranquilizers do not enhance sleep: they change the usual pattern of nighttime sleep by reducing the amount of the needful REM sleep. Stimulants, such as the amphetamines, have the same effect.

How Much Sleep? Research and common experience both indicate that sleep requirements are individual, governed by factors of age, general state of health, current activities, emotional outlook and previous sleeping habits.

Most adults sleep 6 to 8 hours out of 24. But some need more; a few less. Occasionally a person "drugs" himself with too much sleep and fails to get his full measure of living. The people who claim to get along on very little sleep at night usually do some of their sleeping during the day. They take short naps and they have usually mastered the art of relaxation.

The test of whether or not you are getting enough sleep is a simple, practical, and individual one. You are getting enough if you wake up

in the morning refreshed and ready for the new day. The first half hour after arising can be discounted in applying this test, because it takes varying lengths of time for metabolism to rise to a level of full wakefulness.

Occasional loss of sleep will not have harmful effects. Under conditions of military necessity men have often gone 48 to 72 hours without sleep and recovered with only 12 hours of rest and sleep. Even test subjects, who have been kept awake as long as 200 hours, have not suffered significant physiological changes, although they do exhibit some temporary psychological deficits; they become restless, irritable, and unable to add numbers accurately in their heads.

Sleeping Soundly. There is no best position for sleeping. Any position in which you are comfortable will serve. It is the common practice in Western society to sleep in a bed. But there are some primitive people who sleep in a squatting position. The Japanese sleep on the ground or floor without mattresses. Sailors manage to get a good night's rest in hammocks. And, as every college student knows, almost anyone can learn to sleep sitting up.

It must be recognized that some hours of sleep are deeper or "sounder" than others. These 2 to 4 hours of deep sleep, whether they come before or after midnight, are the important ones in the body's recuperative process. The different levels of sleep can be detected in "brain wave" patterns. The factors that make for sound sleep are many and often highly individual. Darkness, quiet, agreeable room temperature, and an accustomed, comfortable bed favor a good night's sleep. So do regular sleeping habits—that is, going to bed about the same time almost every night—and a balanced pattern of living that is free from repeated, abnormal tensions. A good day is the best prelude to a good night's sleep.

Insomnia. Insomnia (sleeplessness) is a common complaint. Many people who make this complaint are getting more sleep than they think; they remember the hours they were tossing about and forget the time they were asleep.

Everyone has occasional sleepless nights, usually after a particularly worrisome day. But persistent insomnia deserves a medical check-up and not frantic self-medication.

Excessive fatigue is sometimes a cause of insomnia; a person may be just too tired to sleep. On the other hand mild exercise, like a short walk before going to bed, may induce sleep.

Eating habits may be a factor in insomnia. One person may be kept awake because he has had too heavy an evening meal, another because he is really hungry. Coffee, tea, and other cerebral stimulants taken late in the day have different effects on different people. Some will not be bothered by them; others will be kept awake. Personal experience is the only test.

You may not be sleeping because your room is too hot or too cold, too noisy or too light. A change to a more comfortable bed and mattress may also help. If the failure to sleep has deep psychological origins, improvement in the physical factors of the sleeping quarters will not help much.

Relaxation of mind and muscles is the key to falling asleep. That is why many of the time-honored technics of getting to sleep often work. These include: leisurely retiring, reading or listening to music before retiring, taking a warm (not hot) bath, counting sheep (or anything else), breathing deeply and rhythmically, consciously attempting to relax the muscles.

The greatest single cause of sleeplessness is simply the fear that one is not getting enough sleep. Sleep needs differ. When you go to bed, feel confident that you will get enough rest, whether you sleep or not.

Sleeping Pills. Sleeping pills are sedative and hypnotic drugs, usually but not always barbiturates. (More information on barbiturates will be found in Chapter 4.) Addiction to barbiturates is possible and overdoses can be fatal, particularly when the pills are ingested simultaneously with alcohol. Bromides and antihistamines (drugs sometimes prescribed for hay fever) also have sleep-producing effects.

The self-prescribed use of sleeping pills—especially the barbiturates—can be dangerous. The sale of barbiturates and some other kinds of sleeping pills without a physician's prescription is forbidden in all states. Those pills that can be bought without prescription contain ineffective drugs or such small quantities that they can't work, except by suggestion.

SUMMARY REVIEW QUESTIONS

1. What does the term mental health mean to you? How do you think it is achieved? What are valid goals of mental health? What are the principal obstacles in the way of reaching these goals?
2. Cast up your own list of "principles of mental health." How does it compare with the advice along this line you have gleaned from other sources? Why do you think you have given somewhat different emphasis to your "advice to yourself"?
3. How close is the relationship between mind and body in the human being? What specific examples can you give to indicate that this is either a very close or a distant and somewhat casual relationship?
4. What is an emotion? How do human emotions originate and how are they usually expressed?
5. What, in your own experience, have been the greatest obstacles to restful sleep? How have you overcome them, or how would you expect to overcome them?
6. How, practically speaking, can you tell whether you are getting enough sleep? Are you getting enough sleep? If not, what do you propose to do about it?

7. Are the following statements sense or nonsense? Why? *What is mind? No matter. What is matter? Never mind. . . . The language of behavior is spoken by every cell in the body. . . . A person can be too tired to sleep. . . . Some people have no emotions at all. . . . Man is born, suffers, dies. . . . And they lived happily ever after.*

Recommended for Further Reading: *The Human Mind* by Karl Menninger, M.D. *Managing Your Mind* by S. H. Kraines and E. S. Thetford. *The Revolution in Psychiatry: the New Understanding of Man* by E. Becker. *Psychology: The Briefer Course* by William James. *Understanding Human Nature* by Alfred Adler.

2

THE UNCONSCIOUS MIND

PERSONALITY HAS BEEN DESCRIBED AS "THE sum total of our ways of behaving, especially toward other people." Our behavior is controlled not only by apparently conscious thought and decision but also by our emotions, which have roots in the past. We are always influenced more or less by our unconscious mind, which is the dwelling place of our emotions and the matrix of our personality structure.

Personality Development

"As the twig is bent, so the tree inclines." "The child is father to the man." In these old proverbs also is summed up a great deal of the best present-day knowledge of normal personality development. This development begins at birth; the behavior patterns of later life are established in the cradle, the nursery, and the elementary school room.

Despite individual differences, personality development follows a fairly consistent and universal pattern. It normally proceeds step by step, stage by stage toward the elusive, relative, and rarely attained goal of "emotional maturity." Physical growth and biological readiness precede the emotional development. Each intermediate stage in personality development must be worked through before a person can go on to the next stage. No one can leap from infancy to adulthood. Arrested and distorted development, however, is all too common. The relationship of the individual with his own family, from earliest infancy onward, is a crucial factor in personality development (see "Function of the Family" Chapter 7).

The Stages of Love. The newborn infant is helpless, dependent on his mother or her substitute for survival, yet he is born with the will to live and love. This innate will to survive, to grow up and enjoy life is the basic font of vital human energy; it has been given the name of *libido*. As personality development progresses, a large part of the libido evolves into more directed and controlled feelings, which we call love. Fully developed, the libido represents all those inner strivings which tend to preserve and extend life—to "heal, cultivate, protect, and inspire" the human personality. But in the infant this love force appears in a crude, undifferentiated, untutored form.

The infant begins by loving himself. This is called *narcissistic love,* after the Greek legend of Narcissus, the handsome lad who fell in love with his own image in a pool. The infant "loves" and finds pleasurable gratification in different parts of his own body in a regularly observed succession. His first libidinal attachment is to his mouth (he puts everything into it), then to his anus, then to his genital organs.

As he becomes increasingly aware of the difference between himself and other people, the infant gradually shifts his love to objects outside himself. The first libidinal shift is to his mother, then to other members of the household. The young child identifies himself closely with his parents, idealizes them, and seeks to imitate them. This is *imitative love.*

There comes a time, usually between the ages of four and seven, when the imitative child wants jealously and intensely to "possess" the parent of the opposite sex. Little boys naïvely say,

"When Daddy is at the office, I'll be Daddy"; and little girls earnestly assert, "When I grow up, I'm going to marry father." This stage of development, which certainly occurs in Western culture with its ideal of romantic monogamous marriage, is called *oedipal love,* after the Greek legend of King Oedipus, who was fated to kill his father and marry his mother.

In later childhood, as the boy and girl become aware that their oedipal longings are impossible of fulfillment, emotional attachments shift outside the home and become centered in "loyalty" to a gang or a "crush" on a friend. The new libidinal attachment is usually to a person of the same sex. This is sometimes designated as *homosexual love.* In late childhood, a period of sexual latency, this is a perfectly natural emotional attachment—not to be confused with adult homosexuality.

In puberty, love attachments return to the opposite sex. But this usually begins as a kind of *idealistic love* for some distant, unattainable personality—as unattainable in reality as was father or mother, but secretly and subtly cast in the parent images. The idealistic yearnings of hosts of teenagers for the same popular and symbolic figure of the sport or entertainment world is a repeatedly observed phenomenon.

The next and final stage in the development of the capacity to love is *heterosexual love,* love for a person of the opposite sex. This is the fulfillment of the normal course of love development. But it does not wipe out all previous love attachments; some self-love, for example, always remains. Nor does it exclude the simultaneous presence in the psyche of anger and fear.

Anger and Fear—"Negative Emotions." Anger, fear, hate, jealousy, and revenge are in a sense protective reaction patterns, slumbering reflexes evoked by threats or suspicions of danger. They mobilize psychic energy and physical resources for that end. But when too frequently or constantly evoked, particularly by imagined danger, and when unchecked in their operation, they can have a destructive effect on personality.

Anger, or aggression, in its many guises is the normal but primitive response to frustration. It is basically the desire to remove by attacking, killing, or destroying anything that threatens the survival of the individual in body or spirit. All too often anger is destructively turned against oneself.

When you are thwarted or frustrated by yourself, others, or circumstances, you cannot help *feeling* angry. But there is a vast difference between *feeling* angry, *appearing* angry, and *acting* angry. You can learn to do something constructive with your mobilized energy. You should neither swallow it (repress it) nor turn it against yourself. For anger repressed will return in some other emotional disguise.

The seeds of anger, like love, are sown in infancy. Frustrations evoking and nourishing anger begin at birth, when the human being is "continually encountering the painful experience that the world is no longer shaped so exactly to his subjective demands as was the maternal womb."

Infants are born with certain instinctual reactions which are sometimes called "fears." However, the face and substance of fear changes as experience enlarges. For example, people get progressively more afraid of snakes as they grow older. One of the most pervasive human fears is that of loss of parental love, or, more abstractly, fear of rejection or social disapproval.

Fear is the emotion associated with flight from danger which threatens survival. Fear and cowardice are not the same thing; one can *feel* afraid and still *act* bravely, which is what most "heroes" do.

Personality patterns, it should now be plain, reflect the constant interplay of positive and negative emotions. In wholesome personality development the "loving" emotions are encouraged to blossom and modify the effects of the negative emotions. Technically speaking, we seek to "eroticize our aggressions." We turn now to consider the unconscious mind, where these things occur.

The Unconscious Mind

The unconscious mind is a paradox. We become aware of it only when and to the extent that it releases memories, thoughts, and feelings to consciousness. It holds and withholds many secrets. We assume the existence of an unconscious mind because it offers the most rational and scientific way of explaining human behavior. This hypothesis has superseded the animistic explanation that a child is "bad" or his father an alcoholic because the Devil is in him.

There are those who cling to "free will" and reason as the fundamental determinants of human conduct. On this score it can be said that we must act as if our wills were free and as reasonably as our unconscious minds will allow us. But there can be little doubt today that individual reason and will are persistently limited by unconscious forces. We are fundamentally driven by our emotional reactions. We can do only what the structure of our personality permits.

For these and other reasons we must now examine the structure of the unconscious mind. It is the major area of psychic processes and hence the central subject matter of mental health and mental hygiene. To use several figures of speech, the conscious mind is only the facade of the unconscious; it is the part of the iceberg that floats above the water; it is just the skin of the apple. The picture of the unconscious mind that we shall present is of necessity generalized and oversimplified. But it is not merely hypothetical; it corresponds with and explains how human beings actually behave.

The structuring of the unconscious mind here set forth is based on psychoanalytic theory, initiated and expounded principally by the Viennese physician Sigmund Freud. It has acknowedged limitations, but it is far from being outmoded.

The most serious criticism of the psychoanalytic formulation of human conduct is probably that it does not give full enough weight to the physiological factors involved. Freud, who began as a neurologist, anticipated this criticism and worked out his theory precisely because there was not enough information at that time on the physiology or pathology (disorder) of the human nervous system to explain the huge backlog of unhappy people and mental illness that confronted him.

The success of recent drug therapy (e.g., tranquilizers and cerebral stimulants) in treating mild and severe mental illness suggests that physiological modifications of the nervous system can favorably modify the events presumed to occur in the unconscious mind. But the new ability to alter and improve the physiological factors in mental illness does not entirely wipe out the psychic factors.

Those who doubt the existence and importance of the unconscious mind must find a better explanation for such questions as: How can a fact be remembered one minute and forgotten the next? Where do dreams come from? Why do so many people feel uncomfortably anxious and guilty about trivial and unimportant events of their past and present experience? Why do patterns of reaction established in childhood persist throughout adult life?

Although other terminology for the structure of the unconscious mind can be and has been used, the well-accepted (Freudian) construct divides it into three interacting parts: the *id,* the *ego,* and the *superego.*

The Id. A newborn baby, helpless though he is, nevertheless has instincts and aptitudes (like the sucking reflex) for survival. This passion for existence, this inherent vital emotional energy we have pointed out can be described as his libido. In a more impersonal term it can also be characterized as the id. All that we can guess concerning the existence of the id we gain from observations of the conduct of the libido. (We have already traced the normal course of libido attachments to "love objects" from early infancy through adulthood.) In the structure of the unconscious mind, therefore, the id can be construed as the uncontrolled source of the inborn tendencies, the instincts, the unconscious striving of the human organism to live and enjoy life.

The id, however, has characteristics which are not in accord with the best in human conduct. Like a child who "wants what he wants when he wants it," the id constantly seeks its own pleasure and gratification. It acts as if pleasure were the only thing in the world that counts. It operates on the pleasure principle exclusively.

This is the way infants and children behave, and it takes education, maturation, and social pressure before they give up the pleasure principle as the chief guide to conduct. Even in adults, of course, the pleasure-seeking drive persists—but it is under greater control.

The id does not distinguish between good and evil. It is illogical; it holds contradictory wishes and impulses at the same time. In a word, the *id is unrealistic.* The human organism which responded solely to its whims, its sexual and aggressive tendencies, would probably not long survive.

The Ego. The ego represents the conscious self. Through it the id is kept in touch with reality —with the external world about it. Through the perceptual apparatus of the human organism, the ego sees, hears, tastes, smells, and feels what is going on about it. The ego acts in terms of the reality principle, which is an important characteristic of adult behavior. The ego gradually develops and gains strength in the course of the individual's growing up and becoming educated in the ways of the world.

But the ego is frequently under pressure to satisfy the id. This it cannot always do, any more than a parent can completely satisfy all the demands of a child. The relationship of the id to the ego has been aptly described as that of the horse to the rider. The rider directs the horse with more or less success. Sometimes, however, the horse is balky. He runs away; he may even throw the rider. In other words, the pleasure principle often defies and sometimes dethrones the reality principle.

The ego is almost the whole of the *conscious* mind and it is the seat of the higher faculties of the mind. However, a large part of the ego is submerged in the unconscious mind. A traffic of sensations, thoughts, and memories back and forth between the conscious and the unconscious passes over the highways and nerve pathways of the ego. Not all thoughts and feelings pass with equal freedom. The ego places barriers— defenses—against unwelcome impulses entering consciousness. We shall have much more to say

about these ego defenses, or mental mechanisms, later on in this chapter.

The important characteristics of the ego, learned in maturation, are that it is in constant touch with external reality; that it can learn by experience; that it can interpose thought between wish and act; that it unifies, modifies, and integrates thoughts and feelings; and that it can be reasonable.

The Superego. Crudely speaking, the superego is the conscience, the small voice within us that warns against temptation and wrongdoing. But the voice we hear is only the conscious part of the superego. A larger part of it is buried in the unconscious, where it frequently bullies the ego and makes itself felt in vague but distressing feelings of guilt and shame. The superego embraces not only our conscious moral standards but also our "ego ideal"—the picture of ourselves as we would secretly like to be and appear to the world.

While the reality principle restricts the ego to what is possible, the superego tells it what is permissible, or what is socially acceptable. The superego is an essential check on asocial or antisocial conduct.

A peculiarity of the superego is that it is often behind the times. Its sternest admonitions frequently remain those that were formed in early childhood principally between the ages of three and six. At this time the child is strongly identified with his parents (or their substitutes). Their least prohibitions and commands, their values and their attitudes, are etched deeply on the young and weak ego of the child, and these feelings become the essence of his superego.

The unfortunate catch in this is that the parents, impelled by their own superegos, too often urge the child to be better than he can be ("a *perfect* little lady or gentleman") and better than they, the parents, are or were themselves.

Conflict in the Unconscious Mind. This can be understood as battles between the ego and the id, the superego and the id, the ego and the superego, and struggles within the id. The focus of these conflicts is on the ego. It must mediate between the id and superego; it must obey the dictates of the superego; it must control the whimsical demands of the id; it must satisfy the needs of external reality; it must guide the entire personality through the shoals and competitions of the real world. Some egos are stronger than others, but no ego can always meet all the demands upon it. It must sometimes adopt compromises, subtle means of self-protection variously called "ego defenses," mental mechanisms, and mental dynamisms.

When the ego is under stress from the id or being "punished" by the superego, the individual whose ego is being hurt suffers from anxiety—a vague but often powerful feeling for which he has no obvious or immediate explanation. He cannot put his finger on the source of the anxiety because it is concealed and disguised in the unconscious mind. The anxiety may express itself in feelings of tension, guilt, inferiority or even physical symptoms (e.g., a headache). There are always some physical reactions to the stress of anxiety. In one sense anxiety may be considered an admission on the part of the ego that it is temporarily unable to cope with its taxing job.

Later in this chapter we shall deal with constructive ways of handling anxiety. At this point we shall set forth some of the mental mechanisms by which the ego seeks to defend itself against otherwise intolerable anxieties generated by conflicts in the unconscious mind.

The Mental Mechanisms

Mental mechanisms (mental dynamisms, ego defenses) operate solely in the unconscious mind. At the time we are using them, or *overusing* them, we are not aware of the fact. In retrospect we can sometimes recognize how our egos were defending themselves, and we are usually acutely aware of the mental mechanisms grossly employed by other people.

It is possible to identify some types of behavior originating in the use of mental mechanisms; childish behavior in an adult, for example, indicates the use of a mental mechanism called re-

gression. Different people habitually use different mechanisms; most people use several. When one compromise fails, the uneasy ego grasps desperately for another.

We must not blame ourselves or other people for using mental mechanisms; they are sometimes necessary to a particular individual to enable him to deal with his real-life situations. We may, however, fairly question the persistent overworking of one or another mental mechanism. This betrays serious unresolved conflicts in the unconscious mind, or, in other terms, an unsettled personality or a troubled person.

Repression. The most important mental mechanism is called *repression;* it is an emotional block that keeps us from remembering something even if we want to. In brief, the ego buries unpleasant memories and associations and frightening feelings. It also inhibits pleasant feelings, which arouse the threat of the id going out of control and prompting socially unacceptable behavior of a sexual or aggressive nature. Repressed material represents emotional reactions that we want to hide even from ourselves. But this repressed, buried, warded-off, hidden material does not disappear. It seeks expression one way or another. Since it is barred from directly entering the consciousness, it usually appears in a disguised and distorted form.

Among the ways in which repressed memories and experiences may assert themselves are dreams, amnesia, purposeful forgetting, slips of the tongue, and the formation of neurotic anxiety symptoms. In dreams we find disguised images of the circumstances that have been repressed into the unconscious. Dreams usually represent wish fulfillments—but of wishes we would not dare harbor in the conscious mind. Very often they are wishes to harm those we love—parents, spouse, children, brothers, and sisters.

Amnesia means loss of memory—forgetting or repressing whole spans of time. Unpleasant war experiences are sometimes thus blanked out. Again, we do not like to look forward to events that threaten pain, difficulty, or embarrassment. So we purposefully forget a medical appointment; we stand up a date we didn't want in the first place. Of great significance is the universal experience called *infantile amnesia*. Almost everyone "forgets" the feelings of frustration, fear, and other experiences that occurred during infancy and early childhood.

Identification. Identification is the process by which the ego gains strength through attachment to another person, group (notably the family), or institution. The infant, as noted, identifies himself first with his mother, then with other members of his immediate family. The young child feels and behaves as though he were the parents themselves. He *uncritically* imitates their ways; he *unconsciously* adopts their traits, habits, ideas, prejudices, and values. When he is angry at them, he may hit himself!

Identification in later life represents the need for belonging to some group or "herd" and being accepted by that group. Even outcasts huddle together for mutual reassurance. Identification is on the whole one of the most satisfactory adjustment mechanisms. However, *overidentification* with one's family, school, or other group may sharply limit one's personal development, inhibit outgoing feelings toward other people, and indicate unresolved inner feelings of a childlike dependency on others.

Idealization. Identification of the young child with his parents gradually turns into idealization of them. The child's own ego ideals, the inner picture of himself as he feels he would like to be, are permanently established in his superego by this process of idealization.

Idealization, as a mental mechanism, is a device the ego adopts to escape the recriminations of the superego. When it substitutes other ideals for the original parent ideals, it always includes at the core of the new ideals some fraction of the original pattern. "Idealistic love," as we have noted, is shaped in the inner image of one's parents.

Like identification, idealization is usually uncritical. This often leads to overestimation of the people toward whom it is directed. We see idealization blissfully at work in young lovers, who refuse to see the least blemish in their beloveds.

Idealization is also employed at the very highest cultural levels—in religious worship and love of God, commonly idealized as Father, all-powerful and all-loving. We attribute to God all that is best in man.

Regression. Regression means reverting to immature and often childish behavior in the presence of current difficulties and frustrations. In terms of overt behavior it is one of the easiest of the mental mechanisms to observe and identify in other people. We all know the boy who won't play if he can't be captain of the team; the girl who sulks or goes into a temper tantrum if she misses a much-desired date; the tennis player who smashes his racket when he loses a match; the "perpetual undergraduate" college alumnus, yelling himself hoarse at a football game; the child who throws himself on the floor and screams at the top of his lungs when he is denied candy.

Regression is a retreat from the complexities of the present to the fancied security of the past. The ego feels more comfortable—for the moment—in seeking an old solution for a present problem.

Projection. We frequently seek to excuse our own failings by blaming them on someone or something else. The student who is failing a college course may sincerely but erroneously believe that the instructor is down on him. The poor workman blames his tools. Auto accidents are always "the other fellow's fault." When the ego rejects responsibility for failure and projects the blame elsewhere, it is employing the mental mechanism of projection.

But the process of projection may be much broader than merely excusing failure. We may, for example, project our own feelings on other people or the world at large. When we feel "blue," we may see the whole world as black. We often attribute our own most undesirable traits to other people. If we are "bad," they are worse. We are most prone to project on others those feelings which trouble us most. Thus, if we feel secretly hostile toward somebody else, we may imagine that he is equally hostile toward us—which may or may not be the case. Seeing others in a distorted image of ourselves may make us unduly critical, sarcastic, cynical, and pessimistic.

Substitution. Substitution and displacement are mental mechanisms akin to projection. We sometimes substitute one love object for another—as does the childless woman who lavishes maternal affection upon a dog or cat. We may also displace our feelings, sometimes because we are afraid to express them toward the person who aroused them. Thus a man may be angry at his boss but displace his anger upon his wife—for some trivial reason. A girl who is angry at her parents may take it out in a quarrel with her boy friend.

Rationalization. Rationalization is perhaps the most widely and frequently used of the unconscious ego defenses. It reflects a built-in bias, of which we are unaware, in favor of ourselves, our feelings, our own opinions, ideas, and prejudices.

Rationalization is the practice of finding and giving plausible and apparently "reasonable" explanations for thought and conduct that stem from quite different motivations than those we openly express. Rationalization is unconscious self-deception. It usually comes as a great shock to find that others do not see us or our points of view as we see them ourselves. We often rationalize our conduct to cover up our less worthy motives—often our jealousies—toward other people. Thus a teacher or mother chastises children "for their own good"—unaware that she is enjoying her own sense of power.

Rationalization is not valid reasoning. To a certain extent rationalization is inevitable. Since all our strongest personal beliefs—and prejudices—are rooted in emotions, it is not surprising that we defend them by rationalization rather than by critical, logical thought.

Some of the most penetrating observations on rationalization were written more than a generation ago by the late James Harvey Robinson in his brilliant book, *The Mind in the Making,* thus:

We are incredibly heedless in the formation of our beliefs, but find ourselves filled with an illicit passion for them when anyone proposes to rob us of their companionship. It is obviously not the ideas themselves that are dear to us, but our self-esteem, which is threatened.

We are by nature stubbornly pledged to defend our own from attack, whether it be our person, our family, our property, or our opinion. A United States Senator once remarked to a friend of mine that God Almighty could not make him change his mind on our Latin-America policy. We may surrender, but rarely confess ourselves vanquished. In the intellectual world at least peace is without victory.

Few of us take the pains to study the origin of our cherished convictions; indeed, we have a natural repugnance to so doing. We like to continue to believe what we have been accustomed to accept as true, and the resentment aroused when doubt is cast upon any of our assumptions leads us to seek every manner of excuse for clinging to them. The result is that most of our so-called reasoning consists in finding arguments for going on believing as we already do. . . .

The "real" reasons for our beliefs are concealed from ourselves as well as from others. As we grow up we simply adopt the ideas presented to us in regard to such matters as religion, family relations, property, business, our country, and the state. We unconsciously absorb them from our environment. They are persistently whispered in our ear by the group in which we happen to live. . . .

The little word *my* is the most important one in all human affairs, and properly to reckon with it is the beginning of wisdom. It has the same force whether it is *my* dinner, *my* dog, and *my* house, or *my* faith, *my* country, and *my* God. We not only resent the imputation that our watch is wrong, or our car is shabby, but that our conception of the canals of Mars, of the pronunciation of "Epictetus," of the medicinal value of salicine, or the date of Sargon I, are subject to revision.

Fantasy and Daydreaming. Unconscious fantasy, often translated into fancy daydreaming, is one of the most subtly dangerous mental mechanisms because although up to a certain point it is useful and constructive, beyond that difficult-to-determine point it can be destructive of the personality. Everyone engages in fantasy and daydreaming; the world properly respects the faculty of constructive imagination, as illuminated by artists in every media.

Fantasy becomes dangerous, however, when we no longer distinguish between what is fantasy and what is reality. In the unconscious mind fantasy is the property of the id, which indulges in wishful thinking just as much as it can without restraint from the ego. It is not strange, therefore, that fantasy plays such a large role in childhood. The child acts out his wishes and fantasies in play, but he is deadly serious about his world of make-believe. The id is overwhelming the ego.

Normal fantasizing has been carried too far when it has become a facile substitute for work and effort needed to bring a vision to reality, when wishful thinking about success supersedes all struggle to attain it.

Conversion. The conversion of conflicts in the unconscious mind into physical symptoms of illness is one of the most commonly employed of all mental mechanisms. Physicians estimate that at least half the patients they see are suffering from complaints in which psychic or emotional factors are the prime if not the sole complaint.

The student who always gets a headache when faced with an examination is displaying a conversion symptom. So, too, is the soldier who suffers from hysterical blindness when he sees his buddy blown up a few feet away from him. Conversion reactions are in fact more common in wartime than peacetime, and they are the explanation of such conditions as hysterical paralysis, convulsions, loss of voice and deafness, "shellshock," "soldier's heart," and "battle fatigue."

Illness becomes a way out of an intolerable situation. Physical pain is substituted for inner anxiety. The patient is unaware of the source of his pain. It is just as real to him as if it had a definite basis in a recognizable bodily defect. For example, a patient with a severe backache of purely psychogenic origin feels just as bad as if X-ray evidence actually showed a fracture in his spine.

Conversion symptoms are often difficult to relieve for the added reason that they offer some secondary gains or benefits to the patient. He gets sympathy because he is "sick"; he may be relieved from the pressure of ordinary duties and responsibilities; he may even collect unearned money because of his "affliction." For example, some people who have been involved in accidents do not recover from their symptoms until they receive a substantial cash settlement from an insurance company.

The "chronic invalid," the hypochondriac always worried about his health, and the neurotic who "enjoys" poor health offer further examples of conversion reactions. There is no accounting for their long lists of vague aches, pains, and other complaints except on a psychological basis. Fatigue is one of the commonest complaints.

Nevertheless actual impairment of bodily functions may result from prolonged unconscious conflicts. Practically any organ or system of the body can be affected by "psychophysiological disorders." Many emotional reactions, for example, are visibly expressed in skin troubles. Other diseases which may be initiated or aggravated by unconscious anxiety include bronchial asthma, peptic ulcer, chronic colitis, and heart disease (especially disease of the coronary arteries). Bodily illnesses wholly or partly of psychic origin are often described as "psychosomatic"—from "psyche" for mind and "soma" for body.

Some Other Mental Mechanisms in Operation. From the descriptions and examples of mental mechanisms already given it should be obvious that hidden struggles and conflicts within the unconscious mind create not only psychosomatic illness but also the wide diversity of personalities whom we meet in real life and in fiction. Without going into the complete details of the psychic processes involved in each, we shall give brief descriptions of generally recognizable "stock characters" whose peculiar behavior patterns are controlled by overworking ego defenses and mental mechanisms.

The Extrovert. He turns to the outside world, to fierce rounds of activity, to careless and unreflective action in order to smother his inner conflicts. "The life of the party" is usually running away from himself.

The Introvert. He substitutes thought for action. He shrinks from his social environment. He finds decision painfully difficult. He looks too long before he leaps.

The Perfectionist. He sets his goals so high that neither he himself nor others can reasonably criticize him for failing to achieve them.

The Specialist. He chooses so odd or unique a line of endeavor that there is little competition in it; thus he escapes the normal competitive struggle.

The "Know-It-All." He covers up his inner sense of inadequacy by an attitude of superiority. He appears too cocksure, dogmatic, and positive about his knowledge and opinions. He knows all the answers, he thinks; but he holds only minor jobs.

Mrs. Grundy. She viciously gossips about and criticizes others to compensate for her own feelings of inferiority. She secretely fears that, given the chance, she would behave worse than those she criticizes.

The Alibi Artist. He cannot face overt criticism. He fears that others will discover and confirm the low opinion he has about himself.

The Isolationist. His unconscious mind has fashioned logic-tight compartments so that some parts of his inconsistent, paradoxical, multiple personality are completely isolated from others. This is the Dr. Jekyll and Mr. Hyde character. A more recent portrayal of the multiple personality is to be found in the well-known psychiatric study entitled *Three Faces of Eve.*

The Symbolist. He performs symbolic acts as a bribe to his superego in order to blot out or undo even more painful thoughts lurking in his unconscious mind. A classic example is Lady Macbeth repeatedly washing her hands in the vain hope of washing away her deeper feelings of guilt about having instigated murder.

The Fetishist. He displaces his strong feelings for a person onto a thing. Afraid to express openly a love for a particular woman, he holds some physical symbol of her—a handkerchief, a lock of her hair—in even higher esteem.

Pollyanna. She persistently looks at the world through rose-colored glasses. She childishly denies that life includes struggle and difficulty. Eventually she is tripped up and overwhelmed by it.

Sublimation. Sublimation means directing, channelizing, and converting basic emotional drives, crude instinctual impulses, into *socially acceptable and useful activities.* It is the true taming of the id by the ego under direction of the superego. Sublimations are the most constructive compromises and the happiest solutions to the inevitable frustrations that life sets before us. Though difficult to achieve, they bring social reward and approval which reinforces and strengthens the ego.

Sublimations take many forms. Some serve for a time; others for a lifetime. The lives of dedicated men and women—scientists, artists, missionaries—illuminate how satisfying and creative sublimation can be.

Most commonly the making of a home and the rearing of a family give the opportunity for the sublimation of feelings to a most socially useful end.

Sublimation is not entirely an unconscious process. Conscious effort enters into it. One deliberately chooses realistic goals and activities which he can, step by step, and in spite of frustrations and difficulties, hope to reach.

Doing the Best You Can. It is important for college students to realize that all roads to mental health do not lead through sublimation and the exercise of initiative and creativity to its highest degree (and often with frustrations beyond the tolerance of the individual concerned). There is another type of mental health, found among many college students, which may be described by the simple phrase of "doing the best you can." Psychiatrists Roy G. Grinker, Sr. and Jr., and John Timberlake, affiliated with the Institute for Psychosomatic and Psychiatric Research and Training of the Michael Reese Hospital and Medical Center, Chicago, have offered an elaborate description of this particular type of "mentally healthy" college student (in the June, 1962 issue of the *Archives of General Psychiatry*).

These doctors offer the following description of a group of 65 goal-oriented and mentally healthy young men attending a small college. (The college is deliberately not identified by the investigators, nor do they assume that the type of mental health that these young men enjoyed is to be considered the prototype for all college students. Indeed for many highly intelligent, artistically or scientifically oriented college men and women the kind of "mental health" they discovered and described in their particular study would be deadly.)

On the surface, the investigators point out, this group of 65 young men were free from psychotic, neurotic, or disabling personality traits.

The students, averaging 18 years of age, came from every area of the United States and Canada, from farms and cities. All were working toward degrees in health and physical education, group work, or community recreation, and had strong convictions and motivations about their career choice.

Through interviews, questionnaires and a behavior rating scale, Dr. Grinker found the following conditions characteristic of this group:

¶ Sound health from birth.
¶ Average intelligence.
¶ Relatively low socioeconomic family circumstances.
¶ Affectionate relationship with both parents.
¶ Parental agreement and cooperation in child-raising.
¶ Definite and known limitations on behavior.
¶ Punishment reasonable and consistent.
¶ Sound early religious training.
¶ Held a job early in life.
¶ Externally oriented rather than introspective, with low degree of creativity.
¶ Ideals of contentment, sociability, doing good, and making friends.
¶ Success sought in achieving limited goal rather than ambition to rise higher socially, earn more, or live better than parents.
¶ Strong identification with father and father figures.

Any one, or all, of these factors may be important in the development of this type of personality. Average intelligence with a capacity for honest and accurate self-appraisal is an antidote to useless and disappointing goal-seeking.

In contrast to the plight of students at many modern universities where an infinite number of goals are possible, this group had a single goal, finishing school and starting their chosen work.

Furthermore, most of the students studied had become associated with this type of work in childhood and felt that the college and the future career for which they were preparing was the "right place" for them.

While this type of adjustment is associated with "stability and a special type of happiness," it is also associated with narrowness and limitations of interest, ambition, creativity, and excitement.

These young men cannot be understood apart from the culture in which they were reared. Parental emphasis on early work, sound religious training, and the ideals associated with doing good as well as parental firmness and interest constitute aspects of an ethic acceptable without rebellion because of the sincere manifestations of love and consistency toward the child.

The subjects became more interested in avoiding failure than attaining great success and "doing the best you can" became the essence of their way of life.

Anxiety

The legitimate question remains: How otherwise than by sublimination can we reduce or minimize the burdens of anxiety inevitably generated by conflicts in the unconscious mind?

Relief of Anxiety. The first step is to understand that anxiety wears many disguises which we have tried to strip away by describing the behavior patterns that result from overworking of the mental mechanisms. The perfectionist, the hypochondriac, the man who continually projects his own failings on others, the woman who always rationalizes her mistakes, and all the rest are motivated by an inner anxiety. This emotion may parade as fatigue, overactivity, homesickness, physical illness, a sense of inferiority, depression, and in scores of other guises. By recognizing that anxiety is the basic motivation for personal conduct which displeases himself and attracts unfavorable reactions from others the individual is in a better position to seek and get help with his problem.

How else do you get rid of anxiety? Essentially by talking it out! University of California Medical School psychiatrists J. Ruesch and A. R. Prestwood[1] made a special study of the problem of relieving anxiety and came to this well-accepted conclusion:

The successful management of anxiety generated in daily life seems possible only through a process of sharing and communication.

The process of communication is essential for healthy functioning. Thus are people able to combine their efforts, to complement and increase their ability to cope with their surroundings. The ability to communicate and hence to share anxiety seems to constitute the process responsible for feelings of personal security on the part of the individual. Alleviation of anxiety comes through personal contacts. This process is basic to all interpersonal relationships from babyhood to old age.

An Age of Anxiety? Anxiety is one of the most common symptoms that a practicing physician encounters in his patients. The range of this anxiety is wide, reflected in patients suffering from simple tension to those with severe mental illness. But is ours really more of an age of anxiety than previous generations? At a symposium on "Anxiety and a Decade of Tranquilizer Therapy" held in New York in April, 1964, Dr. James G. Miller, of the University of Michigan, and Dr. Raymond B. Cattell, of the University of Illinois, expressed grave doubts as to whether this was really an age of anxiety beyond that of earlier eras.

Miller acknowledged the stresses of modern life: the hydrogen bomb, the population and information explosions, the increasing pressures of urban life. On the other hand, he pointed out, fear of sudden death and malignant illness is diminishing because medical research has provided powerful weapons against them.

"Civilization has curbed some of the lawless

[1]J. Ruesch, and A. R. Prestwood, *A.M.A. Archives of Neurology and Psychiatry* (November 1949).

terrors and removed some of the rudeness of life in previous centuries," Miller continued. "Education has reduced superstition and fears arising from ignorance. A pervading sense of potentially malign supernatural powers has receded. There may even be less anxiety now than in the more brutal past," Miller concluded.

Dr. Cattell reported on the results of psychological studies of anxiety. Of ten nations that he had studied, the lowest levels of anxiety were found in the United States and Great Britain, while the highest levels were found in such underdeveloped nations as India. "It would seem that anxiety is higher where standards of living are lower, and where a country has cultural and political crevasses separating its peoples," Dr. Cattell observed. "But with America and Britain lowest on these lists," he continued, "the view that we live in an unusually anxious culture and age is scarcely supported." Interestingly, Dr. Cattell found the highest levels of anxiety in the United States among newspaper editors and writers; the lowest, for professionals, among university administrators.

There are many definitions of anxiety. Dr. Miller, for example, views it as a "signal-like pain." It reports whether a person has adequate processes of adjustment to cope with actual or threatened stress. Abnormal signs of anxiety, he felt, could cause useless distress; but mild anxiety can sometimes be associated with better performance. Dr. Cattell took a sterner view. He described all anxiety as "a lack of confidence, a sense of guilt and worthlessness, an unwillingness to venture, a dependency, a readiness to become fatigued, irritable, and discouraged, an uncertainty about oneself and a suspicion of others, and a general tenseness." He felt that this kind and degree of anxiety does not motivate but rather disorganizes the psyche.

Speaking from a woman's point of view at the symposium, author Marya Mannes called the "destructive anxieties" of this age the "pressures of society and the mass media to make [women] conform to the classic and traditional image in men's eyes and to be not only the perfect wife, mother, and homemaker, but also the ever-young, ever-slim, ever-alluring object of their desire." Miss Mannes also designated the "anxieties engendered by the quest for success [as] relentless, degrading, and corroding. They infect husband and wife and the nature of their love. . . . Whatever is attained is never enough," Miss Mannes continued. "These are the social anxieties which afflict our age," she said.

Dr. Ashley Montague, Princeton anthropologist, described anxiety as "the unspecific fusion of fear and insecurity with uncertainty and helplessness in the face of danger—a generalized fear." He further elucidated, "Fear is usually a response to a specific danger; anxiety is the response to a diffuse, generalized fear. As such, anxiety, like stress, appears to be a concomitant of the very process of living."

There are disagreements on the origins as well as the nature of anxiety. There is (1) a psychoanalytic viewpoint, with many variations; (2) a conditioned reflex theory; and (3) an organic view. In the psychoanalytic view anxiety represents conflict in the unconscious mind, particularly a conflict between instinctual desires and a fear of what will happen if they are carried out. The anxious individual feels trapped between two opposing forces. According to the conditioned reflex theory (originally Ivan Pavlov's), anxiety is a conditioned response or learned habit that follows anticipation of danger. Neurotic symptoms are considered learned patterns of behavior that reduce the anxiety, which Pavlovians feel to be the central and most important motivational force in human behavior. In the organic or biological concept of anxiety, its basis is physical and it is caused by dysfunction of certain structures of the brain.

It should be pointed out that there is such a thing as a "normal anxiety," which is in proportion to the danger that elicits it. When anxiety occurs repeatedly and out of proportion to the threats involved—possibly as a result of unconscious conflicts—a condition of abnormal anxiety is present.

It would be a major, indeed impossible, task to wipe out all the anxieties that afflict the human race. There are available, however, individual treatments for people who are deeply troubled and disabled by their own anxieties. Part of the relief for anxiety comes from "talking it out" either in everyday communication or in professional psychotherapeutic interviews.

In addition to that crucial means of relieving anxiety there are now chemotherapeutic agents —drugs—which aid in the task. This is basically the class of drugs known as tranquilizers, introduced into medical practice in the mid-1950's. According to one definition (by Chauncey D. Leake), tranquilizers are chemical compounds that are specifically useful for the relief of anxiety and are differentiated from other central nervous system depressant drugs by that quality. All of them have somewhat different pharmacological action but their net therapeutic effect on mood and behavior is to reduce anxiety. However, one cannot depend on tranquilizers alone, or any other drug, to dispel his anxieties.

Chronic (Pathological) Fatigue

Closely akin to anxiety, and perhaps another form of it, is the condition often described as chronic, or pathological, fatigue. Chronic fatigue may also be called "emotional fatigue." It is different from the physiological fatigue that follows after strenuous work or exercise.

Chronic, or pathological, fatigue is a symptom that something is wrong with the person who suffers from it. Many people are chronically fatigued without realizing it. This fatigue may be expressed in changed moods, attitudes, and behavior, for example, exceptional irritability, loss of a sense of humor, or even loss of weight, poor appetite, and restless sleep. A constant state of muscular tension—considerably beyond normal muscle tone—commonly accompanies chronic fatigue. This abnormal tension, or hypertonus, arises because the muscles are being constantly stimulated by unconscious motivations to make first this move and then that. However, the stimulus to complete the move is inhibited and countermanded before the muscles can fully obey. These alternating commands keep the muscles constantly on stretch. Fatigue products are never completely enough dispelled, so the feeling of fatigue persists.

External pressures and environmental circumstances are factors in bringing on chronic fatigue. This has been studied particularly in the field of industrial hygiene. Workers become fatigued and less productive when they must work under conditions of poor light and glare, poor ventilation, too much noise and heat, uncomfortable seating, and exposure to dusts and fumes.

Other factors that induce fatigue are excessive hours of work, lack of properly spaced rest pauses, awkward working positions, "speed-up" of work beyond capacity to perform, and the monotony of simple, repeated operations. Workers are less productive also when they are afraid of and hostile toward their jobs and bosses.

Some of the facts discovered in the study of industrial hygiene can be profitably applied by the wise student in eliminating fatigue factors from his own life. He can arrange to do his studying under the best possible conditions of physical comfort and efficiency. Equally important is a rhythm of work balanced with relaxation. A rest pause of five minutes during each study hour is advisable. There should be some regularity in the student's schedule of study, play, eating, and sleeping. Too much extracurricular pressure should be avoided. Procrastination, delay, and overcrowding of hours bring on fatigue and reduce efficiency. Careless students work the hardest.

While fatigue is a symptom of disease, it must also be recognized that fatigue may predispose to disease—for example, the common cold. Sufficient time for recovery from fatigue must be allowed, especially after infectious diseases. Convalescence should not be unduly shortened. For simple fatigue, rest is the sovereign remedy. But in cases of chronic fatigue professional help may be needed, and great effort may have to be exerted to root out its causes.

Why to Stay away from Stimulants. The *wrong way* to fight fatigue is by indulgence in chemical stimulants. The reason? Too often, when taken in sufficient dosage to have any genuine effect, they create a "rebound reaction" and, after a short while, you end up feeling more fatigued than before you took the drug.

Probably the best known and most widely used stimulant drug is *caffeine,* which is the active ingredient in coffee, tea, chocolate drinks, some cola drinks and many nonprescription "stay awake" drugs.

There are, of course, many other drugs known to stimulate the central nervous system, including amphetamines (such as benzadrine) and whole new series of psychic stimulants that were developed in the 1960's. When prescribed by a physician upon proper indications, these are valuable medications.

Many college students, however, have the mistaken idea that they can take these so-called "pep pills" indiscriminately and without harm. "Pep pills" are often used by students to cram for exams or to drive all night to get home or back to college after an exciting weekend. This is a dangerous practice, because all potent stimulant drugs may have side effects (in addition to rebound reactions) and untoward reactions that were not anticipated by the indiscriminate self-medicator. There are better ways than chemicals to deal with fatigue; notably by better organization of one's time, by recreation, relaxation, good sleeping habits, and the control of factors and problems which induce needless psychic stress and muscular tension.

SUMMARY REVIEW QUESTIONS

1. What is the relationship of personality to emotions? To the unconscious mind? How do we judge personality?
2. What is the proper sequential order in which the following types of love appear in the course of normal personality development: idealistic, narcissistic, oedipal, homosexual, heterosexual, imitative? At approximately what age does each appear?

3. What are the two chief "negative emotions"? What is their purpose? How should they be consciously managed?
4. What do you understand by the term *unconscious mind?* What is its relationship to the conscious mind?
5. What do you understand by the id? The ego? The superego? What are the leading or peculiar characteristics of each?
6. How do conflicts in the unconscious mind produce anxiety? What can be done to relieve such anxiety?
7. What is a mental mechanism (or dynamism)? Can you name six and explain briefly what each one means?
8. How do you explain in terms of overworked mental mechanisms (or otherwise) the behavior of "stock characters" described in the following terms: the hypochondriac, the alibi artist, the homebody, the absent-minded professor, the perfectionist, the spit-fire, the sarcastic critic, the extrovert, Lady Macbeth, Pollyanna?
9. Do you believe that we live in an "age of anxiety"? Justify your answer, whether positive or negative.
10. What is chronic, or pathological, fatigue? How does it differ from normal, or physiological, fatigue? In what way, if any, is it related to anxiety?
11. Are the following statements sense or nonsense? Why? *Anyone who is afraid is a coward. . . . It is easy to get angry at those you love. . . . The child is father to the man. . . . Fatigue never hurt anyone. . . . The man who knows where he is going is on the road to mental health. . . . Always do the best you can with what you have where you are.*
12. What do the following terms mean to you: libido, infantile amnesia, repression, fantasy, frustration, emotional maturity, neurotic anxiety, ego defense, fetishist, tranquilizer, stimulant?

Recommended for Further Reading: *Discovering Ourselves* by Edward A. Strecker, M. D. and Kenneth E. Appel, M. D. *Love or Perish* by Smiley Blanton, M. D. *The Undiscovered Self* by C. G. Jung. *Anxiety: A Condition of Modern Man* by Henri Steiner and Jean Gebser. *Psychopathology of Everyday Life* by Sigmund Freud, M.D.

3

ALCOHOL AND ALCOHOLISM

ABOUT SEVEN-EIGHTHS OF AMERICAN COL-lege men and three-fourths of American college women have taken a drink of an alcoholic beverage some time in their lives. However, not more than one boy in five or one girl in ten drinks oftener than once a week. Conversation about liquor among college students far outruns their actual consumption of alcoholic beverages. It would have to. The sale of alcoholic beverages to young people is almost everywhere illegal—and most college students are still minors under these laws. (Legal definitions of a "minor"—a definition often linked with the age at which a young man or woman may marry without parental consent—vary from state to state: under 21 in many states, under 18 in others, for example.) This fact in itself may help to explain why boastful attitudes about the amount of liquor they can "hold" persist among many college boys. Their bragging, incidentally, frequently harks back to a one-time experience.

The right to drink alcoholic beverages is considered an adult privilege; and many younger college boys are fighting to prove that they are already fully grown adults. For this reason alcoholic bravado is often unconsciously equated in the minds of the braggarts with their sexual prowess. When they brag to their dates about how much liquor they can drink, they really mean to say, "See what a man I am!"

Why College Students Drink

Unquestionably a certain number of college students drink liquor on some social occasions.

There are indeed in Western civilization certain socially acceptable occasions (and even rituals) for the use of alcoholic beverages. They are, for example, an integral part of certain religious rites and ceremonies. Very few drink heavily; they would not last long on any campus. Some students continue social drinking for the rest of their lives. Others, after a juvenile fling, subside into abstinence. Some drift into chronic alcoholism, and a few end on Skid Row. There is also a group of college graduates who abstain from liquor during youth but begin drinking in later years.

Drinking is less fashionable and not so "smart" today as it was some years ago on American college campuses—particularly during the prohibition era (1918 to 1933), when college students were directly aping their law-breaking elders.

The attitudes and practices of the administration and alumni of any particular college are very likely to determine student attitudes toward the social acceptability of drinking. If the faculty club has a bar on campus and the alumni club a bar off campus, if cocktails are served at official college functions and faculty parties, if alumni turn up half-drunk at athletic events, it will be rather difficult to convince students that drinking is either socially unacceptable or morally wrong.

As long as beer is seductively advertised on television and "hard liquor" in magazines of intellectual stature, it will be difficult to re-establish the picture of Old John Barleycorn, with a noose in his hand, hauling young men and women down the road to perdition. One swallow doesn't make a drunkard. It is only fair to point out that *attitudes* toward alcohol differ not only in different colleges but also in different sections of the United States. There is general and official agreement, however, that college students should not drink.

Why do college students sometimes drink? Some drink to prove they are "men." Others regard their ability to consume large amounts of liquor as a bid for attention, or a point of superiority to assuage inferiority feelings. Still others drink out of a feeling of rebellion against parents or college authorities.

Curiosity is another impetus toward drinking in college. A few young people feel that they cannot afford to miss the "experience" of getting drunk, unpleasant and risky as it and its after-effects may be. Social pressure is another impulse to college drinking. Many students drink simply because they think it's "the thing to do." Their friends or their fraternity brothers or sorority sisters urge them on. A few college women undoubtedly consent to drinking because they are afraid they will be unpopular or considered "poor sports" if they do not. All such superficial reasons for drinking may, however, lead to a subtle or unconscious desire to utilize alcohol as a means of removing inhibitions related to unconventional behavior.

No amount of exhortation will keep an adult college student from drinking if he is bent on doing it. On the other hand a sober examination of the pros and cons of the facts about alcohol and alcoholism will permit any individual intelligent enough to be in college to make up his or her mind about drinking.

The Risk of Alcoholism. Some authorities, as might be expected, are more vehement than others about the risks of alcoholism. Dr. Marvin A. Block, a Buffalo, New York, physician, for example, and others, have estimated that one out of every 15 teenagers is likely to become an alcoholic. Dr. Block feels that home influences are the decisive factor in whether or not the risk becomes an eventual reality. He calls "kiddy cocktails"—soft drinks served to children in cocktail glasses—"a dangerous procedure." He sees very little alcoholism, however, among individuals who came from homes where drinking was done regularly with meals. Children from such homes, he finds, look upon drinking as part of their home life and rarely go on to excessive indulgence in alcohol in later life—unless their own parents have set them an unfortunate example of excessive and unruly drinking. Dr. Block concludes:

We should teach our young people that not to drink does not affect them socially, that alcohol is not a necessity of life, that some people may drink if they wish, but that to others it will bring harm. If we could teach people that the real sophisticate never drinks excessively, and that to do so means social ostracism, we'd find less and less alcoholism.

Varying Tolerances to Alcohol

It must also be recognized, however, that varying tolerances to alcohol occur among different individuals. An explanation as to why two people of the same weight who drink the same amount of alcohol may react differently to it was given in the May 19, 1962 issue of the *Journal of the American Medical Association* as follows:

An experienced drinker has learned how to counteract some of the adverse effects of alcohol, whereas a novice, faced with the same situation, would be less capable of compensating for the alcohol-imposed handicap.

This is the answer of the AMA Sub-Committee on Alcohol, given in answer to a question submitted to the *Journal*.

Habitual drinkers absorb their alcohol more slowly and oxidize it more rapidly than do persons who rarely take a drink.

Also, the presence of food in the upper gastrointestinal tract tends to retard the rate of alcohol absorption and thus ameliorates the effect of a given dose.

However, the group said, there is little difference among individuals in ability of brain tissue to resist the effect of a given tissue concentration of alcohol.

All persons show some impairment in driving ability at a blood alcohol concentration of 0.10 per cent, and in some this ability is impaired at a level as low as 0.02 per cent. Regardless of tolerance, the fatal concentration is 0.6 per cent to 0.8 per cent.

Showing estimated *per cent* of alcohol in the blood by number of drinks in relation to body weight

Body Weight	Drinks											
	1	2	3	4	5	6	7	8	9	10	11	12
100 lbs.	.038	.075	.113	.150	.188	.225	.263	.300	.338	.375	.413	.450
120 lbs.	.031	.063	.094	.125	.156	.188	.219	.250	.281	.313	.344	.375
140 lbs.	.027	.054	.080	.107	.134	.161	.188	.214	.241	.268	.295	.321
160 lbs.	.023	.047	.070	.094	.117	.141	.164	.188	.211	.234	.258	.281
180 lbs.	.021	.042	.063	.083	.104	.125	.146	.167	.188	.208	.229	.250
200 lbs.	.019	.038	.056	.075	.094	.113	.131	.150	.169	.188	.206	.225
220 lbs.	.017	.034	.051	.068	.085	.102	.119	.136	.153	.170	.188	.205
240 lbs.	.016	.031	.047	.063	.078	.094	.109	.125	.141	.156	.172	.188

The chart defines a blood alcohol percentage of .050 or less as usually innocuous.

OVER .050 but LESS than .150 results in some impairment of JUDGMENT and VISION.

A concentration of .150 or MORE results in increasingly dangerous INTOXICATION.

However, since the passage of time REDUCES blood alcohol concentration, the actual concentration of alcohol in the blood at any given time may be determined by subtracting .015 per cent from the percentage shown on the chart for every hour that elapses since the first drink.

*This has been reproduced from the New Jersey Department of Law and Public Safety pamphlet "Blood-Alco Chart."

(Blood alcohol per cent means the per cent of the chemical substance, alcohol, to the estimated total volume of blood, about 7 quarts, circulating in the entire body. Thus it may be observed that a very small percentage of alcohol in the bloodstream—indeed as little as $\frac{2}{100}$ of 1%— can have significant effects.)

To set the stage for a more exact understanding, let us briefly consider what alcohol and alcoholism really signify, and how many people we are talking about when we speak of drinkers and alcoholics.

Alcohol is essentially a *depressant drug* which affords a prompt, but temporary, escape from the stresses of external reality or inner turmoil. We speak, of course, only of *ethyl alcohol,* the active ingredient in all alcoholic beverages. Alcoholism, therefore, may be described as poisoning with an overdose of alcohol. Drunkenness is the temporary result.

Chronic alcoholism is the outcome of prolonged and repeated use of alcohol to compensate for deep-seated personality problems. It falls within the category of mental illness, although there is also a biochemical approach to the dis-

ease. Some scientific investigators have suggested that alcoholism is a form of allergy; others, that it is a metabolic disease. It is probably fair to say that the causes of alsoholism are multiple and in large measure still undefined.

Well over 90% of 80 million adult drinkers in the United States use alcoholic beverages temperately. They can "take it or leave it alone." Their home, business life, and health are not adversely affected. They are *social drinkers.*

But somewhat over 6.5 million people have gone beyond social drinking and have become what may be loosely termed "alcoholics." About 85% of these alcoholics may be classified as *heavy drinkers.* These excessive drinkers (both men and women) frequently harm themselves physically, psychologically, and socially.

Beyond this group are some 600,000 to 800,000 *chronic alcoholics* (also called *problem drinkers* or *compulsive drinkers*) who no longer have any control over their desire or need for alcohol. They are the true "slaves to drink."

The Pattern of an Alcoholic. The gradual steps by which an individual becomes a chronic alcoholic can usually be recognized. Here, progressively, are some of the warning signs of an insidious drift toward chronic alcoholism:

¶ When you are out drinking with friends, you are always the one who has to have that "last" or "extra" drink.

¶ Your hangovers get worse and worse. You find you are suffering from temporary blackouts. You are plagued with feelings of remorse, anxiety, or guilt.

¶ You discover that drinking means more to you than to other people and you start looking for that alcoholic kick more often than you used to. You begin sneaking drinks at odd times.

¶ You find yourself turning more and more to alcohol. One drink is never enough. You don't want to stop drinking until you are drunk.

¶ You won't admit what's happening to you. You find all kinds of excuses and rationalizations for your drinking. You assert that you can handle your liquor. (The people with whom you associate, however, may not accept your excuses; and you will gradually find yourself excluded from their company.)

¶ You make a great discovery—a cure for hangover; namely, one, two, or more drinks in the morning.

¶ You become a solitary drinker. Alcohol alone is company and pleasure enough for you. But you may feel quite dejected between your sprees. You may begin to brood over yourself. You may feel very self-conscious and afraid of being with other people. At other times you may feel very antagonistic toward and critical of others—often those nearest and dearest to you.

¶ Getting drunk, going on benders, becomes the main goal of your life—even though the results are severe hangovers, terrifying fears, social ostracism, tremors (shakes), and even worse, delirium tremens (DT's). At this point you have become a truly chronic alcoholic. You desperately need the help you should have sought earlier. . . . But you can still be helped, if you make up your mind.

The Effects of Alcohol

The effects of all alcoholic beverages depend upon the amount of alcohol, ounce for ounce,

that they contain. Hard liquors—whiskey, brandy, gin, vodka, and rum—have the highest concentration of alcohol by volume; "100 proof" means the beverage contains 50% alcohol. Light wines run from about 7 to 12% alcoholic content, and beer much less.

A bottle of beer and a shot-glass of whiskey are roughly equivalent in their alcoholic content.

Beer often tends to be fattening. In caloric value and vitamin content a glass of beer is about half as nutritious as a glass of milk. Inasmuch as it is rapidly metabolized in the body, alcohol does have some little food value.

The concentration of alcohol in the blood stream determines its effect. Behavior of the "average" drinker can be correlated with percentages of alcohol in his blood stream approximately as follows:

Blood Alcohol 0.01%. The drinker feels his head clear; he breathes more freely through his nose; there is a mild tingling of the mucous membranes of the mouth and throat.

This primary physiological kick is one of the reasons why alcohol is so commonly regarded as a stimulant. It does stimulate the sensory organs in the mouth and digestive tract. For a few minutes this leads to more rapid circulation of the blood and with it a clearing away of some fatigue products of the body. Hence the drinker "feels better," momentarily. The depressant effect begins when the alcohol in the blood stream reaches the brain.

Blood Alcohol 0.02%. The drinker enjoys a pleasant feeling and is willing to talk freely. He has a sense of warmth and physical well-being. This is the appeal of alcohol to the social drinker. Still there may already be a touch of dizziness, a slight throbbing, and sense of fullness in the head.

Blood Alcohol 0.03%. The drinker has a feeling of mild euphoria. "All's right with the world." He doesn't worry. He has in effect lost the capacity to worry because the depressant effect of the alcohol has already impaired his judgment and memory.

Blood Alcohol 0.04%. The imbiber displays lots of energy. He talks freely—and loudly. But his hands begin to tremble and his movements are a bit clumsy. Beyond this point he is legally intoxicated as shown by "drunkometer" tests.

Blood Alcohol 0.05%. Now the drinker is "sitting on the top of the world." His inhibitions are almost all removed. He says he can "lick anybody in the world"—but he has difficulty in lighting a match.

Blood Alcohol 0.07%. Now the worm has begun to turn. A feeling of remoteness steals over the drinker. His pulse is strong and his breathing heavy. His energy is abated.

Blood Alcohol 0.1%. Now the drinker staggers perceptibly. He talks to himself. He feels drowsy.

Blood Alcohol 0.2%. The drunkard now needs help to walk. He is easily angered. He feels nauseated. His bladder control is poor.

Blood Alcohol 0.3%. The victim is now in a stupor. He does not understand what is said to him. He may sleep and vomit by turns.

Blood Alcohol 0.4%. The patient is now completely unconscious—"out cold." The depressive effect of alcohol has wrought a deep anesthesia.

Individual Differences in Effect. Despite the similarity of effects in terms of blood concentration of alcohol, it should be pointed out that individuals differ greatly in the amount of alcoholic beverages they need to yield a similar degree of intoxication. Heavier people can stand larger doses of alcohol than smaller people. Some may be drunk on one-quarter of the amount of alcohol that it takes for others. A teetotaler will respond to a far smaller dose of alcohol than a chronic alcoholic. As with many other drugs, a certain amount of tolerance to alcohol is developed—which means that the intake doses must be increased.

The circumstances under which alcohol is taken may also modify its effects. It is, for example, more intoxicating on an empty stomach than when taken with a meal. Alcohol is one of the few substances that is directly absorbed into the blood stream from the stomach. Furthermore, it passes more rapidly from the stomach into the intestines when there is no food present to delay this passage. From the intestines also alcohol is rapidly absorbed and carried to the brain.

Some Psychological Effects of Alcohol. Under the influence of alcohol, even in "safe" concentrations, mental processes are altered. Fantasy increases; alertness diminishes. Many carefully devised psychological tests have proved this point—for example:

Thirty to 60 minutes after drinking 1 to 3 ounces of alcohol, reaction time is significantly increased. It takes an experienced auto driver half again as long as normal ($3/_{10}$ instead of $2/_{10}$ second) to get his foot on the brake. A professional typist makes 40 to 50% more errors in her typing. A bricklayer lays only 90% as many bricks as he could while completely sober. Ability to add simple numbers decreases 10%. Capacity to do problems involving mathematical reasoning falls 10 to 20%. Ability to match words with opposite meanings decreases by one-third to one-half.

Throughout all these tests, the subject is usually under the impression that he is doing better than he would when cold sober. He is fooled because his judgment as well as his reaction time is impaired. In an experiment with 20 automobile drivers, all thought they were driving more slowly than usual when the fact was that they were driving faster. Long-experienced British bus drivers, with two shots of whiskey under their belts, were willing to try to squeeze their buses through a gap 14 inches narrower than the bus!

Physiological Effects of Alcohol. In the past, gruesome physiological effects were pointed out as the effects of alcohol. Cirrhosis of the liver, with the showing of a "hobnailed liver" in a bottle, was a prize demonstration. Every ailment to which the alcoholic—or even the moderate user of alcohol—was subject was attributed to this one cause.

Today it is the consensus of medical opinion that the *temperate,* moderate and occasional use of alcoholic beverages has little, if any, residual effect on the health of the user. Statistical records show that moderate users of alcohol live as long as total abstainers. This would indicate that temperate use of alcohol does not result in bodily harm. On the other hand the immediate aftereffects of alcoholic indulgence—hangover, headache, and nausea—and the more frequent risk of accident or contraction of venereal disease while under the influence of alcohol must be accounted as bodily risks due to alcohol.

The continued excessive use of alcohol brings physical and mental deterioration and often untimely death. Excessive drinkers shorten their lives; their resistance to disease, notably pneumonia, is decreased; their nervous and digestive systems are impaired; they are subject to alcoholic psychoses, such as delirium tremens (DT's).

Alcoholics often skip meals and generally neglect their diet. Bloated with liquids, they blunt their normal hunger pangs. Since they eat so poorly, chronic alcoholics often suffer from nutritional deficiencies, especially lack of vitamin B, which exaggerates their nervous difficulties.

Alcohol—Medicine and Drug. Alcohol is sometimes prescribed as a medicine by physicians. Its judicious use is generally confined to elderly patients suffering from chronic disease. It eases their pain and discomfort and gives them a welcome sense of temporary well-being. In small doses it is a spur to appetite.

Alcohol also has the pharmacological effect of a vasodilator; it causes the blood vessels to expand. This is why a feeling of warmth follows alcohol ingestion, and why alcohol is not forbidden—in moderation—to patients suffering from some forms of heart disease or high blood pressure. The therapeutic uses of alcohol are, however, very limited. It is *not* good for snakebite.

Alcoholism as a Mental Illness

In recent history alcoholism was regarded as a sin, or a weakness in the moral fiber. Indignant citizens insisted that the alcoholic could stop drinking if he wanted to. Many drunkards were hopefully lured into "signing the pledge" by earnest temperance workers who had no real idea of the underlying reasons for alcoholism.

Today we know enough about alcoholism to describe it properly as a mental illness, or at least as the primary symptom of an illness.

Here is the testimony of an ex-alcoholic on the nature of the sickness: "I remember—I can never forget—the years in which I suffered from acute chronic alcoholism. They were the most painful years of my life. I suffered constantly, not just one kind of pain, but all kinds of pain. I suffered

physically, mentally, emotionally, financially, and socially—in every department of my life." The writer of these lines is Mrs. Marty Mann, now executive director of the National Council on Alcoholism.

What Makes An Alcoholic? What makes an alcoholic? Why do some people cross the line from social drinking to problem drinking? Since research in alcoholism is still comparatively young, there are no final answers, but psychiatric studies have given some powerful hints.

First, there is the possibility that many chronic alcoholics have physical constitutions which are especially sensitive to alcohol—just as other people are peculiarly allergic (sensitive) to different foods (e.g., strawberries) and drugs (e.g., penicillin).

Second, the psychological reasons for compulsive drinking undoubtedly differ to some extent in each individual case. The personality and the history of each chronic alcoholic supplies the clues to his particular reasons for excessive drinking. Yet there are some permissible generalizations.

Alcoholics are preponderantly males. However, in comparatively recent years there has been uncovered a considerable number of female alcoholics, who use alcohol primarily as a bulwark against loneliness. Women find it easier than men to conceal addiction to alcohol. Three-fourths of known alcoholics are between the ages of 35 and 55. They come from all walks of life, and they exhibit all degrees of intelligence. Many are outwardly jolly and sociable creatures. Others may be just the opposite: dour and sour. They seem to want and need to be popular with their fellow men. Here is the fallacy. Underlying this need, which is a wish to be loved, the alcoholic has a deep, vague, sometimes unknown (to him) feeling of insecurity. It is this dreaded feeling which he tries to drown and deny with alcohol.

The alcoholic suffers from a deep-seated neurosis, whose origin far antedates the excessive drinking. Regardless of the actual circumstances of his life, the alcoholic lives with unconscious, painful, neurotic conflicts. He wants to run away from himself. Alcohol seems to temporarily float him away from his problems and give him respite from his emotional conflict.

The origins of the neurotic conflicts of the alcoholic probably go back to childhood. They often embrace feelings of long-repressed anger against parents who betrayed, rejected, or frustrated him as a child. Alcohol temporarily releases this dreadful inner feeling of guilt, frustration, and insecurity, so the alcoholic resorts to it more and more. His drinking may also represent a secret revenge against his parents.

The alcoholic is not consciously aware that he is responding to a clash of forces in his unconscious mind. Indeed he can rarely be persuaded to recognize that he has inner conflicts. Yet his unspeakable secret terror and his inner burden make the alcoholic in greater need of release than the ordinary person. *The difference is quantitative, not qualitative.* Alcohol does ease emotional tensions; the alcoholic stands in greater and more constant need of such relief. Obviously all neurotics do not become alcoholics. They find other outlets (for example, obesity or gambling) or happier solutions for their inner torment.

Treatment of Chronic Alcoholism. The treatment of chronic alcoholism in the past was generally disappointing. The patient was sobered up, remorsefully "went on the wagon" for varying lengths of time, then plunged into another stuporous alcoholic spree. This cycle was repeated many times. Recent approaches to treatment are much more hopeful. Any alcoholic who really wants to free himself from the affliction of compulsive drinking can probably succeed in this attempt.

The basic approach to the treatment of alcoholism now concerns itself, first, with raising the alcoholic's ability to tolerate the tensions that drive him to drink, and second, with reducing or eliminating his stress situations. The alcoholic often desperately needs psychotherapy to understand himself—but he is not always ready for it. Meanwhile, he usually requires supportive therapy. Here the new tranquilizing drugs, chlorpromazine and meprobomate, for example, are often of great help.

Complete medical care (medical rehabilita-

tion) is also usually necessary, for the alcoholic is likely to be suffering from conditions which place additional stresses on his psychological and metabolic weaknesses. Malnutrition—particularly lack of vitamins—chronic indigestion, fatigue, chest and abdominal pains, and neuritis are common symptoms that require attention. Massive vitamin therapy, particularly with the vitamin B group, is sometimes effectively prescribed.

The aversion treatment, combined with psychotherapy, is sometimes helpful. In one such method the patient takes a drug (like antabuse) which makes him exceedingly sensitive to alcohol. He becomes ill and vomits whenever he takes a drink. This reaction enforces sobriety for many months while the patient is in the process of acquiring an improved attitude toward his inner problems.

In the final analysis, however, the alcoholic requires a high degree of social rehabilitation. He is particularly responsive to his social environment. Here, Alcoholics Anonymous (AA), an organization of recovered alcoholics started in the United States in 1935, has done great service in saving chronic alcoholics. They estimate that 50 to 75% of those who join their ranks and make a real effort to free themselves from compulsive drinking succeed in doing so. The alcoholic can never take another drink if he wants to stay "cured."

Alcoholism as a Social Problem

Even a single episode of intoxication can plunge an individual into folly of far-reaching consequence. However, it is the heavy drinkers and chronic alcoholics who create the social problems associated with alcohol. Crime, accident, and divorce rates are significantly higher among alcoholics than among the rest of the population. Many homes and families are wrecked by the neurotic illness exhibited as alcoholism. The social consequences on wives (sometimes husbands) and children is tragic and enormous.

The cost of alcoholism in the United States, in terms of care and treatment of alcoholics in hospitals and jails, crime, accidents, lost wages, support of dependents and so forth is estimated at well over $1 billion a year. This may perhaps be charged against the $3 to $4 billion a year collected in federal, state, and local taxes on the sale of alcoholic beverages. Actually between 4 and 5% of the national income, a sales figure now over $10 billion annually, is consumed in the purchase of alcoholic drinks.

Alcohol is a traffic hazard of the first magnitude. One of every five fatal auto accidents involves either a drunken driver or a drunken pedestrian. Legal interpretations obscure many of the official statistics on drunken driving, but its frequency is far too great for comfort. The drunken driver is often under the impression that the *other fellow* is on the wrong side of the road.

A past president of the American Automobile Association declared: "A person who has been drinking is fifty-five times more likely to have an accident involving personal injury."

There can be but one safe motto: *If you drink, don't drive. If you drive, don't drink.* You are also well within your moral rights to refuse to ride with a driver who has been drinking.

Prevention and Control of Alcoholism

The prevention and control of alcoholism is still a world-wide problem. It is an ancient and repetitive problem too. The Greeks of antiquity used wine as a weapon of conquest over barbarian tribes in the Mediterranean just as the

IF YOU DRINK**					Effects	Alcohol concentration in the blood	Before you drive WAIT***
Cocktails	OR	Highballs	OR	Beer			
WITHIN FIFTEEN MINUTES					If even one cocktail is taken on an empty stomach, absorption may be so rapid that alcohol piles up in the blood stream for a brief period and produces an exaggerated effect for a short time.	.03%	½ hour
WITHIN ONE HALF HOUR					Warmth—mental relaxation—decrease of fine skills—less concern with minor irritations and restraints.	.06%	1 hour
WITHIN ONE HOUR					Buoyancy—exaggerated emotion and behavior: talkative, noisy or morose. Perceptible loss of fine coordination.	.09%	2 hours
WITHIN TWO HOURS					Clumsiness—unsteadiness—tunnel vision.	.12%	3 hours
WITHIN THREE HOURS					Intoxication: Obvious and unmistakable impairment of bodily functions and mental faculties. Even after considerable alcohol has been eliminated, acute hangover symptoms remain.	.15%	5 hours

*Based on a person of average size—150 lbs. The effects will increase or decrease with corresponding weight differences.

**The body reacts quicker to alcohol taken when the stomach is empty.   ***After finishing the last drink.

Driver WAIT Meter* (Time Allowance Chart)

white man, some 23 centuries later, employed "firewater" to the destruction of American Indian tribes. The Greek philosopher Plato noted that "drunkenness is an important subject and it takes no mean legislator to understand it."

One fact, however, appears to be established by centuries of experience with alcohol: you cannot legislate it out of existence. In 1918, for example, the United States was politically manipulated into passing a national law (actually a constitutional amendment) intended to eliminate any use and all possible abuse of alcohol by legally prohibiting the manufacture, transportation, and sale of all alcoholic beverages. This "noble experiment" was a dismal failure. Bootleggers, moonshiners, racketeers, and their respectable customers nullified the law within a few years. In 1933 the national prohibition laws were formally repealed. The practical control of alcoholism in the United States is still left mainly to police departments. Arrests for drunkenness make up a large proportion of the total arrests in any metropolitan area.

Since chronic alcoholism is an illness, one of the first steps in the prevention and control of this illness is to keep the patients out of jails and put them in hospitals adequately equipped and staffed for this purpose. Such complete programs are rare, although over 3000 general hospitals will now admit patients for the treatment of acute alcoholism. Out-patient clinical facilities must also be made available. All this requires considerable outlay of money and continuing public support. It is, however, a less expensive way of dealing with the problem than jailing drunks.

The full and practical cooperation of the medical profession in managing the problems of alcoholism must also be obtained. This has been difficult to get because alcoholics have always been unsatisfactory and refractory patients for the doctor in private practice. With better methods of treatment, however, the professional attitude is gradually changing. Finally, programs of research and education in the field of alcoholism must be relentlessly pursued to bring the vast problem more clearly into focus.

The individual as citizen can do much to help meet the expensive and often heart-breaking problem of alcoholism. In the last analysis, however, his own temperate use of or abstinence from alcoholic beverages will provide the basis for effective community control. The individual who has a strong personality, inner spiritual resources, and a sensible working philosophy of life rarely needs alcohol to escape rather than face up to the normal stresses of everyday living.

SUMMARY REVIEW QUESTIONS

1. Why do college students sometimes drink alcoholic beverages? Do you consider any or all of these reasons valid?
2. How do you distinguish between social drinkers, heavy drinkers, and compulsive drinkers? Approximately how many people in the United States fall into each of these categories?
3. To what extent do you regard alcoholism as a moral weakness? A sin? An illness? A crime? On what outside opinion or authority do you base your own judgment?
4. What are the immediate effects of drinking alcoholic beverages? What determines these effects and what factors serve to modify these effects? What are the long-range effects of (a) temperate, moderate use of alcoholic beverages and (b) excessive use of alcohol?
5. What are the steps by which an individual gradually descends the scale from social drinking to chronic alcoholism? What are the clues or warning signs by which the stages of this descent can be recognized?
6. Since chronic alcoholism is a sickness, what kind of sickness is it? What makes an alcoholic? How can chronic alcoholics be treated? Can they be "cured?"

7. In what respects is alcohol a social problem? How can this problem be met? Do you believe that chronic alcoholism can be prevented or controlled? If so, how? If not, why not?
8. Are the following statements sense or nonsense? Why? *Anything is worth trying once. . . . Alcohol is a stimulant. . . . Tolerance for alcohol is the same for everybody. . . . If you drink don't drive; if you drive don't drink. . . . "I wonder often what the vintners buy/One-half so precious as the stuff they sell."*–from the *Rubaiyat of Omar Khayyam.*
9. What do the following terms mean to you: ethyl alcohol, 100 proof, blood alcohol, AA, cirrhosis of the liver, "noble experiment," aversion treatment, social drinker, DT's tolerance (to alcohol)?

Worth Looking Into: *Marty Mann's New Primer on Alcoholism* by Marty Mann. *The Neutral Spirit: a Portrait of Alcohol* by Berton Roueché. *Alcohol and Alcoholism,* produced by the Public Information Branch of the National Institute of Mental Health. *The Lost Weekend* by Charles Jackson.

4

DRUG USE AND ABUSE

STUDENT DRUG USE IS INDEED A COMMENTARY on American society, but it is above all an indirect criticism of our society's inability to offer the young exciting, honorable, and effective ways of using their intelligence and idealism to reform our society.

Thus does Kenneth Keniston, of the Department of Psychiatry of the Yale Medical School, conclude a report on "Heads and Seekers: Drugs on Campus, Counter-Cultures, and American Society."[1] This same article begins:

Students who use drugs are usually treated by the mass media as an alien wart upon the student body of America. . . . Few subjects arouse feelings as intense and irrational as does the topic of student drug use; in few areas is there greater tendency to distort, to perceive facts selectively, and to view with alarm. Few topics are treated with so much heat and so little light.

A distinction may be made between drug users and drug abusers. Practically every American *uses* psychoactive drugs—for this list includes aspirin, sleeping pills, stimulants, tranquilizers, anti-depressants, ethyl alcohol, caffeine (in coffee and tea), and nicotine (in tobacco). Any of *these* drugs is subject to abuse, for taken in excess they become poisons. "The dosage makes the poison," runs an old medical axiom.

Drug Users in the College Community

What is new in the pattern is the use by college students (and even occasionally high school stu-

[1]K. Keniston, M.D., "Heads and Seekers: Drugs on Campus, Counter-Cultures, and American Society," *The American Scholar*, 97–112 (Winter 1968–1969).

dents) of new or at least newly recognized drugs which change moods and alter consciousness. Student drug use—and abuse—usually involves hallucinogenic drugs; they produce hallucinations, that is, sense perceptions not based on objective reality. The victim of hallucinations sees, hears, smells, tastes, or feels things that aren't there.

Most commonly used of the hallucinogens is marihuana. Others are LSD, DMT, psilocybin, mescaline, and peyote. Student use of the hallucinogens is increasing. However, it does not reach anywhere near the exaggerated figures that have been used in some debates. A recent Gallup poll arrived at an estimate that only 5 to 6% of all college students have "ever tried" any of the hallucinogenic drugs. Keniston estimates that fewer than 10% of American college students have ever tried such drugs.

Drug use and abuse seems to be more common at colleges and universities where there is a high "intellectual climate"—such as the Ivy League colleges, some of the Big Ten universities, and a few small, liberal arts colleges. At these colleges, a drug use rate (at least one try at the drugs) ranges between 10% to 50% of the student body. Use of drugs is lowest in the vocationally oriented departments of a university; that is, schools of business administration, engineering, agriculture, and education (of teachers).

Keniston divides "drug users" into three separate classes: (1) *tasters,* who have tried a drug no more than three times and do not intend to continue; (2) *seekers;* and (3) *heads.* The *seekers* makes up the largest contingent of college drug users.

Relatively speaking, they have used drugs only a few times, but they plan to continue use in their search for relevance both within and without their college experience. These students can be called seekers because they seek in drug use some way of "intensifying experience, expanding awareness, [and] breaking out of deadness and flatness [of their current pattern of life]."

Heads is shorthand for "pot heads," users of marihuana, and "acid heads," users of LSD and other, less potent, hallucinogens. This is a relatively small group of students who use drugs often, for example, every weekend. To quote Keniston again:

For such young men and women drug use is not just an intermittent assist in the pursuit of meaning, but a part of a more general "turned-on" ideology.

But even among the heads, drug use does not invariably constitute the deeply psychopathological and self-destructive phenomenon it is sometimes said invariably to be. . . . Many students who use marihuana routinely do *not* experience the ominous personal deterioration, the "bad trip," or loss of motivation that is sometimes thought to accompany even casual drug experimentation.

There exists, however, a small but highly publicized group of drug-takers for whom even a single experience with the hallucinogens produces serious ill-effects. Marihuana, rarely, and LSD, more often, can elicit panic states or transient psychotic reactions. The real risk for these students, however, is that they will temporarily drop out of the college scene into some "hippie" subculture. However, many of those who drop out eventually find their way back to the mainstream of society.

In the late 1960's the *New York Times* conducted a nationwide survey on drug usage. The survey revealed that for many students the use of drugs—particularly marihauna—was considered a part of growing up, perhaps "as common as the hip flasks during the Prohibition era." Many students sample drugs simply because they are available. Others want to appear daring or sophisticated. Some do because it is "the social thing to do, like sipping a cocktail." Others say, "It's not addict-

ing, it's cheaper than booze, and the high is better."

The college drug user tends to be rather bright but introspective. He often has deep personal or family problems and appears alienated from the values of his fellow students and his family. However, it should not be assumed that all college drug users fit this pattern.

Some Definitions

By *medical* definition, a narcotic is a drug that will put you to sleep or into a stupor and, at the same time, relieve pain. By *legal* definition, narcotics are a defined group of addictive (habit-forming) chemical substances whose indiscriminate use renders the user useless to himself and often dangerous to society.

In the practice of medicine, narcotic drugs, prescribed by a physician who understands both their effects and side-effects, have a legitimate place. Morphine, the pain-killer, is one of the sovereign remedies in the doctor's bag.

The "true" narcotics are drugs derived from opium, that is, opiates and synthetic substitutes for morphine, such as meperidine and methadone. The true opiates are all derived from the poppy plant, *Papaver somniferum.* Opium itself is a crude, gummy resin which can be smoked in a pipe. The most important drug derived from opium is morphine; the most dangerous, heroin; others are codeine and papaverine. Chemists and pharmacologists have tried for decades to formulate a synthetic drug that would have the painkilling effects of morphine without its addicting property. Hundreds of such drugs have been tried; those that relieve pain also produce addiction.

The opium poppy is now grown in such countries as India, Turkey, China, Egypt, and Mexico, where the climate is hot and dry and where land and labor are cheap. The unripe seed pods of the poppy contain a juice from which crude opium is extracted.

Although cocaine is legally defined as a narcotic under United States law, it is actually a stimulant drug. Marihuana is also regarded as a narcotic, though strictly speaking it is not.

The distinction between true drug addiction and drug habituation has been defined by the World Health Organization as follows:[2]

Addiction is a state of periodic or chronic intoxication produced by the repeated consumption of a drug and involves tolerance, psychological dependence, usually physical dependence, an overwhelming compulsion to continue using the drug, and detrimental effects on both the individual and society. *Habituation* is a condition, resulting from the repeated consumption of a drug, which involves little or no evidence of tolerance, some psychological dependence, and a desire (but not a compulsion) to continue taking the drug for the feeling of well-being that it engenders. Detrimental effects, if any, are primarily on the individual.

However, since these two terms have been used interchangeably, the World Health Organization had suggested that the term "drug dependence" be used, with the modification of the particular drug added. As an example, "drug dependence of the barbiturate type."

Historical Perspectives

The use and abuse of drugs that reach the central nervous system and affect behavior have been known since antiquity. The most widely used of such substances is probably ethyl alcohol.

Still other psychoactive drugs—opium, marihuana, and cocaine—were discovered by prehistoric man. These intoxicating substances were often employed as part of a religious ritual. The Chinese knew about marihuana as early as 2700 B.C.; the ancient Egyptians were acquainted with opium as early as 1500 B.C. There is also a reference to the use of opium in Homer's *Odyssey* (9th century B.C.).

The Greek and Roman physicians of antiquity used opium for its ability to induce sleep and relieve pain. In the early Christian era its use spread to many parts of Europe, and it was fur-

[2] From *Drug Abuse: Escape to Nowhere,* Smith Kline & French Laboratories, in cooperation with the American Association for Health, Physical Education, and Recreation, 1969.

ther used medically to suppress cough and relieve diarrhea, usages which still prevail.

The use of opium either as a medicine or as an intoxicating agent gradually spread throughout the world. American physicians in the eighteenth century used it to relieve pain associated with venereal disease, cancer, gallstones, some fevers, and as a remedy for diarrhea, vomiting, and the pains of childbirth.

In spite of its widespread medical use, physicians were slow to realize the fact that opium was an addictive substance. The same opinion was held about two alkaloids of opium discovered early in the nineteenth century—morphine in 1805, codeine in 1832. Physicians who were aware of opium addiction thought they could remedy the condition by prescribing morphine or codeine. All they did was to transfer patients from one addicting drug to another. The addicts preferred the morphine to the opium—it was ten times as strong!

Another factor that promoted the use of opiates was the invention in 1843 of the hypodermic needle and syringe. This instrument was used widely during the American Civil War to administer morphine not only for relief of painful wounds but also for the treatment of dysentery. As a result, many thousands of soldiers returned to civilian life addicted to morphine. Their addiction was intensified by the fact that opium and its derivatives were freely and cheaply sold in pharmacies and even rural stores; as laudanum (1 grain of opium to 15 drops of alcohol) and paregoric (1 grain to 480 drops).

In 1898 still another alkaloid of opium—heroin—was derived synthetically from morphine. This turned out to be the most powerfully addicting drug of all. At first heroin was used as a treatment for morphine addiction; but the error of this was soon discovered. Heroin has no legitimate medical uses.

The medical viewpoint on the hazards of opium and its derivatives gradually crystallized during the nineteenth century. In general, until late in the century, physicians thought of opiate addiction in about the same category as alcohol addiction. In 1889 one physician wrote, "The use of morphine in place of alcohol is but a choice of evils, and by far the lesser." The use of narcotics spread in America by their use in advertised "patent medicines." There was no control at that time over such medicines, since the first Federal Pure Food and Drug Act was not passed until 1906.

Public opinion did not then harshly condemn opiate addiction. Except for smoking opium in Chinese "opium dens," its use—at least orally—was considered an unfortunate habit rather than an affront to public morals. The use of opiates was more prevalent in the upper classes. Distinguished men of literary and political stature were acknowledged "opium eaters." Among them were Edgar Allan Poe, the American author; John Randolph, an American statesman; Samuel Coleridge and Francis Thompson, English poets; and Thomas De Quincy, who wrote "Confessions of an English Opium Eater."

The risks of narcotic addiction came to be more sharply understood in the early part of the twentieth century. In 1909 a federal law was passed prohibiting the importation of opium or its derivatives except for medical purposes. In 1914 the Congress of the United States passed the *Harrison Act* to control narcotic addiction. It did not make addiction per se illegal but put controls on the production, manufacture, and distribution of narcotics. Physicians were permitted to dispense or prescribe narcotic drugs. (Included among the "narcotic" drugs was cocaine, which is actually a stimulant.)

It soon became evident that private physicians could not succeed in treating narcotic addiction on an outpatient basis because the patients were so unreliable. For a brief time (1919–1923) local and state health departments set up clinics to dispense drugs to addicts as a part of treatment. But this effort also proved unacceptable because it was feared that narcotics were being dispensed too freely, and the clinics were closed.

At this point, the drug addict who could not break his habit turned to the underworld "black market" for his drugs, which had previously been a minor source of supply. The money cost for drugs in this market was high. A large number of addicts therefore became involved in criminal activities to support their addiction.

A number of additional federal laws to control the narcotics traffic were subsequently passed, and many states and cities passed laws and ordinances based on the federal models. The federal laws included:

Marihuana Tax Act (1937). This law provided the same controls over marihuana as the Harrison Act did for narcotics. (Again, marihuana is a hallucinogen, not a "narcotic" in the same sense that opiates are; but the extension of terms of Harrison Act to marihuana has suggested that it is.)

Narcotic Control Act (1956). In the face of increased juvenile use of narcotics after World War II, this act provided heavy penalties for the unlawful sale of narcotics and marihuana to minors. For example, an adult who furnishes heroin to a minor may be subject (for a second offense) to imprisonment from ten years to life, an optional fine up to $20,000, or the death penalty if a jury so directs.

Drug Abuse Control Amendments (1965). These enactments extended the Federal Food, Drug and Cosmetic Act to control stimulant, depressive, and hallucinogenic drugs which may be subject to abuse. Barbiturates, amphetamines, LSD, and comparable drugs are included in these categories.

The enforcement of these antidrug laws was formerly vested in the Federal Bureau of Narcotics, operating under the United States Treasury Department; the Food and Drug Administration (FDA); and the Bureau of Customs. In 1968 these enforcement agencies (except for the Bureau of Customs) were merged into the Bureau of Narcotics and Dangerous Drugs in the United States Department of Justice.

Even as wider and stricter enforcement of laws against narcotics and other dangerous drugs were enacted, a somewhat different picture of the addict appeared. He was regarded not only as a criminal, but as a sick, tortured person, desperately in need of help.

A White House Conference on Narcotics and Drug Abuse, in 1962, helped further to establish this new image. One panel of this meeting referred to the addict as "an inadequate personality . . . unable to cope with the stresses of normal life."

The conference also noted the increase in the abuse of stimulant, depressive, tranquilizing, and hallucinogenic drugs on the part of young people in high school and college.

Heroin

Heroin, variously known as "H," "hard stuff," etc., is the most dangerous narcotic in terms of producing addiction. It is an outlawed drug that has no approved medical use. Addicts may at first take this narcotic orally or by sniffing it. Later, however, they usually inject it into their veins ("mainlining") for quicker effect. The injections or "fixes" are made with a hypodermic needle and syringe, but in a pinch a vein and an eye-dropper to insert the drug often serve a desperate addict.

Probably three-quarters of confirmed narcotic addicts use heroin. They may be "hooked" in a few weeks or even days. No one who begins to use drugs would choose to become an addict. In fact, no one really believes it will happen to *him.* Among the fallacious arguments for "just trying" narcotics are: "You'll get a thrill out of it." "You'll feel good." "It peps up your sex appeal." The truth is that opiates do not increase sex desire; in fact, they are likely to diminish it. And the temporary "good feeling" or "high" is purchased at a high price.

The initial, early effects of the opiate drugs (depending on the dose) are to relieve pain and produce a false sense of well-being (euphoria). Addicts have said that heroin "makes my troubles roll off my mind" and "it makes me feel more sure of myself." But the dosages must be continually increased to achieve this "desirable" end. Soon, however, the user becomes physically and psychologically dependent on the drug; the craving is relentless. At this point the addict does not feel supernormal with the drug. He is miserable and subnormal without it. (Some of his physiological processes cannot function without the drug.) His total preoccupation with getting the next doses of the drug he craves almost always prevents him from either continuing his education or holding a job. His health is likely to be poor, causing his life expectancy to be considerably shorter than that of the nonuser.

One characteristic of addiction to heroin and other opiates or their synthetic substitutes is *withdrawal sickness* (also known as the "abstinence syndrome"). Beginning about 18 hours after the last dose of the narcotic, the withdrawal symptoms occur. These include sweating, shaking, chills, vomiting, diarrhea, and severe stomach pains. These symptoms may remain acute for as long as 36–72 hours. Modern treatments have eased some of the pangs of the withdrawal symptoms, but so-called "cold turkey" withdrawal remains a painful experience.

"Street" supplies of heroin are uncertain as to dosage, since the drug is "cut"—diluted—with milk sugar. Therefore it is possible that in some cases true physiological dependence has not occurred, causing comparatively mild withdrawal symptoms. On the other hand, the uncertain dosage may have a sufficiently high percentage of heroin to cause death.

The addict is almost always in trouble with his family and with the police. At least half the known addicts have police records even before they become addicted. Since an addict may have to spend $75–$100 for a day's supply, he finds that he has no other avenue except crime to raise that amount. Women addicts usually become prostitutes; men become thieves, muggers, and "pushers."

Most addicts begin young. A third of them are under 20, and two-thirds under 30. They are generally found in large cities among socially and economically depressed groups. Of the 60,000 heroin addicts known to the Federal Bureau of Narcotics and Dangerous Drugs, more than half live in New York State, and most of these in New York City. But no age, class, or profession is exempt from the risk.

Chart Listing Drugs, Medical Uses, Symptoms Produced and Their Dependence Potentials*

Name	Slang Name	Chemical or Trade Name	Pharmacologic Classification	Medical Use	How Taken
Heroin	H., Horse, Scat, Junk, Hard Stuff, Harry, Joy Powder	Diacetylmorphine	Depressant	Pain Relief	Injected or Sniffed
Morphine	White Stuff, Miss Emma, M, Dreamer	Morphine sulphate	Depressant	Pain Relief	Swallowed or Injected
Codeine	Schoolboy	Methylmorphine	Depressant	Ease Pain and Coughing	Swallowed
Methadone	Dolly	Dolophine Amidone	Depressant	Pain Relief	Swallowed or Injected
Cocaine	Speed Balls, Gold Dust, Coke, Bernice, Corine, Flake, Star Dust, Snow	Methyl ester of benzoylecgonine	Stimulant	Local Anesthesia	Sniffed, Injected or Swallowed
Marijuana	Pot, Grass, Locoweed, Mary Jane, Hashish, Tea, Gage, Reefers	Cannabis Sativa	Stimulant Depressant, or Hallucinogen	None in U.S.	Smoked, Swallowed or Sniffed
Barbiturates	Barbs, Blue Devils, Candy, Yellow Jackets, Phennies, Peanuts, Blue Heavens	Phenobarbital Nembutal, Seconal, Amytal	Depressant	Sedation, Relieve high blood pressure, epilepsy, hyperthyroidism	Swallowed or Injected
Amphetamines	Bennies, Dexies, Co-Pilots, Wake-Ups, Lid Proppers, Hearts, Pep Pills	Benzedrine, Preludin Dexedrine, Dexoxyn, Methedrine	Stimulant	Relieve mild depression, control appetite and narcolepsy	Swallowed or Injected
LSD	Acid, Sugar, Big D, Cubes, Trips	d-lysergic acid diethylamide	Hallucinogen	Experimental Study of Mental Function, alcoholism	Swallowed
DMT	Businessman's High	Dimethyltriptamine	Hallucinogen	None	Injected
Mescaline	Cactus, Peyote	3, 4, 5-trimethoxy-phenethylamine	Hallucinogen	None	Swallowed
Psilocybin	Mushrooms	3 (2-dimethylamino)-ethylindol-4-ol dihydrogen phosphate	Hallucinogen	None	Swallowed

*Reprinted with permission of the New York Times, January 9, 1968.

Usual Dose	Duration of Effect	Initial Symptoms	Long-Term Symptoms	Physical Dependence Potential	Mental Dependence Potential
Varies	4 hrs.	Euphoria Drowsiness	Addiction, Constipation Loss of Appetite Convulsions in overdose	Yes	Yes
15 Milligrams	6 hrs.	Euphoria Drowsiness	Addiction, impairment of breathing	Yes	Yes
30 Milligrams	4 hrs.	Drowsiness	Addiction	Yes	Yes
10 Milligrams	4–6 hrs.	Less acute than opiates	Addiction	Yes	Yes
Varies	Varies	Excitation Talkativeness Tremors	Depression, Convulsions	No	Yes
1 or 2 Cigarettes	4 hrs.	Relaxation, Euphoria, alteration of perception and judgment	Usually none	No	?
50–100 Milligrams	4 hrs.	Drowsiness, Muscle relaxation	Addiction with severe withdrawal symptoms, possible convulsions	Yes	Yes
2.5–5 Milligrams	4 hrs.	Alertness, Activeness	Delusions Hallucinations	No	Yes
100 Micrograms	10 hrs.	Exhilaration, Excitation Rambling Speech	May intensify existing psychosis, panic reactions	No	?
1 Milligram	4–6 hrs.	Exhilaration Excitation	?	No	?
350 Micrograms	12 hrs.	Exhilaration, Anxiety Gastric distress	?	No	?
25 Milligrams	6–8 hrs.	Nausea, Vomiting, Headaches	?	No	?

Cocaine

Cocaine comes from the leaves of the coca plant, grown in Peru and Bolivia, where the leaves are chewed for their intoxicating effects. Though legally classed as a narcotic, cocaine is actually a stimulant drug. It stimulates the central nervous system and thus temporarily banishes feelings of fatigue. The user becomes excited and talkative. Later he is afflicted with hallucinations and sleeplessness. Addicts to cocaine take it by injection or by sniffing the white power, which is called "snow." (Its takers are referred to as "snow birds.") Occasionally cocaine is mixed with heroin to provide a potent injection called a "speed-ball."

Cocaine is not widely used in the United States. Its original usage as a local anesthetic has been supplanted by synthetic drugs, such as novocaine and procaine.

Cocaine is a highly toxic drug and has been recognized as such even by potential users. Its abuse leads to rapid weight loss, extreme weakness, and mental deterioration.

Barbiturates

Barbiturates are depressant or sedative drugs. Popularly they are known as "sleeping pills," and in drug jargon as "goofballs" or "barbs." They act to relax the central nervous system. Over 2500 barbiturate drugs have been formulated since they were first introduced in Germany in the early twentieth century. However, only about 30 of the known barbiturates are actually in medical use.

Barbiturates have an important place in medical practice. They are widely used to treat high blood pressure, epilepsy, insomnia, and some mental illnesses; to relax patients before and during surgery; and for a host of other conditions. Of all the prescriptions doctors write for psychoactive (mind-affecting) drugs, about one in four is for a barbiturate. There are short-starting, fast-acting barbiturates and also slow-starting, long-acting ones.

In the higher dosages, which the abusers of these drugs habitually take, their effects resemble those of alcoholic intoxication—confusion, slurred speech, staggering; reduced ability to think, concentrate, or work; and finally a deep sleep (coma). Overdoses can be fatal.

Barbiturates are physically and psychologically addicting. Some experts think barbiturate addiction more difficult to cure than narcotic dependency. Convulsions following sudden withdrawal can be fatal.

The combination of barbiturates with alcohol, even in moderate doses, is especially dangerous. The two drugs, working together, synergize each other, and the total result is greater than that of either drug acting alone. Hence barbiturates are a factor in causing auto accidents, and are a leading cause of fatal accidental poisoning in the United States.

Amphetamines

Amphetamines, popularly known as "pep pills" or "bennies", are stimulants to the central nervous system. They are prescribed in proper doses by physicians to combat fatigue and sleepiness and to depress appetite (in people on weight-reduction programs). Self-prescribed and misused, they can be dangerous. Sometimes they are used in connection with depressant drugs, such as barbiturates, to get a chemical "up" followed by a chemical "down." This is a serious misuse of these drugs.

In heavy doses the amphetamines cause jitteriness, irritability, unclear speech, and tension. People on very heavy doses are withdrawn, dull, and disorganized in their thinking. The sudden withdrawal of amphetamines from the heavy abuser can result in deep and possibly suicidal depression.

Amphetamines are misused in various ways. Truck drivers take them to keep awake on long hauls. This dangerous practice may often result in serious traffic accidents. College students sometimes take amphetamines to keep them awake when cramming for exams. There are two dangers in this: (1) the effect of the drug may wear off and they will fall asleep during the examination; or (2) if increased dosages are used, they may cause a degree of intoxication which will make it practically impossible to write an acceptable examination paper.

Amphetamines and similar stimulant drugs do not produce physical dependence the way narcotics do. However, psychological dependence may result. Tolerance for the drug also develops, which means that larger and larger doses are need to obtain the desired effect.

Marihuana

Marihuana is a drug derived from the Indian hemp plant, *Cannabis sativa*. The flowering tops and the leaves of this plant, as well as its somewhat stronger cousin, *Cannabis indica*, are used to make the drug. It has been known and used for several thousand years, all around the world. It is known as "kief" in North Africa, "hashish"[3] in Arabia, "bhang" in India, and "ma jen" in China.

The drug can be taken in various ways—by chewing the leaves, by sniffing it in powder form, by mixing it with honey or candy for eating or drinking, or—as is most common in North America—by smoking it. The dried leaves and tops of the plant are chopped or crushed and fashioned into thin-paper cigarettes. These are called "reefers," "joints," or "sticks." The drug itself is known in the jargon of drug abusers as "pot," "tea," "grass," "weed," or "Mary Warner." The smoke from a marihuana cigarette smells like burnt rope or dried grass and has a characteristic, sweetish odor.

The strength of the drug varies from time to time and place to place, depending how and where it is grown, how it is prepared, and how it is stored. The kind grown in North America— largely in Mexico—is much weaker than the kind harvested in Asia, Africa, and the Near East. Traffic in marihuana is restricted in almost all

[3]The possibly violent result of using this drug may be judged by one of the words derived from it—*assassin*, from "hashish," a stronger form of marihuana. In some Oriental countries young men were deliberately inspired to commit murder by feeding them hashish.

civilized countries but its use continues. Immense quantities are smuggled into the United States across the Mexican border.

Marihuana was introduced into the United States as an intoxicating drug in the 1920's. Its general use was outlawed by the Federal Marihuana Tax Act of 1937 because it was believed to be a narcotic. This was followed by strict laws and enforcement in almost every state. Arrests on marihuana charges in the United States have doubled in the past decade (since about 1960).

Effects of Marihuana. When smoked, marihuana quickly enters the blood stream and proceeds to the brain and nervous system, bringing about changes in the mood and thinking of the user. The effect on emotions and senses varies widely, depending on who the smoker is as well as how much and what kind of marihuana is used. Also involved are the social setting and what results the smoker expects. Marihuana is commonly smoked in a social setting—at a "pot party" or "tea party."

In some respects the early effects of marihuana are like those of alcohol. The first effect is stimulation, during which time inhibitions may be loosened. Soon afterward the smoker drifts into a state of euphoria. His sense of time and distance is often distorted; a minute may seem like an hour. Because it sometimes produces hallucinations, marihuana is classified as a mild hallucinogen. However, it often produces vivid, visual imagery in the user. The drug effect begins about 15 minutes after the marihuana is smoked and may last from two to four hours.

The marihuana user finds it harder to make decisions which require clear thinking—and he is quite responsive to other people's suggestions. He should not be driving an automobile while under the influence of the drug.

The physical effects of marihuana use are less important than the psychological dependence which it induces. The early physical effects may include dizziness, dry mouth, more rapid heart beat, lower body temperature, red eyes, and occasionally hunger, especially for sweets.

Marihuana does not produce the physical dependence that the true narcotics do. Once an optimal amount is taken, the user does not find it necessary to take increased dosages. There are no withdrawal symptoms when the drug is stopped. These facts have led to the opinion that marihuana is "no worse than alcohol." To evaluate this opinion, we must consider the tragic effects that heavy drinking or alcoholism can have on the individual and upon society.

There is a strong consensus of opinion that marihuana produces a difficult-to-cure psychological dependence if it is taken regularly.

In a 1967 study of narcotic addicts from big city areas, it was revealed that four out of five had previously used marihuana. On the other hand, there are immense numbers of marihuana smokers who do not go on to use morphine or heroin. No cause-and-effect link between marihuana and narcotics has been found.

Federal and state laws deal with marihuana as strictly as if it were a narcotic. To *possess,* give, or sell marihuana in the United States is a felony. The federal penalty for a first offense may be 2 to 10 years' imprisonment and a fine of up to $20,000. Young people tempted by marihuana should remember that an arrest or conviction on a marihuana charge can seriously cloud their future educational and employment opportunities.

A new chapter in the marihuana story was opened in 1966 when an Israeli chemist, with United States support, succeeded in synthesizing the active ingredient in marihuana; namely, tetrahydrocannabinol (THC). This new synthetic drug makes it possible for researchers to determine more exactly the effects of marihuana.

LSD and Other Hallucinogens

A hallucinogen, as was already noted, is a drug that causes hallucinations. These are trancelike states of mind in which an individual may see, hear, taste, smell, or appear to touch something that is not really there. In other words, the hallucinogens alter perceptions. For example, a doll might appear as a frightening monster. The drug-taker may also suffer from delusions (false beliefs), and imagine that someone is out to "get" him (a delusion of persecution). The great appeal in taking hallucinogenic drugs is the alteration of the state of mind in the direction of believing oneself a more sensitive, powerful, and important person than he really is.

LSD, lysergic acid diethylamide, is an hallucinogenic drug and, at present, one of the most potent of them. There are 300,000 doses to the ounce! The hallucinogens are also called psychedelic—or mind-expanding—drugs, but this is usually a false designation. These drugs are as likely to constrict consciousness as to expand it. Among the other known hallucinogenic drugs are: psilocybin, derived from a "sacred mushroom" used for centuries by Mexican Indians to produce visions and hallucinations as part of their religious ceremonies; mescaline, derived from seed-pods, "buttons," of the peyote cactus; morning glory seeds; nutmeg; and Jimson weed.

LSD is a late comer to the field of hallucinogens. It was first discovered in 1938 by Albert Hofman, a chemist working in the Sandoz Research Laboratory in Switzerland. Five years later, in 1943, he accidentally discovered its special property of changing sense perceptions, that is, of producing hallucinations, illusions, and delusions.

A spate of research with LSD followed this discovery. There was some early hope that it might prove useful in treating some kinds of mental illness. Two-and-a-half decades and some 2000 scientific papers later, however, the drug still had no approved place in medical practice. Within that time, though, the use of LSD escaped from the field of careful scientific investigation and was taken up by some presitigious persons. The English author, Aldous Huxley, in a book, *Doors of Perception,* published in 1954, praised LSD's unusual properties.

Among the other early proselytes and proselytizers of LSD were two former members of the Psychology Department at Harvard, Timothy Leary and Richard Alpert. They called LSD a "sacred biochemical," which brought mystic understanding. They claimed that normal consciousness is a dim, dull thing in comparison with the aura of understanding and insight that results from taking LSD or any of the half-dozen other psychedelic drugs. Among these may be mentioned DMT (dimethyltryptamine), derived from the seeds of certain plants found in South America and the West Indies.

Lysergic acid, from which LSD is made (by relatively simple chemical processes), is derived from ergot, a fungus that grows on rye and wheat. LSD may be obtained as a pill, a powder, or a tasteless, colorless, odorless liquid in ampules. It is often taken on a lump of sugar, a cookie, or a cracker.

The negative effects of LSD were not recognized until the early 1960's. In 1965, by an act of Congress, it was declared an illegal, dangerous drug. The manufacture or sale of LSD or similar drugs was made illegal. In some states laws were passed making even the possession of the LSD-type of drugs illegal. Taking these drugs is called "taking a trip." Commonly these trips are pleasurable, but sometimes they are horrible experiences verging on panic. It should be noted that LSD is an *unpredictable* drug or at least that it has unpredictable results on some takers. People who have taken it many times may suddenly find themselves on a disconcerting "bad trip." In some instances, hallucinations have continued, or reappeared, over long periods of time after the drug was taken. In some cases, also, LSD has provoked psychotic reactions.

That LSD is a dangerous drug can be adduced from the testimony of physicians who have treated patients for the results of its effects. Dr. Donald B. Louria, president of the New York State Council on Drug Addiction, has said:

There is no other drug used promiscuously under uncontrolled circumstances that is as dangerous as LSD. It is absolutely unpredictable.

In the 114 cases hospitalized by Bellevue Hospital [New York City] in the past 18 months [1966–1967], the average age was 23 years. Thirteen percent entered the hospital with overwhelming panic. There was uncontrolled violence in 12 percent. Nearly 9 percent had attempted either homicide or suicide, none successfully. Of the 114, one out of seven had to be sent on from Bellevue to long-term mental hospitalization,

and half of these had no history of underlying psychiatric disorder.

A study entitled "[College] Student Use of Hallucinogens" was undertaken by Dr. Herbert D. Kleber in the mid-1960's. He noted that 24 percent of those using the LSD-type drug were judged to have adverse reactions. These included anxiety reactions, persistent hallucinosis, worsening of psychiatric symptoms, and psychic dependence on the drug. On the other hand, he reported that half the students who took the drugs claimed that they "had improved their lives." Many people including musicians, who have taken an eight-to-ten hour trip on LSD, have the impression that they are giving tremendously better performances than usual. The playing of a group of musicians under the influence of LSD was tape-recorded. The musicians felt that they were playing more brilliantly than ever before. When they had recovered from their LSD trance and heard their performances being played back to them, they said, "How could we have played so badly!" In short, LSD fools you.

Whether or not LSD has long-range adverse effects on the brain has not been definitely determined, but that it has some danger is suggested by the effects of the drug on test animals. Short-term dangers may also result from the strange effects of LSD. Some users of the drug think they can fly or walk on water, and are injured or killed when they attempt such feats. Recent scientific evidence has demonstrated the damaging effect of LSD on the chromosomes.

Identifying the Drug Abuser

We shall review here some of the signs and symptoms that may be part of the pattern of identification of students in the habit of using dangerous drugs. Sudden changes in behavior always deserve attention. When this altered behavior becomes the new pattern, drug abuse should be considered as a possible factor.

Among the common behavioral signs that may suggest drug abuse in college (or even high school) students are the following:

Significant changes in class attendance; changes for the worse in work turned in; unusual flare-ups and outbursts of temper; unusual activity or indolence; poor personal appearance, since serious drug abusers generally become indifferent to and neglect their appearance as well as their health habits; furtive behavior because the drug abuser fears discovery; wearing sunglasses at inappropriate times to hide dilated or constricted pupils; constantly wearing long-sleeved apparel to hide needle marks on the arms; begging, borrowing, or stealing money or other items, such as radios and jewelry, which can be converted quickly into cash, in order to pay the expenses of the drug habit; frequenting odd places, such as closets, storage rooms, or parked cars, in order to take drugs; and associating with other known drug abusers.

In addition to these behavioral clues common to abuse of all kinds of drugs, each specific category of abused drugs has some special manifestations associated with it, as follows:

The glue or solvent sniffer generally retains on his breath or clothes the odor of the substance inhaled. Furthermore, his nose runs and his blood-shot eyes water. He lacks muscular control, as if he were intoxicated. He may see double or complain of hallucinations. Finding a handkerchief or paper bag with dried plastic cement is a telltale sign of glue sniffing.

The abuser of depressant drugs, notably barbiturates and some tranquilizers, exhibits most of the symptoms of alcoholic intoxication—except that there is no odor of alcohol on his breath. He may stagger and stumble. He is usually drowsy and sometimes falls into a deep sleep in the classroom. He lacks interest in school activities and may appear disoriented.

The abuser of stimulants, especially amphetamines, is characterized by excess activity. He is often irritable, argumentative, and nervous. He has difficulty in sitting still. Because amphetamines have a drying effect on mucous membranes, those who abuse these drugs have bad breath, a dry mouth, and an itchy nose. They can be observed scratching their noses and licking their lips with their tongues. They are often chain smokers; they talk incessantly about any subject at hand; and they frequently boast about going long hours without food or sleep.

The abuser of narcotics (heroin, morphine, and synthetic substitutes) is rarely seen in the classroom. If he is, he will usually appear lethargic and drowsy or display symptoms of deep intoxication. Sometimes narcotic addiction begins by drinking paregoric or cough medicines containing codeine. The presence of empty bottles of such substances in wastebaskets or on school grounds is a tell-tale sign. Other "beginners" in narcotic abuse may inhale heroin in powder form. This leaves traces of a white powder around the nostrils, which become red and raw.

The "mainliner" most commonly uses the veins on the inner surface of the arm, at the elbow. Here scar tissue ("tracks") appears after numerous injections and identifies the narcotic abuser. (Hence he wears long sleeves.)

The narcotic abuser needs equipment, called "works" or "outfit," to "mainline" his drugs. This equipment consists of a spoon with a bent handle or a bottle cap, a small ball of cotton (called "satch cotton"), a syringe or eye-dropper, and a hypodermic needle. Heroin powder is dissolved in a little water in the bent spoon or bottle cap and heated over a match or lighter. The cotton acts as a filter as the narcotic is drawn up through the needle into the eye-dropper or syringe. The "mainliner" must keep his equipment handy. Hence it is likely to be found on his person, in his desk, or in his locker. Finding such an "outfit" is almost a sure sign of narcotics abuse.

The marihuana smoker is sometimes betrayed by the odor of marihuana ("pot")—something like the odor of burning rope—on his breath or clothing. He may also be identified by the possession of marihuana cigarettes, often called "sticks," "reefers," or "joints." These cigarettes are usually smoked in a group situation; after one or two puffs, the joints are passed on to another member of the group.

The marihuana user is difficult to detect unless he is under the influence of the drug at the time he is being observed. He is unlikely to be recognized in the classroom. In the early stages of the marihuana effect, when the drug acts as a stimulant, the smoker is likely to be animated, talking loudly, and bursting into laughter. In later stages he is sleepy or stuporous.

The abuser of hallucinogenic drugs, such as LSD, is not likely to be detected in a classroom. The taking of such drugs, usually called "taking a trip," also usually occurs in a group situation under special conditions. The users generally sit quietly in a dream or trancelike sleep. One member of the group does not take the drug at the time and looks after those others who may be suffering from a "bad trip." Sometimes a user of hallucinogenic drugs may become terribly frightened and seek to escape from the group. Someone must prevent him from taking dangerous or even fatal actions.

Treatment for Drug Addiction

Although there has been some progress, the treatment of drug addiction (or dependence) remains far from satisfactory. Addicts are no longer considered as altogether incurable. The feeling that addiction was largely untreatable arose from the fact that so many patients on opiates went back to drug use after long periods of hospitalization.

The first step in the treatment of the drug abuser is usually detoxification, that is, drug withdrawal. There are several treatment methods, however, in which the patient is carried along for some time on lowered doses of drugs. Sudden withdrawl of addicting drugs is called "cold turkey" and is usually a highly painful process for the addict. Controlled and gradual detoxification is best done in a hospital setting under medical supervision.

The total pattern of treatment, however, goes far beyond detoxification. It includes psychiatric evaluation and treatment, continuing medical supervision, and counseling, especially after the patient returns to the environment from which he has come.

This is the most critical step in the rehabilitation process. The old neighborhood pressure on

the former addict to go back to drugs is tremendous. He needs guidance and support during this period. He may be required to remain in contact with a social caseworker or specially trained probation officer, keep psychiatric as well as other medical appointments, and attend group therapy sessions. This kind of supervision may be needed for several years. Unfortunately, it is rarely available. Hence the "hard core" drug abuser may return to drug use even after a long period of "keeping clean," that is, not taking drugs.

Some Special Treatment Programs. Several kinds of special treatment programs have sprung up in different communities. All of them have interesting possibilities, but they must still be characterized as experimental. For example:

The Methadone Program was initiated in New York City by Drs. Vincent Dole and Marie Nyswander, associated with the Rockefeller Foundation. It provides for carrying along on methadone—a long-acting, synthetic narcotic—former heroin addicts with a history of relapse. The drug is reputed to satisfy narcotic hunger without producing euphoria, the drug-induced feeling of superb well-being.

The British System permitted physicians to carry narcotic addicts along on usually small, maintenance doses of narcotics after all other treatment methods had failed. The treatment was revised in 1968 and patients are now referred to treatment centers.

Synanon consists of a number of residences in the United States where ex-addicts manage the program and admit other addicts to take part in their drug-free project. Once admitted, the ex-addict is expected to work hard toward his own rehabilitation.

Daytop Lodge is another residential facility designed to help ex-addicts take the big step toward transition into community life. Located on Staten Island, in New York, it is directed by Synanon "graduates."

Narcotics Anonymous, modeled after Alcoholics Anonymous, has chapters in many large cities. Spiritually oriented, it relies for its effectiveness on mutual inspiration, discussion, and the therapeutic value of confession.

The California System provides for sending addicts to a rehabilitation center and thereafter to "half-way houses", where outpatients may stay for up to three months. The unique feature of this plan is that all outpatients must submit to periodic tests with Nalline, a synthetic antinarcotic. This drug brings about withdrawal symptoms if the person taking it is using narcotics.

In general, it may be said that methods of treatment which bring favorable community and peer pressure to bear on ex-addicts are more successful than those in which they must go the route alone.

SUMMARY REVIEW QUESTIONS

1. What are the differences between medical and legal definitions of narcotics? What was the public attitude toward narcotics in the United States during the nineteenth century? What changes have taken place in the twentieth century?
2. What are "dangerous drugs" other than true narcotics, as discussed in this chapter? Name four such drugs and describe their origin.
3. How does *narcotic* addiction usually occur? What kind of life does the drug addict live? What is the relationship between drug addiction and crime?
4. What are the effects, physical and psychological, of marihuana? From what and from where does marihuana originate? Is it to be regarded as a true narcotic? What is its relationship to other forms of drug dependence?
5. What are hallucinogenic drugs? Name four and state their origin. What arguments in favor of their use are put forth by the proponents of these drugs? What are the dangers of these drugs, as noted by physicians?
6. Are the following statements sense or nonsense? Why? *Anything is worth trying once . . . . You don't know what living is until you've tried reefers. . . . Barbiturates are not dangerous; doctors prescribe them. . . . Once you're hooked on narcotics, you're hooked for life. . . . Smoking marihuana is no worse than heavy drinking of alcoholic beverages. . . . Overdoses of sleeping pills are frequently fatal. . . . There can be no harm in "taking a trip" with LSD once in a while.*
7. What do the following terms mean to you? psychedelic, heroin, "snow," barbiturate, amphetamine, psychic dependence, "cold turkey," "mainlining," "bad trip," "pot party," hallucinogen?

Worth Looking Into: *Drug Abuse: Escape to Nowhere* published by Smith, Kline & French Laboratories. *Confessions of an English Opium Eater* by Thomas de Quincy. *Drugs on the College Campus* by Helen H. Nowlis. *The Drug Scene* by Donald B. Louria.

PART TWO PERSONAL HEALTH

5

PHYSICAL FITNESS

GOVERNMENTAL CONCERN WITH THE PHYSICAL fitness of its youth has often, but not always, been stimulated by military considerations. Rejection rates of young men deemed medically unfit for military service have aroused considerable alarm about the "flabbiness" of American youth.

In response to this widespread attitude, President John F. Kennedy, in 1961, appointed a President's Council on Youth Fitness and issued a Presidential Message on this subject incorporating their recommendations.

He further defined physical fitness as ". . . a broad quality involving medical and dental supervision and care, immunization and other protection against disease, proper nutrition, adequate rest, relaxation, good health practices, sanitation, and other aspects of healthful living. *Exercise* is an essential element to achieving physical fitness."

In this chapter we shall pay particular attention to exercise as a means of achieving those desirable physical qualities of strength, stamina, and endurance.

It should be noted that there is a more limited standard of physical fitness than the one quoted at the beginning of this chapter. In this narrower concept physical fitness is equated with ability to meet standardized physical fitness tests, and emphasis is placed upon neuromuscular development through strictly defined periods of "vigorous activity" and rigorously outlined sets of exercises.

There is no achieving physical fitness or personal fitness simply by talking about it. The muscles of the body, supported by its other organs, must be put to work or into play in order to attain measurable increases in physical fitness. (Maximum oxygen intake per unit of body weight provides one such objective measurement.) It has been adequately demonstrated that 8 to 12 weeks of rigorous physical conditioning for the "normal" but relatively inactive individual will significantly augment his physical fitness, as measured by the oxygen intake and other tests. Very few college students are prepared to sacrifice 2 or 3 months of their life solely to achieving a measurably high degree of physical fitness. Other more gradual and educationally coordinated methods are in order.

Physical Education is Part of a Great Tradition

One of the opportunities of college life is to learn how to improve and maintain physical fitness for a lifetime. The primary responsibility for this teaching is usually charged to the department of physical education, although other departments may share in the task.

It is significant to realize that physical education in its broad sense is part of the great tradition of education and learning. It has an ancient classical and a chivalric background too. Greek sculpture evoked the ideal of the strong, graceful body; Olympic games their interest in physical fitness. Training for knighthood in the Middle Ages included that phase of physical education which we would today call physical training. The battle of Waterloo, said the victorious Duke of Wellington, was won on the playing fields of Eton. The rise of modern Germany, following the Napoleonic wars, was linked with the development of the gymnastic *Turnverein* (turners or tumblers) movement. The memoirs of World War II's Field Marshal Montgomery are full of analogies from the world of sports.

The tradition of the dance, which is part of physical education combined with esthetics, goes back farther and earlier than any of the rest. Dance is among the most ancient of art forms. Understanding the meaning of dance forms helps us to perceive the cultures in which they originate.

Physical education, is an integral part of human learning. Its primary though not its only goal is to help students attain and maintain that degree of physical fitness which leads to academic and later-life accomplishments. Today the subject area of physical education draws upon the same scientific disciplines that are the basis of the art of medicine and other academic subjects catalogued as biology, psychology, nutrition. Physical education in college has important practical aspects, such as the supervision of athletics and the provision of sports programs for many (or most) students. In conducting these and other programs in which "learning by doing" is the basic methodology, physical education provides for the mental health, social and recreational needs of students. It should be understood therefore that physical education does not preach or teach exercise for its own sake; it simply uses this as one of many modalities for helping students to develop their total personalities. This is in the best academic tradition.

Are You Physically "Underdeveloped"? You may not care whether you are physically "developed" or "underdeveloped." Or you may possibly be afraid that you are *not* up to standard in physical fitness and development when in fact you are above it. The President's Council on Youth Fitness has developed three standard screening tests for "physical fitness." If you take these tests you can quickly and easily classify yourself as up to, above, or below par in physical fitness, defined as physical strength, flexibility, and agility.

The three screening tests are (1) *pullups,* testing arm and shoulder strength (there is a modified pullup for women), (2) *situps,* testing flexibility and abdominal strength, and (3) *"squat thrusts,"*

probing your agility. The tests are fully pictured and described on pages 56 & 57.

If you are at the "freshman stage" of personal and physical development (age 17), you should make at least the following "passing" scores on the three tests:

Men	Women
3 pullups	8 modified pullups
14 situps	10 situps
4 "squat thrusts" in 10 seconds	3 "squat thrusts" in 10 seconds

Advantages and Values of Physical Fitness

Underlying most current discussions on the advantages and values of physical fitness is the assumption that the conditions of American civilization have generally reduced the need for physical activity almost to a vanishing point. Machines do most of the work that used to be done by human muscle power. To mail a letter, one jumps into an automobile and drives around the block. The basic argument here is that better programs are necessary for assuring the adequate amount of physical activity that used to be part of everyday living. (A busy housewife or a farmer still gets plenty of daily physical activity!) For many people, and some college students, however, "regular exercise, adapted to one's physical potentialities, represents a return to the wisdom of the ages" (Jean Mayer).

The best reason for developing the strength, stamina, and endurance that mark a high degree of physical fitness is the personal satisfaction one gets in doing it. The immediate reward is a sense of physical and mental well-being. As C. B. ("Bud") Wilkinson has put it: "We now recognize [physical fitness] as a quality which contributes to our social and intellectual effectiveness. We are awakening to the realization that man's physical function is subtly related to his mental, moral, and spiritual processes. What affects one affects the other."

Another, less appreciated outcome of programs of physical fitness, physical education, and *dance* is that it develops one's *kinesthetic* intelligence. (*Kine* means movement; *esthetic,* beautiful. The word as a whole may be taken to mean "pleasure in movement.") In the conclusion of a brilliant essay, based on studies of "stylized" (that is, volitional) human movements and inquiring into the nature of movement as a significant form of human experience, Drs. Eleanor Metheny and Lois Ellfeldt declare:

Kinesthetic intelligence is one of the significant forms of human intelligence and kinesymbolic knowledge makes a unique contribution to man's comprehension of reality by adding to the store of meanings that are the basis of the significance man finds in his life as a human being. . . . In this context physical education—as we prefer to call it, "movement education"—can be identified as one of the forms of liberal education, comparable with music and the other non-verbal arts as a source of one of the kinds of meaning that enrich man's comprehension of reality as he knows it.

This point may perhaps be emphasized by an anecdote about the great Russian physiologist, Ivan Pavlov. When asked why he spent so much time working in his garden, he answered: "To give joy to my muscles."

Participation in athletics, sports, and games requires at least a minimum degree of physical fitness or physical readiness; yet more desirable qualities are developed *through* participation. Dr. Leonard A. Larson, of the University of Wisconsin, has stated:

The team is a miniature society, containing all the elements of democratic human relations, ranging from respect for the individual personality to group self-government.

Physical education and athletics draw upon and contribute to the philosophies of American culture and contribute to some of the important goals of education: the development of confidence through achievement, understanding of human relations, knowledge and care of the body, and preparation for effective use of increased leisure time. Opportunities in these areas should be offered to all individuals from their early years, when they may begin the foundations for sports participation throughout their lifetime.

Another potent set of arguments for physical fitness and physical activity is that they may decrease a tendency toward the onset of certain diseases and thus increase human longevity. In particular, it is argued that long-term exercise may have a protective effect on the cardiovascular (heart and blood vessels) system and possibly reduce the level of cholesterol in the blood serum. Two distinguished physicians, Dr. Hans Kraus and Dr. Wilhelm Raab, have written a useful book on the role of physical *in*activity as a causative factor in the origin of a variety of diseases. The book is titled: *Hypokinetic Disease.* The term "hypokinetic," coined by Dr. Kraus, is from Greek roots and means "caused by insufficient movement or motion." An American heart specialist, Dr. Joseph B. Wolffe, of Philadelphia, confirms their point, with which many physicians would agree, thus:

After more than three decades of experience as a cardiologist, I am convinced, from empirical as well as clinical observation, that there is a direct correlation between the sedentary, pushbutton character of our culture and the constantly rising incidence of coronary artery disease and other forms of cardiovascular disturbance. . . .

We, of both the medical and non-medical disciplines . . . are duty-bound to imbue the present and growing generation with knowledge for fitness—for *total* fitness, physical, moral, intellectual and emotional. . . . Too many sectors of our leadership reveal a tragic myopia on the subject of fitness. . . . Even among some educators there is a compulsion, in our mechanized, materially oriented era, to place all emphasis on the physical sciences, on mathematical and technological training, at the expense of the healthy development of the nervous, cardiovascular, and other systems of the body so vital for successful coping with one's environment.

Exercise: How Much? What Kind?

A great variety of graded programs and corresponding tests for physical fitness, in its narrower sense, have been developed and applied. For example, a complex series of rating scales for physical capacity (fitness) are included in the *5BX (Five Basic Exercises) Plan for Physical Fitness,* a program originated and promulgated by the Royal Canadian Air Force. The *5BX Plan* and its companion program for women, *XBX,* a ten exercise plan, became internationally popular in the early 1960's. The use of *5BX* and *XBX* pro-

Three Screening Tests for Physical Fitness (arm and shoulder strength, flexibility and abdominal strength, and agility)

IA: Pullups—Men

Equipment.—A bar of sufficient height, comfortable to grip.

Starting position.—Grasp the bar with palms facing forward; hang with arms and legs fully extended. Feet must be free of floor.

Action:

1. Pull body up with the arms until the chin is placed over the bar.
2. Lower body until the elbows are fully extended.
3. Repeat the exercise as many times as you can.

Rules:

1. The pull must not be a snap movement.
2. Knees must not be raised.
3. Kicking the legs is not permitted.
4. The body must not swing.
5. One complete pullup is counted each time you place your chin over the bar.

To pass: 3 pullups.

IB: Modified Pullups—Women

Equipment.—Any bar adjustable in height and comfortable to grip. A piece of pipe, placed between two stepladders and held securely, may be used.

Starting position.—adjust height of bar to chest level. Grasp bar with palms facing out. Extend the legs under the bar, keeping the body and knees straight. The heels are on the foor. Fully extend the arms so they form an angle of 90 degrees with the body line. Brace your heels if necessary to prevent slipping.

Action:

1. Pull body up with the arms until the *chest* touches the bar.
2. Lower body until elbows are fully extended.
3. Repeat the exercise as many times as you can.

Rules:

1. The body must be kept straight.
2. The chest *must* touch the bar and the arms must then be *fully extended.*
3. No resting is permitted.
4. One pullup is counted each time the chest touches the bar.

To pass: 8 modified pullups.

II: Situps (Men and Women)

Starting Position.—Lie down on your back with your legs extended, feet about one foot apart. Your hands, with fingers interlaced, should be grasped behind your neck. Keep your heels on the floor. This can be accomplished by having a partner hold your feet down (as shown in the illustration), or by placing a heavy sofa cushion or gym mat on your feet, or by putting your feet under the edge of a low sofa.

Action:

1. Sit up and turn the trunk to the left. Touch the right elbow to the left knee.
2. Return to starting position.
3. Sit up and turn the trunk to the right. Touch the left elbow to the right knee.
4. Return to the starting position.
5. Repeat as many times as possible.
6. One complete situp is counted each time you return to the starting position.

To pass: Men—14 situps.
　　　　　Women—10 situps.

III: Squat Thrust (Men and Women)

(You will need either a partner or an automatic timer to time yourself in this exercise.)

Equipment.—A stopwatch, or a watch with a sweep-second hand.

Starting Position.—Stand at attention.

Action:

1. Bend knees and place hands on the floor in front of the feet. Arms may be between, outside or in front of the bent knees.
2. Thrust the legs back far enough so that the body is perfectly straight from shoulders to feet (the pushup position).
3. Return to squat position.
4. Return to erect position.

Scoring.—Your partner gives the starting signal, "Ready!—Go!" On "Go" you begin. Your partner counts each squat thrust. At the end of 10 seconds, he says, "Stop".

Rule: You must return to the erect position of attention at the completion of each squat thrust.

To pass: Men—4 squat thrusts in 10 seconds
　　　　　Women—3 squat thrusts in 10 seconds

grams, as outlined in slim printed manuals, was claimed to have eliminated "desk-bound flabbiness" in many parts of the world.

The *5BX* plan presents a graded series of relatively simple calisthenic exercises which are to be self-administered in only 11 minutes a day and can be done without equipment other than the determination to keep up with them. Since all exercise is (by definition) physical effort, and since the human animal often resists such effort, the eventual value of *5BX,* like Walter Camp's "Daily Dozen" of the 1920's, cannot be judged.

Over half of the *5BX* time is devoted to "running in place" (stationary run) with various intermittent kicks and leaps. Also included are various bending and stretching exercises, starting from the erect position and from several floor positions.

It takes a great deal of motivation and willpower to keep up a solitary program of calisthenic exercises. It has also been demonstrated that the presence of spectators or, even more so, participation in a group or class steps up performance of muscular tasks.

How much and what kind of exercise to take each day is a question that has confronted you, and that you have answered, from the time you were learning to walk. When you were a toddler, exercise was the main business of your life. You considered it play. You have been making decisions about exercise, whether work or play, all through your education. Some exercise was probably forced on you—in the form of household chores and compulsory "gym" classes. But basically you have been deciding for yourself how much physical activity and what kind of exercise you were willing to seek or accept. We may divide this exercise into three categories: (1) the inescapable exercise of *daily living;* (2) exercise accepted by reason of *occupation;* and (3) exercise chosen for *recreation.* As a college student you are still making these daily decisions about exercise, and you will continue to do so for the rest of your life. By studying the facts about exercise, physical fitness, and physical education, you will be able to make more rational choices.

Perhaps the only bit of general advice that can be given is this: take *enough* exercise, with pleasure, to feel that your body is toned up to a pitch of well-being. But do not take so much that physical fatigue constantly overburdens your capacity for the enjoyment of life. A moderate amount of exercise daily is far better than sporadic bursts of physical activity.

The amount and kind of exercise you take will be determined by your own motivations, or necessities. You can exercise (1) for fun, (2) to keep in shape, (3) to do your job, (4) to gain strength, (5) to improve your figure or physique, or (6) to reduce. You should know that exercise *alone* will not take off weight, although it may be employed (especially as "spot" exercises) to change body contours. Nor will exercise *alone* maintain health, although it is a step in the right direction.

Regular exercise in moderation keeps the body flexible and supple. The abdomen, for example, can be kept reasonably flat and smooth by bending and stretching. Exercise also keeps up "muscle tone." A further advantage of regular exercise is that it stimulates the general physiology of the body, especially the functions of the circulatory system, the respiratory system, and the excretory system.

Vigorous exercise can be considered useful up to about the ages of 35 to 40. Increasing age should be no bar to *some* regular physical activity. Older people should be encouraged to take exercises within the range of their physical capacities.

We have by no means reached a complete pushbutton stage of civilization, but the ever-increasing introduction of labor-saving devices, linked with a growth of specialization of occupation among the white collar classes, is producing a more sedentary civilization. There is a limit to the amount of sitting a person should do for his own good. On the other hand there is evidence, adduced by Raymond Pearl and others, that lifetime occupations which demand continuous output of physical energy tend to shorten life.

The "student life" can be an extremely sedentary occupation, and students must often be urged to make special efforts to tone up their muscles and bodies generally by taking some agreeable exercise. Curiously, the students who protest most about compulsory physical education are usually the ones who need it most.

Respect the Fatigue Point. For a different group of college students and adults the problem of exercise resolves itself into the problem of not overdoing it. A rule of thumb for this group is: exercise to the point of mild fatigue, but not beyond it.

The amount of fatigue produced is probably the best measure of the amount of exercise that ought to be taken. On this score a statement prepared by the American Association for Health, Physical Education, and Recreation offers sound guidance.[1]

"The ability to recuperate after exercise is a good guide at any age. Recuperation should be reasonably prompt. If (1) breathing and heart rate are still greatly accelerated at the end of ten minutes after exercise, and if (2) there is marked weakness or fatigue persisting after a two-hour rest period, (3) restlessness with broken sleep after retiring for the night, or (4) a sense of definite fatigue the day following, the exercise has been too severe or too prolonged for that person in his present stage of physical training and strength."

Choice of Exercise for Recreation. The best choice of exercise is that which gives the most satisfaction. Many factors must be considered to determine suitability of physical activity, but one should certainly like the sports he chooses. There is little to be gained in teaching a girl who wants to go swimming how to swing a pair of Indian clubs instead.

Exercise should be fun! Exercise is part of the normal desire for play that inhabits the human psyche. In young children play and exercise are nearly synonymous.

Several important studies have shown that sports and games are definitely better than calisthenics and apparatus work in conditioning men for physical fitness. Wilbur's study of college freshmen, for example, indicated that games were better than formal gymnastics in building strength in the arms and shoulder girdle, in establishing body coordination, agility, and control, and in reaching a higher degree of general physical fitness.[2]

Recreation has been defined as "activity for pleasure." It achieves relaxation of mind and muscle. The range of recreational exercises is far broader than most people think. Here are some of the possibilities: walking, swimming, dancing, skating, rowing, canoeing, fencing, bicycling, horseback riding, tennis, squash, handball, softball, volleyball, badminton, skiing, sailing, hunting, pingpong, archery, bowling, fishing, gardening, croquet, shuffleboard, horseshoe pitching, hiking, jogging, climbing, and golf. How many of these recreations have you tried? All of these can be coeducational if desired.

Walking is the most flexible and natural of all forms of exercise. Dancing also is a beneficial form of exercise, especially folk-dancing and "modern dance." Social dancing has its place too. It is believed that the rhythms of dance can afford release of emotional and psychosexual tensions rather than unduly heightening them.

There is an advantage in learning sports and obtaining reasonable proficiency at games that you can play for fun for many years after college.

A contrast between work and play activity is also advisable. People whose occupations are generally sedentary and indoors should choose games and sports that take them out of doors and offer opportunity for the exercise of trunk, leg, and arm muscles. Conversely, the man who stands on his feet all day should select recreations that require a minimum of leg work.

Two New Exercise Hobbies. The late 1960's saw the introduction of two new exercise hobbies: jogging and aerobics.

Jogging has three meanings: (1) a steady or an easy-paced run alternating with breath-catching periods of walking; (2) a kind of running, generally a slow regular trot that has been described

---

[1]Committee report, *The Role of Exercise in Physical Fitness,* American Association for Health, Physical Education, and Recreation (Washington, D.C., 1943).

[2]E. A. Wilbur, "A Comparative Study of Physical Fitness Indices as Measured by Two Programs of Physical Education; the Sports Method and the Apparatus Method," *Research Quarterly* (October 1943).

as the next step up from walking; (3) an entire program of physical fitness, as set forth in a book by William J. Bowerman, track coach at the University of Oregon, W. E. Harris, M. D., a heart specialist, and others. They have provided a detailed instructional guide to jogging, which is one effective kind of physical fitness program. Among the advantages of jogging as a pleasant form of exercise are that it is free, easy, relaxing fun; it can be done alone or in groups; and it is especially good for the heart and lungs.

Schedules are at the heart of the jogging program. It moves from the short and simple to the gradually more difficult. Train, don't strain, say the originators of the system. Here, by way of example, is the schedule for the first week's program for men and women in less than average physical condition:

Week I

Pace 1 equals 110 yards at 55 to 60 seconds, or 25 to 30 seconds, for 55 yards.

Monday, Wednesday, and Friday
(Total distance ½ mile)

			Pace
(1) Jog 55 yards	Walk 55 yards	4 times	1
(2) Jog 110 yards	Walk 110 yards		1
(3) Jog 55 yards	Walk 55 yards	2 times	1

Tuesday, Thursday, Saturday, and Sunday
A 5 to 10 minute walk and some easy stretching exercises.

From this primary program, the distance, speed, and amount of jogging are gradually increased. By the final (twelfth) week of jogging for men or women of better than average physical condition, the following schedule has been reached:

Week XII

Pace 4 = 110 yards at 25 to 30 seconds
Pace 5 = 110 yards at 20 to 25 seconds

Monday
(Total distance 4 to 5 miles)

			Pace
Jog 110 yards	Walk 110 yards	2 times	4 or 5
Jog 880 yards	Walk 110 yards	2 times	4 or 5
Jog 330, 220, 110 yards	Walk as needed	4 times	4 or 5
Jog 110 yards	Walk 110 yards	3 times	4 or 5

Jogging is not a competitive sport. It is a simple method of training for improved physical condition. You should, therefore, avoid overtraining and strenuous *daily* jogging. Work hard one day and rest the next.

Aerobics. Aerobics is the second of the recent plans put forward for increasing physical fitness. It has been described in some detail by the man who developed it, Major Kenneth H. Cooper, M.D., of the U.S. Air Force Medical Corps.

The key to the concept, he states, is oxygen. Aerobics means literally "with *oxygen.*" It is the antonym of the word "anaerobic" which means "without oxygen." (Certain bacteria can live only in an anaerobic environment.)

The human body can store food, but it cannot store oxygen. Cutting off his oxygen supply for a few minutes will cause a man to die.

In some bodies, Major Cooper points out, the means for delivering oxygen is weak and limited in resources. Hence the energy demands of the body surpass the body's capacity to produce it.

Most, if not all, people can produce enough energy to perform daily activities. However, when they are forced into more vigorous exercise, they can't keep up. They become "winded" and fatigued at very low levels of effort. The aerobic pattern of exercises which Major Cooper recommends has the special virtue of building up the cardiovascular and respiratory systems of the body so that they will supply oxygen in whatever amount it is needed.

The aerobic system is a *point* count for different physical activities. You have to make 30 points a week to keep up with the system. You win points by exercising within a definite time limit. The categories of exercise are: running, swimming, cycling, walking, running in place, and engaging in fast games of handball, squash, or basketball. Cooper provides standards against which you may gauge your own condition. What is the distance, he asks, that you can cover in 12 minutes running or running and walking?

Answers to Some Practical Questions about Exercise. *What good are reducing exercises?* They help to distribute body fat, cutting down hip measurements, for example, but they are of little value for losing weight. You would have to walk or scrub floors for about half an hour to work off as many calories as you get in a slice of bread. You would have to chop wood hard for about an hour to get rid of the caloric energy in a malted milk (around 500 calories).

Dare a woman exercise during her menstrual period? Yes, but not too strenuously. Both violent exercise and extreme fatigue should be avoided.

What about exercise after illness or accident? Follow your doctor's orders and advice. Present practice is to avoid abuse of bed rest and get patients, including surgical, obstetrical, and even heart patients, back on their feet as soon as possible. However, some infections (notably virus infections, such as hepatitis) leave their victims in a weakened condition for a long time and prohibit anything but minimal physical activity even though the patient thinks he "feels fine." The acute or convalescent stages of most diseases interdict vigorous exercise.

What about exercise and meals? Among the effects of exercise are changes in the distribution of the blood and depression of gastric secretion. These effects are related to the excitement of competition as well as to sheer physical activity. Heavy exercise immediately after meals, therefore, appears to interfere with digestion.

Therapeutic Exercise The range of exercise is wide and certainly not just recreational or solely for physical development or for training in sports and dance. The experts in rehabilitation, physical therapy, and corrective physical education have developed large batteries of specialized exercises and apparatus to retrain, strengthen, and restore to normal (or nearly normal) and useful function muscles ravaged by a disease, such as poliomyelitis, or by an accident.

Therapeutic exercise as an adjunct to other methods of medical treatment has been developed to a point where once hopeless, bedridden invalids are again able to walk, work, and live almost normally. This field of rehabilitation as a "third phase of medicine" was pioneered and enhanced in veterans' hospitals during World War II, especially by Dr. Howard Rusk. "Dynamic therapeutics," including therapeutic exercise, often achieves heartening results with shattered human bodies. Corrective and therapeutic exercise is administered under close supervision for definite, graded, medical purposes; and it serves high ends. It is not, however, the type of exercise a healthy young adult would normally undertake for pleasure.

Isometric Versus Isotonic Exercise. No current discussion of exercise would be complete without some exposition of isometric exercise and comparison of it with isotonic exercise. Isometric exercise, under that name, gained popularity in the 1950's and 1960's. In some respects it is a rationalization and amplification of certain body-building techniques introduced almost two generations ago to help create the image of the heavily muscled male physique. Isometric exercise has also been commercialized and undignified to the extent of advertising it as "instant exercise," promoted with such promises as "Imagine a 6-second exercise that helps keep you fit better than 24 pushups!"

The essence of isometric exercise is the practice of muscular *contractions* to the utmost of one's ability—maximum, all-out bursts of effort for a brief period of time, usually 6 to 15 seconds. You push, pull, press, or lift against an object that does not move. This object might be as simple as a door-frame;[3] it could also be an isometric

[3] "Isometric Exercises To Build Your Strength "in *Your Guide to Physical Fitness,* 16 pp., n.d. Distributed jointly by the American Football Coaches Association and the Tea Council of the United States (16 E. 56th St., New York 22, N.Y.).

rack,[4] a spring dynamometer for elbow flexion exercise,[5] a back dynamometer for spine extensor exercise,[6] bar bell or other weights too heavy to lift, or a fellow-student on your back.

Because of the lack of or little movement connected with them, isometric exercises are also called "static" exercises. In this they are in contrast to the better-known types of calisthenics, described as "dynamic," "ballistic," or "isotonic" exercises, all of which involve considerable free body movement. A simple example of the difference between isometric and isotonic exercise can be put this way:

Suppose your car is stuck in the mud. To release it, you get out and push against the back frame or bumper of the car as hard as you can, using (contracting) primarily your back and leg muscles. So long as the car does not move, thus requiring repeated contractions of a few sets of muscles, you are doing an isometric exercise. However, as soon as you manage to push hard enough to start the car moving out of the mud, you have crossed over from an isometric to an isotonic exercise. You are also moving many more muscles.

The principal and unquestioned outcome of isometric exercise is to increase the *strength* of the muscles exercised; it does so by an increase in tension; but exactly why the increments of strength increase as a result of tension has not been settled. Neuromuscular performance is not augmented along with the increase in strength, and may even be diminished.[7] Isometric training

did not improve performance in either the high jump[8] or the broad jump,[9] under controlled experiments. It has been concluded that there is a certain limited specificity to improvements in muscular proficiency achieved by isometric training. One investigator reports: "For example, if elbow flexion strength is tested with the elbow at the waist and also with the elbow overhead, then an [isometric] training program instituted with the elbow exercised at the waist, the result afterward will be an increased strength of the performance with the elbow at the waist, but no increase with the elbow overhead."[10] For training of athletes and for general physical conditioning isometric exercises are used along with isotonic exercises, skill trials, and other methods (sometimes graded resistance).

If they work, the isometric exercises increase the muscular strength factor in relatively little time. They do not always work, however, because the person doing them cannot always be sure that he is exerting maximum effort in his contractions. This subjective factor may be why some investigators have found an insignificant increase or no increase in muscular strength attributable to isometric contractions.

However, it is also possible that sufficient time to permit adequate test of the exercises has not been allowed. A person's rate of strength improvement, in isotonic as well as isometric exercises, depends primarily on the extent to which he *overloads* his muscles. It may be that in many reported studies of isometric exercises the overload principle has not been adequately applied. The work done per unit of time is the critical variable in extending muscular strength and also muscular endurance. Isotonic exercises are superior to isometric in developing muscular endurance; for the isometric exercises constrict blood and oxygen supplies.

There was a great burst of popularity for iso-

---

[4]F. A. Lindeburg, D. K. Edwards, and W. D. Heath, "Effect of Isometric Exercise on Standing Broad Jump Ability," *Research Quarterly,* **34**: 4, 478–483 (December 1963).

[5]G. T. Adamson, "Effects of Isometric and Isotonic Exercise on Elbow Flexor and Spine Extensor Muscle Groups," p. 172 in *Health and Fitness in the Modern World,* a collection of papers presented at the Institute of Normal Human Anatomy in Rome, Italy. Chicago: The Athletic Institute (in cooperation with the American College of Sports Medicine), 1961.

[6]*Ibid.*

[7]W. Harrison Clarke, "Development of Volitional Muscle Strength as Related to Fitness," p. 200 in *Exercise and Fitness,* a collection of papers presented at the colloquium on exercise and fitness sponsored by the University of Illinois and the Athletic Institute, December 1959. Chicago: The Athletic Institute, 1960.

[8]Richard A. Berger, "Effects of Dynamic and Static Training on Vertical Jumping Ability," *Research Quarterly,* **34**: 4, 419–424 (December 1963).

[9]Lindeburg, Edwards, and Heath, *loc. cit.*

[10]Laurence E. Morehouse, "Physiological Basis of Strength Development," in *Health and Fitness in the Modern World, op. cit.,* p. 193.

metric exercises in 1953, when two German investigators, Th. Hettinger and E. A. Mueller, announced that a single 6-second a day contraction against two-thirds strength resistance would increase muscle strength by 5% a week, by 50% in ten weeks![11] Later studies have not verified this percentage gain, and a more realistic figure is said to be nearer 2% per week.

The apparent simplicity and quick results of isometric exercises, as reported by the early investigators, have attracted considerable research attention. Some negative results have occurred; for example, decrease in muscular strength, muscular pain and damage. Pierson and Rasch reported the injurious consequences of maximal (twice a day) isometric arm exercises, undertaken experimentally by 15 upperclass medical students, 11 of whom soon developed sore arms.[12] On the other hand some investigators, notably Flint, consider isometric exercises safer than conventional "ballistic" (body-movement) exercises, especially for children.[13] With controlled static (isometric) movements, she believes, there is less risk of going beyond the limits of extensibility of the muscle. Pain would stop the movement before any injury occurred whereas ballistic movement cannot always be stopped the instant pain is felt.

Isometric exercises play an important part in another field of usefulness, namely in *corrective* physical education, physical therapy, and rehabilitation practice.

Collegiate Sports and Athletics

The incessant motions of the human body reach their summit of strength and endurance in competitive athletics and their peak of grace in ballet dancing. There are some interesting borderline events, like bullfighting and figure skating, which are both esthetic and athletic.

The interest in sports and competitive games, especially among young men, is nearly universal. Early American Indians had their lacrosse and other games; soccer teams draw millions of spectators in Europe; and American colleges and universities have their football and other varsity teams. Interest in athletics would persist whether it was formally under the jurisdiction of universities or outside their scope—as in professional sports.

College athletics, however, periodically come under fire as being "overemphasized." While abuses are possible, colleges and college students appear to have far more to gain than to lose by maintaining a high interest in varsity-athletic and intramural-sports programs. Sports for all is a better program than athletics for a few, but both programs could be carried through in most colleges and universities.

There are values in intercollegiate athletics beyond the direct benefits of the comparatively few varsity athletes engaged. They provide a rallying point for "school spirit," which means a sense of belonging to a recognized group. They help bridge the gap between successive generations of college men and women, for alumni are often as much interested in college teams as undergraduates. Something also can be said for college sports, as William James put it, as "moral substitutes for war." When 50,000 or more people of all ages, on a brisk Saturday afternoon, concentrate on the outcome of an intercollegiate football game and feel with one another in victory or defeat, a psychotherapeutic event of some magnitude occurs.

Athletics, sports, and dance undoubtedly increase the physiological capacities of those who engage in them, particularly heart, lung, and muscle power. The trained athlete is capable of supporting the following changes in his circulatory system during vigorous competition: the stroke volume of his heart may be increased threefold; the total output of the heart may be increased tenfold; his heart rate may double; his blood pressure may increase by half; the total volume of his blood (and the red cells in it) may increase by perhaps 10%.

[11] Th. Hettinger and E. A. Mueller, "Muscle Testing and Muscle Training," *Muskelleisting und Muskeltraining, Arbeitsphysiologie,* 15: 2, 111 (October 1953).

[12] W. R. Pierson and P. J. Rasch, "The Injurious Consequences of Maximal Isometric Arm Exercises," *Journal of the American Physical Therapy Association,* 45: 582–583 (1963).

[13] M. Marilyn Flint, "Selecting Exercises," *JOHPER,* 35: 2, 19–23 (February 1964).

All these changes are for the purpose of supplying blood and oxygen to the active muscles. In times of sustained, vigorous output of energy the skeletal muscles may demand 15 or more times as much oxygen as they need at rest.

The respiratory system of the trained athlete is also more capable of meeting the demand of the tissues for more oxygen, that is, of satisfying the "oxygen hunger" that accompanies vigorous exercise.

Muscle Training and Efficiency. In training muscles for quick reaction and for strength, the principle of overload can be applied. Thus, a batter usually swings several bats before he goes to the plate, but he hits with only one. Constant practice is essential for the attainment and maintenance of muscular efficiency at specific tasks. This is as true of small muscles as of large ones. A famous pianist once said, "If I fail to practice one day, I know it. If I skip practice two days, the critics know it. If I don't practice for three days, the public knows it." Grace of body requires regular, though moderate, exercise of the muscles.

SUMMARY REVIEW QUESTIONS

1. Give at least two definitions of "physical fitness." Describe valid tests, if any, for physical fitness as you have defined it.
2. What are the values and advantages of physical fitness?
3. What is the best criterion for determining when you have had enough exercise? Why is it such a good criterion?
4. Of what great traditions in education is physical education a part?
5. What are two or three of your favorite recreations? How would you rate them (highest first) in terms of their "energy cost?"
6. What are isometric exercises? Give some examples. How do isometric exercises differ from isotonic exercises?
7. What are the arguments for and against intercollegiate athletic competitions? How do athletics, sports and dance increase physiological capacity?

Worth Looking Into: *Youth Physical Fitness* (Blue Book) by the President's (John F. Kennedy) Council on Youth Fitness. *How To Be Fit* by Robert Kiphuth. *Guide to Physical Fitness* by Justus J. Schifferes. *5BX Plan for Physical Fitness,* from the Royal Canadian Air Force. *The Alabama Student* (and other essays) by Sir William Osler.

6

NUTRITION, DIET,
AND WEIGHT CONTROL

AMERICAN COLLEGE STUDENTS TODAY ARE probably the best nourished group of human beings who have ever lived. They have benefited physically by the startling advances that have been made in science and technology since the beginning of the twentieth century. These advances have included the sciences of nutrition and agronomy (scientific agriculture). Agronomy has given us such a plethora of foods in the United States of America that in the mid-1960's the government was still paying farmers *not* to grow certain plant and animal crops, and it held in storage around 8 billion dollars worth of excess agricultural products accumulated over the previous decade.

In the United States, well-stocked supermarkets lie within easy driving distance of practically any family, and packaged or refrigerated food delicacies from all parts of the world are available to any table. Much of our conversation about food concerns itself with how to diet and lose weight Eating places are the most common commercial enterprises in the country; cookbooks, next to Bibles, are the most staple items of the book publishing business.

We may sometimes forget that a vast number of the people in the world, and still some in the United States, are struggling just to get enough to eat.

An International Congress of Nutrition[1]

The Sixth International Congress of Nutrition convened in Edinburgh, Scotland, in August 1963. A review of this meeting by Krehl and Hodges will give a hint of the present breadth and complexity of the science of nutrition and also of the advanced subjects of research with which experts in the field are concerned. As the reviewers say, "The science of nutrition is a very diffuse subject, since it cuts across a number of basic disciplines. . . . The breadth and scope of nutrition is so great that it is impossible for one individual to encompass the entire field."

Two key themes at the nutrition congress were (1) the relationship of food supply to the world's present population explosion; and (2) the relationship of diet to disease, especially coronary heart disease—a relationship which implies a closer application of nutrition principles in medicine. But the congress also covered such topics as proteins and amino acids, vitamins, minerals and trace elements, lipids (fats), the

---

[1]"Sixth International Congress of Nutrition in Retrospect," reported by W. A. Krehl, M. D., and Robert E. Hodges, M. D., in Borden's *Review of Nutrition Research,* **24**: 4 (October–December, 1963).

65

nutrition of ruminant animals, animal production, plant genetics, endocrinology, nutrition in pregnancy, and early growth.

Later in this chapter we shall provide a simpler description of the fundamentals of nutritional science; but this early presentation of the jagged edges of front-line research should serve as a challenge to understanding the subject.

Food Supply. "The threat of hunger and malnutrition in a world undergoing a population explosion is the great threat and challenge to the future of man," affirmed Lord Boyd Orr, honorary president of the congress. He pointed out that the present world food supply would have to be nearly doubled to eliminate hunger and malnutrition, and that the chief increases would have to be in the expensive, protein-rich foods. If the world population actually reaches 6 billion by the year 2000, as sometimes predicted, the world food supply will have to be increased *fourfold,* Boyd Orr said. He believes that it would be possible to meet the demand by the extension of agricultural methods presently in use in the most technically developed countries, an optimistic point of view. Should these agricultural methods prove inadequate, however, he looks to biological and chemical methods applied to synthetic food production to provide a supplement to natural foodstuffs. Boyd Orr has long been an advocate of good nutrition and progressive agriculture as means of resolving key international problems.

Nutrition of the Preschool Child. The executive director of UNICEF told the congress what nutrition can do to better the lot of the world's children. He pointed out that the death rate of children from birth to one year in the technically underdeveloped areas of the globe is five times as high as in developed areas; and the death rate of preschool children, one through four years, in the developing countries sometimes 40 times as high as in the more fortunate areas. The quantity and quality of food available to the young child is a dominant factor in these statistics. To relieve the plight of children in many countries it is recommended that a "crash" preschool protection program be inaugurated—to supply protective foods within economic reach of the population.

Diet and Disease. The 1963 congress also debated dietary factors in causation of cardiovascular disease. There seemed little doubt in the minds of most nutritionists that diet in some elusive way is related to the etiology of coronary heart disease. But there were positive differences as to the degree of this relationship and the nutrients most responsible. For example, the Canadian Heart Foundation, accepting the premise that high levels of cholesterol in the blood significantly increase the risk of coronary heart disease, has recommended that people generally, and especially males, should consider the desirability of replacing about 50% of their intake of animal fats with unsaturated fats of vegetable origin. Other nutritionists questioned whether such a sweeping dietary change was justified.

A South African investigator reviewed the relationship of dietary protein to atherosclerosis (the accumulation of fat particles on the inner lining of the arteries), a presumed primary cause of coronary heart disease. One suggestion in his paper was that really long-term nutritional studies, beginning at birth and running 60 to 70 years, might have to be initiated to prove the debatable points in the relationship of diet to chronic and degenerative diseases. A Russian scientist, reporting animal (rabbit) experiments, claimed that vitamin C and nicotinic acid inhibit the development of atherosclerosis while vitamin D tends to increase it. Other nutritionists reported on changes in carbohydrate intake as a factor in reducing blood cholesterol. Among recommendations were (1) shifting the source of carbohydrate from readily available sugar to cereal starches, and (2) maintaining a larger intake of cereals (breadstuffs) in proportion to fat. A report on the milk and meat-eating Masai tribe of East Africa demonstrated that in this population, at least, a high intake of animal fat bore no relationship to increased blood cholesterol or atherosclerosis.

Proteins and Amino Acids (the building blocks of protein). Some points made and questions raised at the congress on this topic were the following:

A high-protein diet increases work capacity and favors increased productivity. For optimal growth, the diet must contain sufficient carbohydrate and fat so that the balanced protein is drawn on only minimally as a source of calories. At low protein intake levels the addition of certain amino acids may lead to amino acid imbalance and impaired growth. New research tools are needed to evaluate in a quantitative way the amino acid needs of different levels of calorie intake. More definitive measures of protein nutrition than determination of nitrogen balance are needed. What is the role of "protein reserve" in the body cells toward maintaining a nutritive balance?

Vitamins. The importance of vitamin B_6 (pyridoxine) in human nutrition was reported on by several investigators. After 21 days on a pyridoxine-deficient diet most of 11 healthy male subjects had abnormal electroencephalograms. On the characteristically high-protein American diet, a daily intake of about 2.0 milligrams of pyridoxine is recommended as optimum. Isotopes have proved valuable in nutritional studies. With radioactive vitamin D, it was possible to get a much more exact picture of its distribution in body tissues. Vitamin D is apparently destroyed in the liver. Isotopic techniques have also provided a clearer picture of calcium metabolism and recommendations for daily intake.

Minerals and Trace Elements. Several studies on mineral and trace element metabolism were reported at the congress. For example, the importance of metallic enzymes in cellular function was pointed out. These catalytic enzymes contain a metal atom firmly incorporated in their structure and essential to their activity. There is a *zinc*-containing enzyme which splits peptides. It was noted that the trace element, selenium, apparently exerts an activity comparable to that of fat-soluble vitamin E.

The brief summary of the Sixth International Congress on Nutrition presented above certainly does not cover all aspects of research in nutritional science now going on in the world. It should strongly suggest, however, the kinds of research upon which our present knowledge of nutrition is based. It is obvious, however, that a broad consideration of the subject of food and nutrition demands attention to social and psychological factors as well as to the findings made through physiology and biochemistry.

Food Prejudices

Unprejudiced normal appetite is the best guide to nutrition. Man and rat are omnivorous creatures; they eat everything. Even some of the things we call prejudices or superstitions about eating have a sensible basis, sometimes deep in folk-wisdom. For example: On a particular island in the South Pacific, it was observed that all food was liberally sprinkled with pepper made from a pepper tree that grew in front of every household. Indeed, the marriage ritual of people on this island absolutely required that the girl to be married must take shoots or seeds from the pepper tree in front of her mother's house, plant and grow them in front of her own. When a scientific analysis of the diet of these people was made, it was discovered that the pepper tree was the only source of vitamin C on the island.

Some personal food prejudices also have a reasonable basis in physiology and psychology. When a person says he doesn't like milk—or eggs, or chocolate, or onions—he may well know by personal experience that this particular food or beverage does not agree with him. He may indeed have a slight or pronounced allergy to it. Allergy to cow's milk, for instance, occurs both in infancy and later life.

Generally speaking, it is a good idea to avoid foods that you can still taste for several hours after eating—foods that "repeat on you," as the saying goes. It is also understandable that you may resist foods that were forced upon you at some time earlier in your life. You may secretly feel that you are swallowing your pride with every mouthful, and this masked resentment is a detriment to digestion. On the other hand you may learn to like foods that you formerly disliked—sometimes because you have discovered their nutritional value.

The child who cries for candy, ice cream, or

soda pop may sometimes be expressing a real need for the extra caloric values that they make quickly available or for the love and affection the giving of them represents. The disgruntled, crying child may also be lacking other nutrients —often minerals—in his diet.

We must also reconcile sex differences in attitudes toward food. Woman has traditionally played the role of food-giver in the household; indeed, this may be considered an extension of the mammary function. As food-giver, woman holds a position of power in the household and psychological implications of this fact should not be overlooked. To give (or withhold) food is in the final analysis to have the power of life or death, and even in subtler ways it is a means of controlling members of a family.

Food Fallacies. There remains, nevertheless, a vast amount of food prejudice and faulty eating habits arising from sheer ignorance, foolish fads and fashions, and from faulty and even fraudulent advice and advertising about food.

Some examples of nonsense preached in the name of nutrition are: "Eat raw foods only," "Don't mix carbohydrates and proteins at the same meal" (the stomach mixes them beautifully), "Molasses and yoghurt guarantee a ripe old age," and the like.

Half-truths and misstatements about food find millions of willing believers. This is a field in which the "big lie," told with a straight face, readily flourishes. People are more gullible about food nonsense than about almost anything else. They can be easily sold on the "magic" powers of one food or another. Here are some more of the lies about food that you are likely to encounter. *Don't believe them!*

"You are what you eat." Nonsense—you are also what you breathe and what your heredity determines you shall be.

"Fish is brain food." So is all other food.

"An apple a day keeps the doctor away." The apple-growers get sick and call physicians.

You may also hear such nonsense as: celery is a tonic, onions will cure a cold, garlic is good for heart disease, only "organic" foods supply proper nourishment, tomatoes are poisonous,

corn is hogfood. Don't believe it! You may also be urged to buy "health foods" (at fancy prices), daily vitamin pills (at even fancier charges), or "reducing foods." Save your money!

All pure foods are health foods when included in a scientifically sensible eating plan. A wide variety of common foods will supply all the vitamins you need. There are no "reducing foods." The amount not the kind of food is what counts in any diet safely designed to effect weight loss. Knowledge of the scientific facts about food and nutrition will fortify you against any of the food fallacies and myths you may henceforth encounter.

The Science of Nutrition

Nutrition is a comparatively young science. It dates back only to 1833, when a backwoods American army surgeon, William Beaumont, published at his own expense a thin classic volume entitled *Experiments and Observations on the Gastric Juice and the Physiology of Digestion.* The experiments were performed on a half-breed Indian, Alexis St. Martin. He had suffered a gunshot wound in the abdomen and it had never completely healed over. Beaumont tied different articles of diet to silk threads and introduced them into the Indian's stomach through the unclosed wound. He pulled the strings out again at suitable intervals of time and observed what had happened to the foodstuffs. He thus demonstrated that digestion was essentially a chemical process.

Intense research in nutrition since Beaumont, especially in the 1920's, has established some 50 to 60 chemical substances as essential to the nutrition of the human race. It is not necessary to know all their names, for the ingestion of a wide variety of common foods will deliver them all in adequate quantities.

Food and nutrition are not the same subject, although they are intimately related. Food does not become nutrient until it is eaten, digested, and absorbed through the alimentary system and delivered by way of the blood stream to the tissues and cells of the body which require these various nutrients for their function. A sick person can be "fed" by dripping purified essential nutrients into his veins (intravenous feeding). The more important use of the science of nutrition, however, is as a guide for selecting and eating foods which give the normally working organs of the body what they need for highest function.

The functions of food in the human body are obvious: to supply energy for muscle and other tissue function, which goes on all the time, to provide substance for the growth and repair of body tissues, and to insure a supply of all the nutrients, for example, vitamins and minerals, needed to regulate and control the complicated metabolic processes of the body. Water is equally essential. The energy requirements of the human being are provided by the combustion (oxidation) of the end products of carbohydrate, fat, and protein digestion.

When we are talking about proteins, carbohydrates, fats, and vitamins we are talking a chemist's language. These are not foods—like bread, meat, or butter—but rather chemical classifications of the ingredients in foodstuffs. Carbohydrates are so named because they contain definite proportions and arrangements of carbon, oxygen, and hydrogen. Proteins contain also nitrogen, which is their distinguishing chemical element, and sometimes other basic elements like sulfur or iron. By dealing with foodstuffs as organic chemical compounds we can better understand their function and effect in the human body.

Food Components

We now turn brief attention to "food components," that is, the specific needs for water, protein, carbohydrates, fats, vitamins, and minerals in the human diet.

Water. The human body is two-thirds water. We may readily conclude, therefore, that water is the prime requisite of the living person. Without it none of the other elements in food would be of any use. Water holds all the other elements in solution, both in and outside the body cells. The blood and lymph are principally water. The entire metabolism of the body requires water for its processes. A loss of 10% of the body's water is serious; a loss of 20% (as by extreme perspiration or bleeding) is scarcely tolerable.

The body excretes about 2 quarts of water a day. Most of it passes off through the kidneys as urine. However, sizable amounts of water are also lost through the skin by sweating and through the lungs in the process of breathing. Water is also expelled in the feces. The rate of water excretion is not constant. Hot weather, fever, or excessive exercise, for example, will increase the rate of water loss from the body, which strives, however, to maintain a water balance.

The powerful sensation of thirst is the mechanism by which the body makes known its water demands. Abnormal thirst, of course, may be a sign of disease (diabetes). If you follow your own sensations of thirst, your water intake will probably be adequate.

Various estimates have been cast up as to how much water a person should drink a day. The right answer to this question is simply, "Enough"—as guided by your thirst. Additional water will be taken in as part of the foodstuffs eaten, and about a half pint will be created as a result of the oxidation of these foods in the body.

The water content of most foods is very high, especially in fruits and vegetables, many of which contain over 80% water. Fish foods are 75% water and many meats, such as beefsteak, are over 50% water. Ham and eggs are about half water; bread is more than a third water; butter contains comparatively little water (about 15%).

Under conditions of summer heat, where extreme sweating occurs, the replacement of fluids should be supplemented with the intake of salt (sodium chloride), which is intimately associated with the body's water metabolism. The extra salt may be taken in salt tablets or by generous salting of food.

Protein. Protein is the protoplasmic stuff of which living animal tissue is made. It is manufactured in and by the animal body. The building blocks of protein are the so-called amino acids, all of which contain nitrogen. Animals get their amino acids primarily from plants—though carnivores like lions and omnivores like rats and men get the largest share of their protein requirements by eating other animals. The corn-fed hog is the most efficient machine yet designed for the manufacture of protein.

Protein is essential to any human diet. No protein, no life! Indeed, the word, protein, adapted from the Greek by an early investigator, Mulder, means, "to take first place." The animal body uses the end-products of protein digestion to build and repair all of its essential cells and tissues.

Plants are capable of synthesizing amino acids by withdrawing nitrogen from the soil and the atmosphere. All animal proteins eventually derive from plant proteins. In the human diet it appears advantageous, however, that at least one-third of its protein requirements be met by animal proteins, for they are the complete proteins that contain all the essential amino acids. Plant proteins are incomplete.

The human diet is adequate in protein when the combination of animal and vegetable proteins makes up about 10 to 12% of the diet.

There are many sources of protein in the mixed human diet. Among the richest sources of complete proteins are milk and liver. Other good sources of protein are meat (especially beef which has 50 to 90% protein exclusive of water), fish (which is 6 to 25% protein), eggs, cheese, nuts (especially Brazil nuts), and some vegetables like peas, beans (especially soy beans), and lentils. Cottage cheese is the least expensive protein food; lamb chops the most expensive—when figured in price per pound of protein.

There is a strong argument for including proteins in breakfast menus. They are digested more slowly than carbohydrates and most fats. Hence their presence in the digestive tract often prevents annoying midmorning hunger pangs.

The vegetarian gets some proteins from vegetables, if he is a strict vegetarian, or from animal-derivative products, such as milk and eggs, if he is not so strict. The need for some complete proteins cannot be obviated.

Amino Acids: How They Got Their Place in the Diet.[2] It took about a half a century of research to discover and demonstrate the essential amino acid requirements of man. German chemists, Kossel and Kutscher, at the turn of the twentieth century, found a quantitative method for separating the basic amino acids, arginine, histidine, and lysine. Emil Fischer at the same time discovered techniques which put in the hands of biochemists reasonably adequate tools for the study of proteins. Two distinguished American chemists, Thomas B. Osborne and Lafayette B. Mendel, then picked up the trail and proved, about 1914, that certain amino acids cannot be synthesized by living cells out of materials ordinarily present and must be supplied in a preformed state. This set the stage for thousands of animal experiments (largely rats) and eventually for the quantitative investigation of human requirements. In 1949 W. C. Rose was able to publish a list of the eight amino acids essential, or indispensable, to man and define the minimum daily requirement of each. He set a recommended daily intake at twice the minimum daily requirement. The eight indispensable amino acids for man and their recommended daily intake in grams is as follows: tryptophan, 0.5; phenylalanine, 2.2; lysine, 1.6; threonine, 1.0; valine, 1.6; methionine, 2.2; leucine, 2.2; and isoleucine, 1.4.

Analyses of U.S. dietary habits, food purchases, and per capita consumption of proteins containing the eight essential amino acids reveal that the possibility of anyone in the United States experiencing an amino acid deficiency would be very remote indeed—except, of course, in extremely impoverished areas.

Carbohydrates. Carbohydrates are energy foods. They are the chief source of the fuel which the body burns to meet its energy requirements. In the average, normal American diet about half the requisite calories should be supplied by carbohydrates. Fats are also fuel foods, but much richer in energy, weight for weight. It should be

[2] "A Half Century of Amino Acid Investigations," W. C. Rose, *Chemical and Engineering News*, **30**: 23, 2385–2388 June 9, 1952.

pointed out that fats and carbohydrates play somewhat interchangeable roles in the body metabolism. Both contain the same basic chemical elements—carbon, hydrogen, and oxygen— though in greatly varying proportions and chemical structures. The carbohydrate requirement is the most elastic food need of the body. It is the easiest to cut down without losing nutritional essentials.

All human beings ingest a certain amount of cellulose, which is a tough plant fiber. In reasonable quantities this supplies "roughage" for the diet and aids the processes of digestion and excretion. Excessive amounts of "roughage," such as bran, act, however, to irritate the alimentary canal and should be avoided.

The common sources of carbohydrates are familiar: potatoes and other "starchy" vegetables (which may contain from 3 to 20% carbohydrate); bread, cake, spaghetti, macaroni and all other products made from cereal grains (of which wheat, containing about 70% carbohydrate is the most common); candy, sweetened drinks and all other forms of ingesting sugar.

Carbohydrates are in general the cheapest foods and can usually be produced at the least expenditure of land and labor. That is why the masses of most lands have taken some adaptable cereal grain as their staff of life. Even in the United States the price per pound of such staples as flour and sugar is substantially lower than that of meat or butter.

Fats. Like carbohydrates, fats play their principal role in human nutrition by helping to satisfy the energy requirements of the body. More than that, however, they are often the vehicle of other food substances, such as fat-soluble vitamins, needed by the body. In addition they form substances (lipids) which insulate nerve tissue. For optimum nutrition, approximately 25% of a person's total caloric needs should be derived from fats. Fed in excess, fat is neither appetizing nor assimilable and the body balks at it.

Fat-free diets are sometimes prescribed in the treatment of certain diseases, notably acne and heart disease. The fact remains, however, that the animal body can synthesize most if not all its needed fats out of carbohydrates and proteins. The cow, producing butter fat, does this lavishly every day.

The human dietary gets its fat supply from three principal sources: animal fats, dairy products, and plant oils. Among the plants the nuts and seeds are the richest sources of fats and oils. Peanut butter and peanut oil are vegetable fats. Olive oil is one of the most anciently used of vegetable fats. Margarine is hydrogenated vegetable oil; its nutritive qualities, if certain fortifiers are added, are equivalent to those of creamery butter. Claims have been made in recent years that "unsaturated" (soft) fats are to be preferred over "saturated" (hard) fats in the human dietary (for prevention of hardening of the arteries). These claims are not proved.

Fried and fat foods in the human diet often appear indigestible because the fats have been *overcooked.* It becomes difficult for the fat solvents in the digestive tract, such as bile, to break down these particles for full digestion.

Vitamins and Minerals

More nonsense has been written and spread about vitamins than about any of the other dietary essentials. The history of the discovery of vitamins provides a fascinating tale of scientific discovery and the commercial manufacture of synthetic vitamins literally by the ton was a triumph for modern industrial chemistry. However, diet which takes in a variety of common foods will supply all the necessary vitamins, since they are widely distributed in nature. Except in the case of clearly demonstrated vitamin deficiency, it is not necessary for the individual who eats a varied diet to get his daily vitamins from pills. The need for vitamin supplements in reducing diets or in the presence of illness or following surgical operation is something else again.

The recognition of a whole class of vitamin deficiency diseases must be chalked up as one of the major victories of twentieth century medical science. Many disease entities are now known to be caused by a lack of specific vitamins in the diet and to be curable by the administration of those vitamins in some item of food or in synthetic form. For example, lack of vitamin D causes rickets; of thiamin (vitamin B_1), beriberi (polyneuritis); of ascorbic acid (vitamin C), scurvy; of niacin, pellagra. All these are clearcut cases. The diseases were known and described long before vitamins were discovered and named.

Only when vitamin depletion or deficiency has gone a long way can the diagnostician put a sure finger on it. Physicians have sometimes prescribed vitamins in vague and obscure ailments because "they can't do any harm and they might do some good." People who prescribe vitamins for themselves are often taking only a "sophisticated faith cure." One general observation about vitamin deficiences now seems clear. The deficiency is rarely that of a single vitamin; it is much more likely to be a multiple vitamin deficiency. As they actually operate in the human body, we may now think of vitamins as components of its complicated enzyme system.

It is not enough simply to have vitamins in the diet; the body must be able to absorb and utilize them. For these reasons the official estimates of human vitamin needs—so far as they can be determined—are usually on the generous side. (See table of Recommended Daily Dietary Allowances on pages 76 & 77.)

In the history of science vitamins were employed on an empiric basis without any knowledge of their actual existence. The ancient Egyptians, for example, knew that eating liver would enable them to see better at night. We know that liver contains stores of vitamin A, whose absence from the diet tends to cause the condition of night-blindness (xerophthalmia). Again, the discovery that scurvy could be prevented by taking small amounts of lemon juice and cured by larger amounts was made as early as 1593 by the English sea dog, Captain Hawkins. Today we know that citrus fruits are very rich sources of ascorbic acid.

The word "vitamin," a misnomer, was invented in 1911. Casimir Funk, a Polish chemist, working in London, took great masses of rice hulls and endeavored to extract from them by chemical methods the substance that would cure beriberi. He got a white, crystalline compound that he christened—wrongly but luckily—"vitamine." His theory was that the compound contained "amines," a class of chemical compounds, and that it was vital to life. Neither of these facts turned out to be correct. Nor was Funk's compound a pure product. Nevertheless, the name caught on and stuck. (Later it lost the final "e.")

There was great value, however, in Funk's easily stated hypothesis that lack of vitamins was the cause of a number of deficiency diseases. It was on this assumption that a great volume of nutritional research was undertaken. The vitamin field turned out to be far more complicated than anyone had imagined. At first it seemed useful and possible to identify vitamins simply by the use of letters of the alphabet. Now we know that there are probably more vitamins than there are letters of the alphabet, and it has become the general practice, except in a few instances, to refer to vitamins by their chemical names. Thus vitamin B_1 has become thiamin; vitamin B_2 or G, as it was variously designated, is now known as riboflavin; and vitamin C is ascorbic acid. There are at least a dozen vitamins in the B complex.

Important Vitamins. From the practical standpoint of human nutrition, only a few vitamins have to be seriously considered in diet planning, namely A, C, D, and three members of the B complex—thiamin, niacin, and riboflavin. Other known vitamins include: pyridoxine, pantothenic acid, choline, biotin, inositol, para-aminobenzoic acid, folic acid, vitamin B_{12} (probably concerned in blood formation), vitamin E (possibly concerned with the integrity of the neuromuscular system), and vitamin K, essential to normal blood clotting. Vitamins are distinguished as fat-soluble—vitamins A, D, E, and K—and water soluble—most of the others. Some are heat-labile and therefore easily destroyed by cooking; most are heat-stable. The functions and principal dietary sources of the more important vitamins are as follows.

Vitamin A was once known as the "anti-infective" vitamin. It appears to aid somewhat in resistance to infection by preserving the integrity of the epithelial tissues. The formation of "visual purple" in the retina of the eye requires vitamin A.

Excellent sources of vitamin A are fish oils (e.g., cod-liver oil), liver, milk, egg yolks, spinach, lettuce, broccoli, mustard and dandelion greens, green beans, carrots, yellow sweet potatoes, Hubbard squash, and such fruits as peaches and apricots.

Thiamin (vitamin B_1) is essential for carbohydrate utilization, normal appetite, and intestinal function. It is the lack of this vitamin which creates the disease beriberi. The body does not store thiamin as effectively as it does many other vitamin substances. By far the best single source of thiamin is dried brewer's yeast.

Riboflavin (vitamin B_2 or G) appears to be necessary for normal growth and for the integrity of mucous and epithelial tissues. Its absence from the diet is usually most evident in cracks in the skin, on the face, lips, tongue, and about the eyes.

Milk is the most common source of riboflavin in the human diet. Other rich sources are liver and kidneys, dried brewer's yeast, lean meats, fish, chicken, beet and turnip greens, carrots, eggs, and peanuts.

Niacin, also called nicotinic acid, was originally identified as the vitamin substance necessary for prevention of pellagra. This disease is characterized by digestive disturbances, usually diarrhea, skin eruptions, mental depression, loss of appetite, sore tongue, and loss of weight. The disease was once extensive among the poor of the southern part of the United States. The addition of fresh fruits and vegetables and milk to their diet, which had been rather strictly limited to "salt pork, hominy grits, and molasses," soon began to wipe out the pellagra belt.

The best sources of niacin in the human diet are liver, dried brewer's yeast, salmon, kidney, lean meats, poultry, peanuts, milk, spinach, lettuce, whole-wheat bread, enriched bread, green cabbage, and peas.

Ascorbic acid (vitamin C) is one of the most delicate of the important vitamins—that is, most easily destroyed by heat and oxidized by standing. Extremely water-soluble, it is often lost in cooking water. The body does not store this vitamin well, so it must be constantly replenished. Ascorbic acid prevents (and cures) scurvy and all the subclinical, mild manifestations of this disease, such as bleeding gums.

Citrus fruits—grapefruit, oranges, lemons, and limes—are the best sources of vitamin C. However, many other *fresh* fruits and vegetables, notably tomatoes, contain generous amounts.

Vitamin D, sometimes called the anti-rachitic vitamin or the "sunshine vitamin," prevents rickets in infants and children. It is essential to the proper absorption and utilization of calcium and phosphorus by the body. It is important to normal tooth formation. Without sufficient vitamin D, children are subject to bone deformities, pot bellies, restlessness—the syndrome of rickets.

Adult men and women, except pregnant women and nursing mothers, have little if any need of vitamin D supplements in their diet. The human body manufactures adequate supplies of vitamin D for itself when sufficiently exposed to the ultraviolet rays of the sun.

Overdosage with vitamins is not common, but it is possible and may have deleterious effects. Overdoses of vitamin D can cause hypercalcification (overhardening of bones), and too much vitamin A can stunt bone growth in a child. Vitamin C is perhaps the "safest" vitamin.

Minerals in the Body. About 4% of the total weight of the body is made up of inorganic or mineral elements, chiefly calcium and phosphorus. Still, there is enough iron to make a good size nail and enough sodium for a small shaker of table salt. In general, the minerals are regulators of metabolic processes. The fourteen so-called mineral elements deemed essential in human nutrition are calcium, phosphorus, iron, sodium, zinc, copper, potassium, sulfur, manganese, magnesium, cobalt, iodine, fluorine and chlorine. "Trace amounts" of other minerals, such as aluminum, silicon and nickel, are also present.

From the standpoint of human diet, however, we must give the most important consideration to the three mineral elements which are most likely to be lacking in the American diet—namely calcium, iron, and iodine. When these elements are supplied from natural food sources, the other mineral elements needed are also likely to be present. A good variety of common foods supplies required minerals in adequate quantities. The body stores and utilizes them well.

Calcium plays many roles. It is essential to the growth, development, and maintenance of bones and teeth. It is necessary to the clotting of the blood. It helps to regulate the heartbeat, to maintain the acid-base balance in the body, and to control the irritability of the neuromuscular system.

Calcium is needed throughout life, but is most important in the early years. The richest source of calcium in the human diet is milk—mother's, cow's, goat's, camel's, or mare's. Another good source is shellfish.

Phosphorus likewise is essential for the development of the bony structure of the body and the regulation of acid-base balance. In many respects calcium and phosphorus play complementary roles. Phosphorus plays an added role in carbohydrate and fat metabolism. Phosphorus is widely distributed in many foodstuffs, often in the form of phosphates. If calcium intake is adequate, phosphorus usually comes along with it.

Iron in the human body is concentrated largely in the blood and blood-forming organs, chiefly the bone marrow. It is an essential constituent of hemoglobin, the crucial element in the red blood cells. It is needed for the transport of oxygen by the red blood cells.

Actually, the amount of iron required by the body is small—only a few specks, equivalent to the daily intake of about 12 milligrams. Variety meats, like liver, are the best sources of iron.

Copper, as a dietary essential, usually goes along with iron, but only about one-quarter as much is needed. *Sodium* and *potassium* are another pair of minerals that complement each other's effects in cell and body metabolism; they are importantly concerned with water balance. Sodium is found in common table salt, along with chlorine that appears as hydrochloric acid in the stomach juices. *Iodine* is essential for the manufacture of thyroxin by the thyroid gland. Iodine is found in seafood and it is added to common table salt in the form of potassium iodide.

The Balanced Diet

If you eat a wide variety of common foods, the chances are that you will be eating wisely. Your nutritional needs can be as readily satisfied by the breadth of your taste for many kinds of food as by the sharpness of your arithmetic in calculating daily food allowances. Your weight will depend not on the kinds but rather on the amounts of food you eat.

Malnutrition, sometimes called "hidden hunger," is the outcome of prolonged failure to include essential food components in the diet. Except in the presence of disease conditions which warrant direct medical attention, malnutrition can easily be prevented by regularly (although not necessarily daily) eating so-called protective foods. These include tomato or citrus-fruit juices ($\frac{1}{2}$ cup a day), milk (at the rate of a pint a day), whole-grain cereals, one raw fruit or vegetable, and some inexpensive fat (for example, peanut butter).

Wise selection of a tasty, well-balanced diet of food and drink is a genuine aid to healthier living, improved personal appearance, and a better outlook on life. Furthermore, as research on the dietary needs of pregnant (and prepregnant) women is increasingly showing, proper choice of diet has an important bearing on the future of the human race.

The six essentials or components of the nutritionally adequate, or "balanced," human diet are water, protein, carbohydrates, fat, vitamins, and minerals. *A good variety of common foods supplies them all in adequate quantities.*

Food Selection: "The Essential 4"

Many valid systems of food selection, aimed at optimum nutrition, are based upon the scientific knowledge of human nutrition summed up in the Recommended Daily Dietary Allowances table on pages 76 and 77.

One such system, now designated as the "Essential 4" food guide, is centered around protective foods and omits specific groupings for fats, oils, sugars, and syrups on the ground that these are usually eaten in combination with the "essential" foods and that their nutritional contribution is mainly in calories.

The "Essential 4" food guide suggests that *daily* food intake include "servings" from each of the four following food groups:

1. *Milk group*—milk, cheese, ice cream.

2. *Meat group*—meat, poultry, fish, eggs, dry beans and peas, nuts.

3. *Vegetable-fruit group.*

4. *Bread-cereals group.*

Let us apply these groupings to the matter of shopping for food or selecting meals at an eating place.

1. Milk Group (2 plus servings a day). This grouping might also be labeled "dairy products" or "milk and milk products."

Some milk or milk products should be taken daily. The "serving" is an 8 ounce cup or glass. In terms of fluid whole milk the recommended amounts are: children, 3 to 4 cups; teen-agers, 4 or more cups; adults, 2 or more cups; pregnant women, 4 or more cups; nursing mothers, 6 or more cups.

In place of fluid whole milk may be substituted fluid skin milk, buttermilk, evaporated or condensed milk, dry milk, cheese—cottage cheese, cream cheese, cheddar-type cheese, natural or processed—or ice cream. The milk equivalent of ice cream and cream cheese is about half that of fluid whole milk, volume for volume; that of cottage cheese, about two-thirds. A 1-inch cube of cheddar-type cheese is equivalent to $\frac{2}{3}$ cup of milk.

2. Meat Group (2 servings a day). This grouping might also be labeled "protein foods," for it contains many foods beyond meats which are valued for their protein content—notably poultry, fish, eggs, nuts, and some high-protein vegetables. Another label for this grouping might be the "main-course" dishes—for these are the foods which generally comprise the main course of a meal and establish its price or cost.

Two or more servings a day should be chosen from this group. Count as a serving: 2 to 3 ounces of lean, cooked meat, poultry or fish—all without bone; 2 eggs; 1 cup of cooked dry beans, dry peas, or lentils; 4 tablespoons of peanut butter.

3. Vegetable-Fruit Group (4 servings a day). These are usually the "side-dish," salad, appetizer, and sometimes dessert courses of a meal.

Four or more servings of fruits and/or vegetables a day are recommended. Count as a serving: $\frac{1}{2}$ cup of vegetables or fruits or such portions as are ordinarily served—i.e., one medium apple, orange, banana, or potato; half a medium grapefruit or cantaloupe. Fruits and vegetables are reasonably interchangeable in this system. You could eat 4 servings of fruit and no vegetables; or vice versa; or 2 and 2; or 3 and 1 either way—provided, however, that you include 1 serving, every day, of a good source of *vitamin C* (ascorbic acid) or 2 servings of a fair source; and 1 serving, at least every other day, of a good source of *vitamin A*.

4. Bread-Cereals Group (4 servings a day). This grouping includes many items that are sometimes designated as "energy foods." It might also be called the "grain-food" group. It includes many low-cost carbohydrates which supply calories and satisfy hunger. However, if these breads and cereal foods are whole grain, enriched, or restored—as they should be and their *labels* will tell—they also furnish worthwhile amounts of thiamin, niacin, iron, and protein to the diet.

Four or more servings a day from the bread-cereals group should be taken. This means 3 slices of bread and 1 serving of cereal, or 5 slices of bread and no cereal. Count as a serving of cereal: 1 ounce of ready-to-eat cereal, $\frac{1}{2}$ to $\frac{3}{4}$ cup of cooked cereal.

Included in this group are bread, crackers, ready-to-eat and cooked cereals—including rice, cornmeal, grits, and rolled oats—macaroni, spaghetti, noodles, and dumplings. Biscuits, muffins, cake, cookies, and other baked goods made with whole grain or enriched flour can also be counted.

Other Foods. You are not through eating when

RECOMMENDED DAILY DIETARY ALLOWANCES,[a] REVISED 1968, FOOD AND

Designed for the maintenance of good nutrition of practically all healthy people in the U.S.A.

	Age[b] (years)		Weight		Height				Fat-Soluble Vitamins		
	From Up to		(kg)	(lbs)	cm	(in.)	Calories	Protein (gm)	Vita-min A Activity (IU)	Vita-min D (IU)	Vita-min E Activity (IU)
Infants	0–1/6		4	9	55	22	kg × 120	kg × 2.2[e]	1,500	400	5
	1/6–1/2		7	15	63	25	kg × 110	kg × 2.0[e]	1,500	400	5
	1/2–1		9	20	72	28	kg × 100	kg × 1.8[e]	1,500	400	5
Children	1–2		12	26	81	32	1,100	25	2,000	400	10
	2–3		14	31	91	36	1,250	25	2,000	400	10
	3–4		16	35	100	39	1,400	30	2,500	400	10
	4–6		19	42	110	43	1,600	30	2,500	400	10
	6–8		23	51	121	48	2,000	35	3,500	400	15
	8–10		28	62	131	52	2,200	40	3,500	400	15
Males	10–12		35	77	140	55	2,500	45	4,500	400	20
	12–14		43	95	151	59	2,700	50	5,000	400	20
	14–18		59	130	170	67	3,000	60	5,000	400	25
	18–22		67	147	175	69	2,800	60	5,000	400	30
	22–35		70	154	175	69	2,800	65	5,000	—	30
	35–55		70	154	173	68	2,600	65	5,000	—	30
	55–75+		70	154	171	67	2,400	65	5,000	—	30
Females	10–12		35	77	142	56	2,250	50	4,500	400	20
	12–14		44	97	154	61	2,300	50	5,000	400	20
	14–16		52	114	157	62	2,400	55	5,000	400	25
	16–18		54	119	160	63	2,300	55	5,000	400	25
	18–22		58	128	163	64	2,000	55	5,000	400	25
	22–35		58	128	163	64	2,000	55	5,000	—	25
	35–55		58	128	160	63	1,850	55	5,000	—	25
	55–75+		58	128	157	62	1,700	55	5,000	—	25
Pregnancy							+200	65	6,000	400	30
Lactation							+1,000	75	8,000	400	30

[a] The allowance levels are intended to cover individual variations among most normal persons as they live in the United States under usual environmental stresses. The recommended allowances can be attained with a variety of common foods, providing other nutrients for which human requirements have been less well defined.

[b] Entries on lines for age range 22–35 years represent the reference man and woman at age 22. All other entries represent allowances for the midpoint of the specified age range.

Water-Soluble Vitamins							Minerals				
Ascorbic Acid (mg)	Folacin[c] (mg)	Niacin (mg equiv)[d]	Riboflavin (mg)	Thiamin (mg)	Vitamin B_6 (mg)	Vitamin B_{12} (μg)	Calcium (g)	Phosphorus (g)	Iodine (μg)	Iron (mg)	Magnesium (mg)
35	0.05	5	0.4	0.2	0.2	1.0	0.4	0.2	25	6	40
35	0.05	7	0.5	0.4	0.3	1.5	0.5	0.4	40	10	60
35	0.1	8	0.6	0.5	0.4	2.0	0.6	0.5	45	15	70
40	0.1	8	0.6	0.6	0.5	2.0	0.7	0.7	55	15	100
40	0.2	8	0.7	0.6	0.6	2.5	0.8	0.8	60	15	150
40	0.2	9	0.8	0.7	0.7	3	0.8	0.8	70	10	200
40	0.2	11	0.9	0.8	0.9	4	0.8	0.8	80	10	200
40	0.2	13	1.1	1.0	1.0	4	0.9	0.9	100	10	250
40	0.3	15	1.2	1.1	1.2	5	1.0	1.0	110	10	250
40	0.4	17	1.3	1.3	1.4	5	1.2	1.2	125	10	300
45	0.4	18	1.4	1.4	1.6	5	1.4	1.4	135	18	350
55	0.4	20	1.5	1.5	1.8	5	1.4	1.4	150	18	400
60	0.4	18	1.6	1.4	2.0	5	0.8	0.8	140	10	400
60	0.4	18	1.7	1.4	2.0	5	0.8	0.8	140	10	350
60	0.4	17	1.7	1.3	2.0	5	0.8	0.8	125	10	350
60	0.4	14	1.7	1.2	2.0	6	0.8	0.8	110	10	350
40	0.4	15	1.3	1.1	1.4	5	1.2	1.2	110	18	300
45	0.4	15	1.4	1.2	1.6	5	1.3	1.3	115	18	350
50	0.4	16	1.4	1.2	1.8	5	1.3	1.3	120	18	350
50	0.4	15	1.5	1.2	2.0	5	1.3	1.3	115	18	350
55	0.4	13	1.5	1.0	2.0	5	0.8	0.8	100	18	350
55	0.4	13	1.5	1.0	2.0	5	0.8	0.8	100	18	300
55	0.4	13	1.5	1.0	2.0	5	0.8	0.8	90	18	300
55	0.4	13	1.5	1.0	2.0	6	0.8	0.8	80	10	300
60	0.8	15	1.8	+0.1	2.5	8	+0.4	+0.4	125	18	450
60	0.5	20	2.0	+0.5	2.5	6	+0.5	+0.5	150	18	450

[c] The folacin allowances refer to dietary sources as determined by *Lactobacillus casei* assay. Pure forms of folacin may be effective in doses less than ¼ of the RDA.

[d] Niacin equivalents include dietary sources of the vitamin itself plus 1 mg equivalent for each 60 mg of dietary tryptophan.

[e] Assumes protein equivalent to human milk. For proteins not 100 percent utilized factors should be increased proportionately.

you have taken the indicated number of servings of the "Essential 4" foods. Depending upon the choices you have made among them, you will still be one-third to one-half short of the daily calorie allowance for an average adult. The deficit can be made up by additional servings of the "Essential 4" foods or by butter, margarine, other fats, unenriched refined cereal products, sugar, and sweets. This additional food will serve to round meals out and to provide additional nutrients. The "Essential 4" food guide is only the *foundation* for an adequate diet. Its minimum number of specified servings together provide most, but not all, of the nutrients needed for good nutrition.

Faulty Eating Habits. Faulty eating habits result not only from poverty and food prejudices but also from emotional stress or sheer carelessness. Skipping breakfast because you are in a hurry to get to class or to the office is a faulty eating habit. The digestive system is "at rest," actually in its normal condition, when it is working on food. Too long an interval between meals may put needless stress upon it. A certain regularity in mealtimes is desirable, though this does not have to be made a rigidly monotonous rule. Eating the same food—often at the same place—every day is another faulty eating habit; a one-track diet is usually a poor diet. Overspicing foods is another habit to be avoided. Here is a simple test for a food ignoramus: he puts salt on his food *before* he tastes it.

How Many Meals a Day? The common American meal pattern has been set at three meals a day, but this is simply a matter of custom and convenience. Other countries, peoples, and climes have evolved different patterns. On the European continent, for example, a "first" and "second" breakfast were once common. Natives of Liberia deem one meal a day sufficient. Industrial workers are more efficient when they have five meals a day instead of three. The midmorning and midafternoon "coffee break" for worker or student and the "late snack" before going to bed are now common and sensible American customs. Eat when you like provided that you get the same general balance of nutriments as given by the conventional three-meals-a-day pattern. The best time to eat is when you are hungry. It is a mistake to engorge a heavy meal when your appetite says "No." The great danger of eating outside of scheduled mealtimes is that it promotes a tendency to ingest far more calories than you need.

Weight Control

Almost everyone at some time would like to add or take off a few pounds. A young woman is usually interested in losing weight to improve or keep her figure. Many young men want to gain weight to step up their physical or athletic prowess. Older people strive to keep their weight down to help resist the degenerative diseases. Within limits one can control his weight. A certain amount of weight consciousness is a good thing, but constant worry about weight is unhealthy. For the most part you must accept a weight appropriate to your body frame just as you accept the color of your skin, hair, and eyes.

Body Build. Body weight is crucially determined by body build. You inherit your body build, whether it is tall and slim, short and stocky, or in between. The breadth of your shoulders, the thickness of your bones, your tendencies to slow or rapid fat metabolism, and possibly the peculiarities of your endocrine system descend to you from a long line of ancestors. Nutritional practices cannot change your "destined" body frame and organs, although lack of nutritional essentials may deform or disorder potential structure and function.

Although no amount of wishful thinking can change your body frame, it is possible, to control—within limits—the amount of flesh, and particularly the amount of body fat, that is suspended from that frame. Some of this control lies definitely within the scope of medical treatment; a lesser part may be achieved by personal effort. Gradual increase in body weight from childhood through maturity is a normal and expected process. Long-continued *failure* to gain weight at this time of life demands medical investigation.

Sudden or radical *change* in weight, whether up or down, is often a sign of disease.

So-called standard height, weight, and age tables have long been in vogue. These have their uses, but they do not tell you what is a normal or optimum weight for you. The tables are only averages, based on measurements of many thousands of people. Few people hit the mathematically calculated standard figure. The range of the normal is very wide. Your best weight may be as much as 10% under or 10% over the calculated standard for your height and age. Beyond that 10% limit, however, which is the common definition of overweight, a medical evaluation of your weight is called for. In terms of your body frame it may still be normal for you.

Overweight. Records of life-insurance companies indisputably show that death rates are higher than average among obese, overweight people. Doctors have long observed that obesity is associated with increased incidence of diabetes, gallstones, high blood pressure, some forms of heart disease (coronary artery disease), and their complications. But nobody has yet proved that overweight is a *cause* of these diseases.

Many overweight individuals can profit from losing weight. Some cannot and some may even be harmed by trying. The doctor treats the whole patient, not just his excess fat. Serious attempts at extensive weight reduction should not be started without a physician's advice.

A person becomes overweight when he takes in and holds on to more calories than he puts out. Technically, he has a positive caloric balance. The aim of any weight-reduction treatment or regimen is to achieve a negative caloric balance. To this end a reduction in food intake is usually the safest and most effective means. Any diet low in calories but adequate in proteins, vitamins, and minerals is a reducing diet. Vitamin and mineral pills may sometimes be necessary and prescribed; in themselves they do not take off any weight.

The use of thyroid substance to take off pounds

WHAT SHOULD YOU WEIGH?

Women[a]	Weight (Indoor Clothing)			Men	Weight (Indoor Clothing)		
Height with Shoes	Small	Medium	Large	Height with Shoes	Small	Medium	Large
4' 10"	92– 98	96–107	104–119	5' 2"	112–120	118–129	126–141
11"	94–101	98–110	106–122	3"	115–123	121–133	129–144
5' 0"	96–104	101–113	109–125	4"	118–126	124–136	132–148
1"	99–107	104–116	112–128	5"	121–129	127–139	135–152
2"	102–110	107–119	115–131	6"	124–133	130–143	138–156
3"	105–113	110–122	118–134	7"	128–137	134–147	142–161
4"	108–116	113–126	121–138	8"	132–141	138–152	147–166
5"	111–119	116–130	125–142	9"	136–145	142–156	151–170
6"	114–123	120–135	129–146	10"	140–150	146–160	155–174
7"	118–127	124–139	133–150	11"	144–154	150–165	159–179
8"	122–131	128–143	137–154	6' 0"	148–158	154–170	164–184
9"	126–135	132–147	141–158	1"	152–162	158–175	168–189
10"	130–140	136–151	145–163	2"	156–167	162–180	173–194
11"	134–144	140–155	149–168	3"	160–171	167–185	178–199
6' 0"	138–140	144–159	153–173	4"	164–175	172–190	182–204

[a]If you are a woman between 18 and 25 years of age, you should subtract one pound for each year under 25.

While these "new" desirable weight tables are "actuarially sound," and represent average normal patterns of weight, you may still be within a normal weight range for yourself if you are 10% over or 10% under the figures given above. Beyond that range you owe yourself a medical check-up for professional diagnosis and possible assistance in your personal weight-control program. (Tables from Metropolitan Life Insurance Company.)

is inadvisable and may be dangerous. Appetite-killing drugs are of doubtful value.

It is one thing to lose weight, quite another to keep it off. Most people who diet strenuously to lose weight regain poundage—return to what is perhaps their "normal weight"—soon after they stop dieting. The best way to keep from becoming overweight is to eat sensibly, exercise reasonably, and live happily from childhood on.

Few people achieve that way of life. A high percentage—probably 75%—of overweight people are anxious people. They use food as a tranquilizer to allay their anxiety. Quite often this anxiety can be traced to the development of unhealthy attitudes toward food and eating in earlier years of their lives. For example, some families regard eating as a chore—to be finished up as quickly as possible. In others, food is used as a reward or a punishment; children are given certain foods (candy, apples, oranges, popcorn, for example) if they are "good," or sent to bed without dinner because they have been "bad."

Some people have unhappily learned to turn to food as a substitute for love and acceptance or as a consolation prize in lives. (Prison riots are often touched off by a decline in the quality of meals.) Some people use their teeth on food as weapons of defense or offense. They overeat either to armor themselves with fat against a too-demanding world, or to become "big as a house" so they can't be pushed around. Some fat people refuse to admit they are overweight; they simply see themselves as big and strong.

Food is intimately connected with the emotional and social circumstances of life from birth. If the helpless infant is not fed by his mother, he dies. It is not surprising, therefore, that distorted attitudes about food and eating often arise early in life or that overweight from overeating is a common result. It is not the only possible outcome. Underweight and many disturbances of the digestive system result from distorted attitudes and emotions about food.

The problem of *weight control is more of a psycho-somatic problem* than the "diet faddists" care to admit. The motivations for weight control must be strong and long continued. There are no quick miracles—no drugs, no pills, no salves, no baths, no electric belts or queer exercise machines—that can permanently "take off those pounds of unsightly fat." There is no royal road to the optimal weight. Even with the best of medical advice, the persistent cooperation of the individual is requisite.

Calories and What They Mean. In the simple mathematics of weight control the key is the calorie: the amount of heat required to raise 1 kilogram (2.2 pounds) of water 1 degree centigrade (from 15 to 16 degrees centigrade). This is the definition of the large calorie, as used in nutritional studies, and it was originally written with a capital "C." There is also a small calorie, used in other physical measurements, which is just one-thousandth ($\frac{1}{1000}$) as large as the nutritional calorie. The popular phrase, "Count your calories," simply suggests that you reckon the number of heat units that you pop into your mouth with your food.

The caloric value of any foodstuff can be easily determined. Experiments reveal that carbohydrates and proteins, weight for weight, yield the *same* number of calories. Fats produce $2\frac{1}{4}$ *times* as many calories as do equal weights of proteins and carbohydrates. In other words:

Fats produce	9 calories per gram
Carbohydrates produce	4 calories per gram
Proteins produce	4 calories per gram

Expressed in pounds, this set of figures means that 1 pound of protein or carbohydrate will yield 1814 calories while 1 pound of fat will yield 4082 calories.

If you want to calculate your own caloric intake, the following table of ratios will be helpful:

Fat: 2¼	Water ⎫
Carbohydrate: 1	Vitamins ⎬ :0
Protein: 1	Minerals ⎭

You must remember, however, that nutrient values of food cannot be judged by gross weight because different foodstuffs contain greater or lesser amounts of *water*.

What price water? It is a question that can be profitably asked when buying food. Butter, as noted, contains only about 15% water, but bread carries twice as much (30 to 35%) and beefsteak three times as much (45 to 50%). The differing percentages of water present explain why you will get the same amount of food energy from a $\frac{1}{2}$-ounce pat of butter as from a medium-sized potato (5 ounces), a large orange (10 ounces), or 33 large lettuce leaves.

The energy requirements of human beings, in terms of calories, are not constant. They vary with weight, age, sex, occupation, and presence or threat of disease. Many interesting calculations have been made concerning the daily caloric requirements of people doing different kinds of work or performing different kinds of exercise. Thus we find that a male student—sitting at his books for ten hours a day—would consume merely 2500 calories. Moderately active, he would need an extra 500 calories. If he were a football player, he would use up 5000 calories a day on game and practice days. The woman student needs about 2100 calories a day. When she becomes a housewife doing her own work, she will need an extra 400 calories a day. If she takes a job as a waitress, her daily caloric requirement will rise to 3000. It must be recognized that all these figures are estimates and averages around which many individual factors play.

Basal Metabolism. Your body expends energy—uses up calories—even while you are asleep, for obviously there is a great deal of internal work that must be done. Energy must be found to keep up the body temperature—man being a warm-blooded animal—to perform the functions of breathing, circulation of the blood, digestion and other metabolic processes, and to keep up the muscle tonus.

The amount of energy that the body must expend to get all its internal work done is designated as its basal-metabolic energy or, more simply, as its basal metabolism. The basal-metabolic *rate* of an individual can be measured, and remains at a surprisingly constant level in adults. Endocrine-gland disorders, especially overactivity of the thyroid gland, can, however, greatly increase the basal-metabolic rate.

Basal metabolism is usually somewhat lower in women and in older people. In the sedentary man about three-fourths of his caloric intake goes to maintain his basal metabolism. The "average" (154-pound) man requires about 1775 calories a day just for this purpose.

How to Lose Weight

The sum and substance of all scientific advice on weight control is simply this: If your intake of calories is greater than your output of calories, you will gain weight. If the output is greater than the intake, you will lose weight.

In a general way you have a "natural weight," just as you have a "natural height," based in the main on your genetic inheritance, your constitutional diathesis, and the general state of your health. The big problem is not really to take off weight but to keep it off. Your emotional attitudes toward food may well stand in the way of maintaining your "natural weight."

Although you have probably heard or read of scores of reducing diets, there are really only three basic systems for safely reducing your daily caloric intake. Though they go under many names, we shall describe them as (1) the Essential Four System, (2) the Fraction System, and (3) the Caloric Number System. All of them require the exercise of some willpower for which there is no obtainable substitute.

1. *The Essential Four weight-reducing system* means restricting your daily food intake to the servings of the four essential food groups (dairy, meat [protein], fruits and vegetables, cereal grains) without supplementation of other servings. This system assures you all the protective foods you need and gives you (depending on your actual bodyweight) somewhere between 50% and 80% of daily caloric requirements necessary to maintain your current weight.

2. *The Fraction System for losing weight* means that you eat a balanced, low-calorie diet by cutting down normal servings, or portions, to a fraction ($\frac{1}{4}$, $\frac{1}{2}$, $\frac{3}{4}$) of their usual size. This is the

theory behind most diets advertised as "eat what you want and get (or stay) slim."

3. *The Caloric Number System for weight loss* is operated as follows:

a. Pick the desirable weight for yourself from the tables "What Should You Weigh?" on page 79.

b. Multiply that number by 15, if you are moderately active; by 13, if you lead a very sedentary life; or by 17 if you are exceptionally active physically. This will give you your own caloric number; that is, the number of calories that you must ingest daily to maintain your desirable weight.

c. If you want to lose weight, deduct 20% to 25% from your caloric number and limit your daily caloric intake to that number of calories. Roughly speaking you will come out with a 1000, a 1200 or a 1500 calorie a day diet.

More drastic dieting than this should not be undertaken without medical supervision. If you reduce your calories by about 500 to 600 a day, you can expect to lose about a pound a week. It often takes a week or two of reduced food intake, however, before your dieting program begins to show effect on your weight. So don't be discouraged if you seem to be making slow progress during the first few weeks of your dieting regime.

Some Practical Hints for People on Weight-Reducing Diets.

¶ Avoid those high-fat, high-calorie "tempting treats" listed in the table of High-Calorie Foods on page 83.

¶ Eat slowly and in small bites. If you don't wolf down your food, small portions will seem bigger than they are and keep down hunger pangs.

¶ Drink water freely—before, during, and after meals. That will help to give you a "filled up" feeling.

¶ Go light on salt, which may tend to give you a "waterlogged" feeling, but be generous to yourself with other spices (which don't contain countable calories).

¶ Practice some appetite-killing habits: (1)

take a cup of hot bouillon or half a cup of skim milk before dinner, (2) remove yourself from the smell as well as the sight of tempting foods; (3) stem hunger pangs at any time of the day by nibbling on low-calorie, high-bulk foods; for example, vegetables like raw carrots, celery, lettuce, and endive; fruits like watermelon, honeydew melon, apples, and grapefruit (unsweetened); breadstuffs like a slice of Melba toast or a rye wafer or two; no-calorie beverages like hot (or iced) coffee or tea (without sugar or cream); and high-protein, low-calorie foods like cottage cheese and fruit gelatin.

¶ Space your food intake generously through your waking hours. You don't have to stick to three meals a day. Eat midmorning, midafternoon, and bedtime snacks of the low-calorie variety as long as you don't exceed your desirable daily caloric intake for a "reducing" diet.

NO-CALORIE AND LOW-CALORIE FOODS

Eat freely, even on a reducing diet.

Pickles (dill, sour, "bread-and-butter")
Cucumbers
Onions
Radishes
Watercress
Salad greens (e.g., lettuce, endive)
Soups (hot or jellied, such as consomme, bouillon, and chicken)
Parsley
Lemon or lime juice, slices, sections (without sugar)
Celery
Green peppers
Cranberries (unsweetened)
Gelatin (unsweetened)
Rennet tablets
Spices and flavoring agents (e.g., salt, pepper, paprika, vinegar, mustard, horseradish, celery and onion salt, mint, sage, cinnamon)
Chemical sweeteners (e.g. saccharin)
Black coffee, without sugar
Tea, hot or iced, without sugar
Lemon and lime drinks, without sugar

HIGH-CALORIE FOODS

Avoid these foods when you want to *lose* weight. Eat them freely when you want to *gain* weight.

	Number of calories
Malted milk (usual fountain size)	450 to 500
Fruit or chocolate sundae (large)	325 to 350
Fruit or chocolate ice cream soda	300 to 325
Lemon meringue pie (3-inch slice)	300
Mince, blueberry, cherry, and other rich and fancy pies (3-inch slices)	300
Beef hamburger on bun (3-inch patty)	300
Cheesecake (2½-inch slice)	250 to 300
Avocado pear (½ of a 4-inch pear)	250 to 275
Hot dog (frankfurter) on roll	250
Iced cupcake (medium)	250
Waffle (griddle cake, 6-inch diameter)	200
Candy bar (chocolate almond, 5-cent size)	200
Peanut butter (tablespoon)	100
"Hidden calorie" foods (depending on number or size of helping)	100 + or −

Potato chips	Olives
Potato salad	Nuts
Salad dressings (with oil)	Fried foods

Reducing Exercises. Contrary to popular opinion, vigorous exercise is not by itself an effective means of losing weight. Moderate exercise, in conjunction with careful dieting, may sometimes prove beneficial, but even this is not always the case, for exercise often sharpens appetite. So-called reducing exercises have more value in helping to redistribute body fat about the contours of a plump figure that they do in helping to get rid of the fat.

Swimming is probably the best of all recreational exercises for weight reduction. The reason is twofold: first, considerable energy is actually expended (about 125 calories in a fifteen-minute swim); and second, the metabolism of the body is forced to speed up in order to counteract the cooling effect of the water on the body temperature. Of course there are limits both to the length of time one should stay *in* the water (not over an hour) and to the temperature of water in which it is safe to swim.

If you actually want to lose weight, you will encourage yourself by keeping a record of your success. Weigh yourself twice a week under the same conditions (same time of day, same scale, same clothes) and make a chart of your progress.

Do not expect miracles. You will gradually lose weight if you can resist excess food.

Gaining Weight. If you want to gain weight, you should reverse the processes suggested for losing weight. In other words, *eat more*. Underweight is generally considered a sign of ill health, and often it is. On the other hand, it must be remembered that some people may be naturally slim or even "skinny" as a result of their inherited body build. No matter how much they eat, they cannot put on weight.

The obvious causes of underweight are wasting illness—particularly hyperthyroidism, diabetes, or infections producing fever; overactivity—restlessness, lack of sleep, constant running around—in short, the "social whirl"; actual lack of food because of poverty or abnormal social conditions such as war and famine, and loss of appetite. These conditions must be corrected before weight gain can be expected as the result of consuming more calories. Lack of appetite may in itself be an expression of some underlying illness.

Psychology of Obesity

Many studies on the relationship of psychologic factors to obesity have been made. One of the best studies was made by Dr. Hilde Bruch, who noted that fat children were the ones who most often became obese adults. Dr. Bruch has written:

Deposition of fat is not a passive process; it is more than a mechanical sequel of positive energy balance. Storage of fats is regulated through the [autonomic] vegetative nervous system and is controlled through impulses from the midbrain.

Thus an individual can give material expression to the inner picture of his own self. Through accumulation of fat tissue the child [or child grown up adult size] aggrandizes his physical appearance . . . Overweight in the child is an active process, expressing the child's effort to achieve growth and self-realization, though in a distorted way.

Although every person, thin or fat, has his own unique personality pattern, there appear to be some common inner characteristics of people who are or grow fat.

The truly fat person, the chronic or compulsive eater, is rarely the happy-go-lucky, food-loving individual that he is often pictured to be. Almost always he is suffering from one or more inner emotional conflicts. He is making use of food in large quantities to overcome the discomfort of his inner struggles. He often employs the resultant obesity as a weapon of offense or in defense of his ego.

Fat children and fat adults may seem passive or submissive, but these appearances are usually deceptive. They have a stubborn determination to control their family environment by being helpless or dependent. They raise a fuss when there is any frustration or delay in meeting their incessant demands. When they meet rejection at school or in later life, they resort to overeating for comfort and compensation.

Many fat people are preoccupied with tales and incidents of crime and violence; their fantasies are engaged by these subjects. They may also have a secret fear of their own feelings of violence and aggression. Because they think of themselves as "big," many fat men have avoided fights all their lives because they imagine that they might kill someone. In retaliation, they attack their food.

Many fat people have a false image of their own bodies. They equate size and strength. To lose body substance—as by going on a reducing diet—means loss of strength or power and may give them a sense of emptiness. One patient put it this way: "I felt I had to eat a lot so my skin would be kept full; I didn't want it hanging loosely around my body."

The fat person frequently views himself as "something special." He does not want to give up this image of himself, even though it is a false and damaging image when viewed realistically. In secret he fantastically misinterprets and overrates his importance, and never is able to live up to his exaggerated expectations. He feels—falsely—that he suffers from one undeserved defeat after another. To him this is an intolerable condition. He seeks a primitive kind of solace through overeating. He turns even his realistic successes into failures because they do not come up to his overwrought expectations.

Fat people often fight back against the demands imposed on them from within or without by refusal to make any effort at all. This is an important reason for their lack of initiative and activity, especially physical activity. In some cases it is more difficult to change their established pattern of inactivity than to change their eating habits! This points up the value of exercise in many programs of weight reduction.

The fat person is certainly not the only one who has psychic conflicts and neurotic problems, but he is the one who seeks to resolve his problems through overeating. He uses food for psychological purposes in a number of ways—to regain comfort, to allay anxiety, to find reassurance, to serve as a symbol of security, and at the same time to express and keep down his hidden aggressive impulses, hostility, anger, and envy. It is not surprising, therefore, that he should often view with alarm the prospect of giving up what has to him so many meanings and does so much for him.

In general we can say that people consistently overeat because they are satisfying hungers other than those for food. Their appetites are regulated by emotional—and, as we shall shortly see, by social—responses rather than by any strictly physiological need for food. Their unmet psychological needs have taproots in childhood, and they have become careless, impulsive, or compulsive eaters.

External Factors in Obesity. In a series of studies on obese and normal subjects, Dr. Stanley Schacter, of Columbia University, observed that internal and external cues to eating affected the eating behavior of obese persons differently from the way they affected normal people. He noted the following facts:

Obese and normal subjects do not refer to the same bodily state, as measured by gastric motility, when they use the word "hunger." The actual state of the stomach has nothing to do with the eating behavior of the obese. In one so-called "taste" experiment, the obese ate slightly more when their stomachs were full than when they were empty.

Fear markedly decreased the amount of food normal subjects ate but had no effect on the amount eaten by the obese. There is good reason to believe that the eating habits of the obese are relatively unrelated to any internal control (hunger pangs) but are in large part activated by external factors or cues (sight or smell of tasty foods). These external cues to eating affect the eating behavior in obese subjects considerably more than they do that of normal eaters.

In the choice of eating places, it seemed more plausible that obese persons would seek out good restaurants and avoid bad ones. This indeed proved to be the case when studied in Columbia University students.

In general, as variously tested, it turned out that the obese are relatively insensitive to variations in the physiological correlates of food (true hunger pangs) but highly sensitive to environmental food-related cues (the sight of someone else eating).

Nutrition Nonsense

It would be unfair to end this chapter without a warning to be continually on the alert for nonsense about nutrition.

In the 1960's nutrition nonsense in the amount of about $1 billion a year was being foisted upon the American public. At the 1962 annual meeting of the American Medical Association two experts on sound nutrition and good medical practice voiced warnings that are worth repeating and remembering:

Fredrick J. Stare, M.D., of the Harvard Medical School, called upon health and medical authorities to stop "pussyfooting" on problems of food quackery and speak out clearly against the nonsense that is issued in the name of nutrition. He pointed out that nutrition quacks display a curious ambivalence, seeking medical approval while at the same time condemning sound medical opinion.

Quacks exaggerate small symptoms and turn normal physiological events (such as everyday fatigue) into signs of illness. In other words, by using the power of suggestion they try to make people feel sick so that they can take credit for "curing" them.

Dr. Arthur M. Master, a distinguished New York cardiologist, went even further in his warnings, criticizing physicians for letting their medical judgment be swayed by fad diets that have captured the fancy of the public and their individual patients. Dr. Master said that several fads in treating heart disease had become so popular that physicians who were not convinced of, and even doubted, their value nevertheless felt constrained to prescribe them. In the "nutritional nonsense" surrounding the treatment (and theoretical prevention) of heart disease, he pointed a skeptical finger at popular concepts of cholesterol and fat in the diet and of salt restriction. (He also warned against the misuse of anticoagulant therapy.) Dr. Master said these diet fads are based on "data insufficiently tested and controlled" and may be of serious significance since they raise implications of considerable change in the dietary habits of the nation.

Many people are trying to avoid all cholesterol and fat in their diet. This may be dangerous nonsense because, as Dr. Master asserted:

There is no conclusive proof that the incidence of coronary disease and thrombosis is directly affected by the amount of cholesterol and fats in the diet. Although in general blood cholesterol is higher in coronary disease, a normal or even low figure is common in such persons. Actually no true standard of normal blood cholesterol has been established.

Dr. Master also designated as still "open to debate" the enthusiastic emphasis on polyunsaturated (soft) fats in the human diet. (It may be recalled that this was also the position taken at the Sixth International Congress on Nutrition.) That soft fats by themselves lower blood cholesterol, as once asserted, has been disproved. Lowered cholesterol is the result of avoiding undue amounts of saturated (hard) fatty acid foods. Consuming larger amounts of soft fats may therefore be both unnecessary and harmful. On the cholesterol controversy Dr. Master offers this summary: "Surely in the present inadequate state of our knowledge it is essential to avoid the extreme anxiety so many people have been thrown into concerning blood cholesterol or foods containing a little fat." (Recent research findings have suggested that the increase in *triglycerides* in the blood serum may be a better index of disease than the cholesterol levels. Dietary fats are composed chiefly of triglycerides.)

In conclusion, when you hear nonsense about nutrition preached by quacks who draw threadbare robes of science about them, remember that the real experts are extremely skeptical about such unwarranted nutritional claims. The human body, when prejudices of appetite have been eliminated, remains the best of all indicators of human food needs.

SUMMARY REVIEW QUESTIONS

1. Is the food supply of the United States adequate? Why or why not? How does it compare with the food supplies of other nations? What are the principal lacks, if any, in the world's food supply?
2. What food prejudices, if any, do you have? How do you think they arose? What are some of the common myths about food (name at least four)?
3. What six vitamins and what three minerals are most apt to be lacking from the ordinary American diet? What role in nutrition do each of these elements play?
4. What was the origin and what is the present range of study and research in the science of nutrition?
5. What are the six essential food components? What role in nutrition does each one (or group) essentially play?
6. What are the functions of food?
7. What risks to health do you see in overweight? Underweight? Losing weight?
8. In the process of losing weight, which three of the following methods would you choose or recommend as the most sensible and effective and why? (*a*) Taking vitamin pills. (*b*) Exercising. (*c*) Reducing food intake. (*d*) Consulting a physician. (*e*) Taking drugs. (*f*) Talking out your problems.
9. Describe the essential features of the three basic systems for losing weight. (*a*) The Essential Four System. (*b*) The Fraction System. (*c*) The Caloric Number System. What do you consider to be the advantages and disadvantages of each?
10. Are the following statements sense or nonsense? Why? *Fluoridation of public water supplies is a racket. . . . You are what you eat. . . . Never drink water with your meals. . . . Fish is brain food. . . . Ceremony is the sauce to meat. . . . Fat people are always jolly. . . . Americans run a great risk of amino acid deficiency in their diets.*

Worth Looking Into: *Recommended Dietary Allowances,* 7th revised edition, 1968, a report of the Food and Nutrition Board of the National Academy of Sciences, National Research Council. *Teeth, Health, and Appearance* by the American Dental Association. *Everybody's Book of Modern Diet and Nutrition* by Henrietta Fleck and Elizabeth Munves. *Essentials of an Adequate Diet* from the U.S. Dept. of Agriculture. *Reduce and Stay Reduced* by Norman Joliffe, M.D. *Your Emotions and Overweight* by Elizabeth M. Dach. *Mayo Clinic Diet Manual, 1961* from the Mayo Clinic.

PART THREE FAMILY LIVING

7

EDUCATION FOR FAMILY LIVING

A FAMILY CAN BE DESCRIBED IN MANY WAYS. First of all, it is a group. (We speak of families of nations and languages as well as of families composed of human beings.) A human family is a group of people tied together by physical factors, such as common ancestry, residence in the same household, or by legal bonds, such as marriage and adoption. The family is the tangible link between the generations of mankind, past, present, and future. In some cultures, such as the Chinese, little distinction in conversation is made between the living and the dead members of the family.

What Is a Family?

The family may also be viewed as a social entity, the fundamental unit of all stable human societies, a cultural pattern, a legal entity, an economic arrangement, a political fact, and a biological process. The relationship of the individual to the family is tinged with all these points of view. Since we have all grown up in families, we tend to take these complex relationships pretty much for granted. It is only when we analyze the functions and operations of the family that we begin to realize how one or more of these interrelationships may be out of joint and that disjointedness the root of discontent and personal unhappiness on the part of individual members of the family.

The pattern of family organization in the United States today is different from the patterns that appear in earlier times and in other cultures. Historians and anthropologists supply us with many other observed patterns of family organization. We have, for example, the matriarchy, common to certain primitive[1] tribes, in which the mother is the dominant and legally central figure. In the patriarchy, which reached a stage of classical development in ancient Hebrew, Greek, Roman and Germanic cultures, the father was the undisputed head of the household and often held absolute power of life and death over its members. There are still matriarchal and patriarchal features in many modern American families; but the ideal of romantic, monogamous marriage has tended to make the modern family more of an equal partnership between mates. Within the last century the rights of children have been increasingly recognized. We must not fall into the error, however, of believing that the family as we know it today is the final stage of its development. It is still evolving. Indeed, especially rapid changes in the patterns of family living have taken place in recent years along with the accelerated tempo of scientific and technological developments throughout the world.

---

[1] Primitive, as the anthropologists now use it, means non-literate, possibly preliterate; or cultures that are transmitted through an oral rather than a written tradition. Primitive cultures differ greatly; they range from the Eskimos and Australian bushmen, with hunting and gathering techniques, through complex agricultural societies like the Inca and Aztec. Primitive peoples are not intellectually or "morally" inferior to residents of more advanced cultures; they are human beings (*Homo sapiens*) in the full sense of the word. We of the modern world are not the lineal descendants of primitive societies, some of which are contemporary, though we have inherited and borrowed from some of these cultures.

The Function of the Family

The family serves many functions essential to the survival both of the individuals who make it up and of the society of which it is a part. Broadly speaking, these functions can be placed under four general headings: satisfaction of personal drives and desires; perpetuation of the race; transmission of culture; and personality development of children.

The family satisfies the personal needs, aspirations, desires, and drives of the individuals who make up the family. This applies particularly to the man and woman who come together to create a family. Marriage may be described as the birth of a family. It is also the normative pattern of sexual adjustment within any society. However, providing a socially approved pattern for the fullfillment of sexual needs and desires is only one part of the much larger pattern of marriage and family living.

If sexual outlet were all there was to marriage, probably few people would be found willing to take all the risks of founding, rearing, and launching a family. There are a few people, of course, who look on marriage simply as a necessary evil; they seek only tolerance or safe-keeping from their spouses and expect little intimacy or response. In general, however, a time of marriage is a time of hope. The founders of a family look to the building of a home and the enlargement of the family circle through children as the surest means of satisfying their deepest emotional needs and their highest social aspirations.

The family perpetuates the race. It provides the physical and social environment through which the human infant can be protected and reared to a state of maturity so that he or she can continue the process of procreation.

There is one important biological fact that helps to explain why the institution of the human family has developed in its own particular way. The human infant has a longer period of helpless infancy and childhood than the young of any other species. The infant must be fed and protected from the elements by its parents or other adults for many months before it is capable even of locomotion. Years must pass before a child can get for himself the food necessary to his survival. Social and environmental factors of dependence also emerge.

The family is the mechanism or medium through which the culture (or way of living) of a society is transmitted from one generation to the next. In this sense the family is the first and most powerful of educational agencies. We get our basic ideas of "right" and "wrong" from observing and hearing in childhood what actions the older members of our families approve and disapprove. Later in life we often lose track of this simple connection and look to some abstract ethical concept to explain our behavior.

The patterns of speech, belief, feeling, and action that guide our conduct are learned from other human beings, and primarily from the members of our family. For example, there is no biologic instinct that teaches us to respect the person and property of other people. The concepts of private property and sanctity of person are ideas that have arisen historically in the minds of men; the newborn infant has to learn them. That teaching takes place primarily within the family circle. Soon, of course, playmates and unrelated adults also influence his conduct. As the child grows up, he is admonished not to take other people's things and not to strike other people without provocation. If he persistently fails to heed these admonitions, he is punished.

The culture of any community is a complex thing. It is a pattern of responses to a wide variety of specific symbols, rituals, and tools. Although we are impressed with tiny fragments of a culture, such as the Western custom of tipping the hat to women, or the Chinese habit of eating with chopsticks, a culture pervades the whole life of the individual reared in it. Folkways, customs, mores, taboos, and laws, both written and unwritten, subtly influence the individual's conduct every moment of his life. We see this more clearly, perhaps, through the study of the cultures of primitive and preliterate peoples, such as South Sea Islanders and American Indians. Yet the weight of our own culture continually bears down on us, creating the climate of opinion which dictates many of our actions.

Cultures change—but slowly. Part of the reason for this is that the "design for living" whose rightness or wrongness strikes closest to our hearts was inculcated in early childhood. In the broadest sense we have all picked up the pattern of our culture from our families.

Our ideals and our prejudices grow from a common stalk, the family in which we were brought up. The attack on the social problems that perennially challenge the conscience of the world—war, poverty, unemployment, vice, and crime—can probably best be made through sharper consideration of the problems of the family. The happy family is the model for the stable nation.

The family molds the personality of the child. To a lesser extent it also reshapes the personalities of all who are party to it. The influence of the family pattern upon the personality of the child begins almost at the instant of birth. Having become a part of the family, the infant must immediately begin to adjust to it. In this process his feelings will inevitably be involved; how he reacts to the process of being acclimatized to family life begins inexorably to set the mold for his future course of life and personal conduct.

From the very beginning of his life the baby is expected to do what the family, and especially the mother, thinks proper. Such demands do not coincide with the baby's drives and instincts. But he is compelled to accede to the family's wishes. Though "self-demand" is increasingly the rule, nevertheless the child must usually eat on mother's schedule, whatever it is. He will be weaned when mother decides it is time. He must go to the toilet when mother says so. Growing up immediately conflicts with the "physiological autonomy" of the child.

His aggressive emotional drives are also restrained. He is not allowed to grab, punch, and strike as he wishes. A strain of resentment against such thwarting is built up, and some hostility consequently takes root. If love is withheld from an infant, a feeling of insecurity takes over. The child's personality grows in a multitude of moments of deep feeling and inner reactions to those

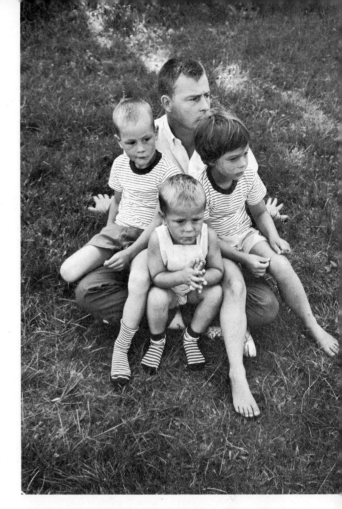

FATHER AND CHILDREN, U.S.A. 1970's . . . The profile of the American family has changed greatly since World War II. Young people marry earlier, and at a higher rate. Family chores, once considered "women's work," are more generally shared by husband and wife. (Photograph by Ken Heyman)

feelings. In adult life these childhood feelings are forgotten or repressed while the deep reaction patterns continue. The individual who has been severely compelled to conform to the family dictates laid upon him in early childhood often reacts with a warped pattern of conduct in later life.

Family Equilibrium

Every family has its own way of getting along. This applies both to the relationships between the members of the family and to their relationships with people outside the family. It is a common pattern, for example, that individuals within the family—such as husband and wife, brother and sister—may criticize one another devastatingly but will fall vehemently upon any outsider who disparages one of the group.

The family evolves; its relationships change as the members of the family grow older and as new members, infants or adults, are added to it. A family is never a static, finished thing like a cut flower or a fly in amber. It is always a growing, changing organism. We may properly speak of the dynamics of family living and seek to understand this process as it applies generally and to our own family constellations.

No matter how poorly a family gets along, it always moves in some direction. We can think of this as a family equilibrium—a balance of needs, hopes, interests, traditions, and interpersonal relationships—through which every family continues to operate. As seen from the outside, all families are in a state of equilibrium; the family is making some sort of adjustment, be it good or bad, to the society in which it is enmeshed. Inside the family circle, however, things may be in a sorry state with open or threatening hostilities between family members on every side. The results of such unresolved hostilities may be very serious and lead eventually to a "broken family."

It will be useful to understand the factors that keep a family in equilibrium, that permit it to make adjustments as it rolls along. The first of these is *imitation;* this takes place at all times within a family circle. It is easy to see how children imitate their parents and sometimes their older brothers and sisters in speech, gestures, eating habits, food preferences, sex prejudices and modesties, and even symptoms of illness. We are often astonished, for example, when a child answering a telephone speaks in a tone of voice that mimics and is mistaken for that of a parent.

A second factor that we encounter in observing the dynamics of family life is *identification.* This goes further than imitation in that it suggests a strong need, whether conscious or unconscious, on the part of the imitator to be like the family member with whom he identifies. A typical example is the tomboy girl, who wants to be like her brothers. The wish to identify one's hopes and aspirations with those of some other family member usually fastens upon the powerful or winning characteristics of that member, such as his or her appearance, position of authority, financial success ("the rich uncle"), or social triumph ("the sister who married so well"). However, there are also distorted identifications in which a weakness rather than a strength is imitated. A daughter, for example, may insist on having "sick headaches" just like her mother.

Profile of the American Family. The American family is flourishing, as the following brief statistical "profile" indicates:

In the United States today close to 95% of the population lives in families, with an average of $3\frac{1}{2}$ persons per household. However, something over 1 million married couples (out of a total of around 38 million) do not have their own households. These are mainly young newlyweds who share living quarters with their parents.

Almost one-half of American married couples have a child before the third year of marriage and about three-fourths start a family within the first five years. Around 3.5 million babies are now being born every year in the United States. This means a lower birth rate than in the fifties and early sixties.

Americans are marrying earlier than in any previous generations. The median age of American husbands at first marriage is just a little over 22 years and that of wives just under 20 years. Over 70% of the men and women in the United States are (or have been) married before they are 25.

Influence of Modern Family "Constellation." The shape and size—we might also say the constellation—of the family of which you are a part will both reflect and in a way create the population picture of the United States in the 1970's and later. By 1967 the U.S. population had passed the 200 million mark, and the Bureau of Census noted that it would continue to increase.

The composition (or proportion) of the American population is also constantly shifting, with significant effects on family living. During the 1960's, the population at ages 18 to 24—the college generation—and at ages 65 and over increased substantially. (This means, among other things, that you encounter more difficulty in getting into college and fiercer competition for jobs from the older generation at the termination of your college career.)

During the sixties, also, a slight decrease occurred in the early-adult, mostly high productive generation, aged 25 to 44, while the proportions of the population (and by inference, individual families) in the 45 to 64 age brackets—the "established" families—and the proportion of people under 18 (youth, children, and infants) remained about the same.

Marriage: The Normative Pattern of Sexual Behavior. Marriage is the name we give to the social institution which upholds the family and permits it to function to the best interests, as far as society can judge them, both of the individuals who make up families and of society as a whole. Marriage is defined by a cluster of laws, customs (mores), habits, and traditions, some written, some unwritten, with both civil and religious sanctions. In primitive societies they are enforced by strict taboos; in the United States they are upheld by public opinion. One must note that as societies and cultures change, laws (or at least the interpretation and enforcement of them) change.

In any society marriage is the normative pattern of sexual behavior. This behavior is condemned or condoned to the extent that it is judged to threaten or support the institutions of marriage and the family. Sexual function is universally regarded as going to the very root of the marriage relationship. Without it there would be no need for marriage.

Social Control of Sexual Behavior

It cannot be denied that the sexual drive in the human species is at times imperious and aggressive. Furthermore its consequences affect lives other than that of the individual involved.

From the earliest recorded times and among the most primitive peoples, therefore, sex has been regarded both as necessary and dangerous, and subject to social control.

The Historical Background. There are a few possible combinations of mating between male and female. These include *monogamy*, which is the exclusive right of one man and one woman to each other; *polygamy*, which means multiple or plural marriage, but is sometimes construed as the exclusive right of one man to several wives; *polygyny*, which is the right of one man to more than one woman—for example, to hold concubines in addition to a wife or wives; *polyandry*, which is the right of one woman to several husbands at the same time; *group marriage* (also called complex marriage), which defines the sexual rights of one group of men to a specific group of women. No society has ever tolerated complete sexual license, or the right of any man to any or as many women as he could get hold of.

Among primitive societies monogamy is exceptional and polygamy is often legitimate, sanctioned by law and custom. Marriage at the earliest possible time is the general rule; it is expected just as soon as biological readiness is established.

In antiquity the strong feelings surrounding the sexual drive caused many primitive tribes, groups, and nations to endow it with magic powers. Hence there arose a number of so-called "fertility cults," usually worshipping a female deity, a symbol of fecundity, who was implored to bring increase to fields, flocks, and families. Evidence of such fertility religions is found in studies of ancient Egypt, Crete, Persia, and parts of Asia Minor.

But there is also to be found in ancient history a tradition of asceticism—the idea that sexual abstinence creates special virtue, especially among those who perform holy offices. The concept of asceticism stood in opposition to the fertility cults of the ancient world. It made its way into Western culture through the Old Testament and the preaching of the prophets of ancient Israel against "the abomination of the heathen." Early Christianity also found itself in the position of opposing the fertility cults. Old Testament attitudes on asceticism were emphasized by St. Paul in the New Testament.

The ascetic ideal came to America in the seventeenth century with the Puritans, "the people of the Book," who left us the heritage of the "New England conscience." The Puritans followed the strictest interpretations of the Bible, even including the ancient Hebrew law prescribing the death penalty for adultery of women.

Over the centuries public opinion, however, seems to swing between what might be described as liberal and conservative poles of permissiveness toward different outlets of sexual behavior. Victorian society, both in England and the United States, generally tolerated segregated districts of prostitution, but would not permit a "nice" woman to show her ankle. Two generations later women were permitted to wear the briefest bathing suits, but most of the "red-light" districts had disappeared. In the United States today public opinion upholds romantic monogamous marriage both as the norm and the ideal.

There is a long history of individual and organized community rebellion against sex restrictions. But it is, on the whole, a history of failure, for society will not long tolerate threats to marriage and family structures.

The Inner Censor. The social control of sex expression is actually achieved in two ways: one open, one hidden. Laws, customs, taboos, and religions present open and obvious controls, intermingled with promises and threats, stated prohibitions, and generally known, even if unstated, permissions.

The real censor of sexual behavior, however, rests in the unconscious mind. Most frequently we obey laws, observe customs, and accept moral codes because something inside us tells us, often commands us, to do so. That something, hidden from other people and operative even when they are not around, is sometimes labeled "the still, small voice of conscience." More exactly, it is the *superego,* formed in childhood, which operates both in the conscious and unconscious minds.

Managing Sex Impulses

While there is at any time a consensus of public opinion about sexual conduct, there remains a wide range of individual attitudes and personal opinions within this consensus.

It must be recognized that every individual has his own particular attitudes toward sex. These attitudes arise from family background, from the total civilization or culture in which one is reared, from the stress of different historical eras, and from economics pressures.

The mid-Victorian (nineteenth century) attitudes toward sexual matters are certainly not the same as those of the mid-twentieth century. The economic stresses and dislocations of widespread military conflicts in the twentieth century have also had the effect of changing sex mores.

The codes of sexual morality set down in the Old and New Testaments, and forming the basis of the moral codes of Western Judaeo-Christian civilization cannot be held as the only possible codes for all peoples of the world—for example, the believers in the Koran, which permits polygamy, and the followers of some of the prominent religions of the Far East.

Even within the confines of Western civilization there are wide ranges of opinion concerning sexual morality and propriety. To some members of Western culture sex is "a joke"; to others, perhaps the majority, it is something "holy" or "heavenly." The divergences of opinion on this subject that you are likely to encounter are sharply illuminated in the two following quotations, each written and published by an eminent American physician.

1. [Sex] is the master joke of the universe. It is so magnificent a joke that the very stars rock with the echo of the laughter it arouses. That is just why it has attracted all those masters of the art of words from the beginning of time—the great comedians, Aristophanes and Rabelais and Cervantes and Shakespeare and Sterne and James Branch Cabell. It is because it is a joke that it is holy. It is because it is a joke, not because it is holy, that it keeps us fascinated even

after we have found out about it.—*Logan Clendening, M.D., in The Human Body.*

2. I shall make no apology for the way the world is made and for the process that brought us all into existence. If one person says that it was God, and another insists that it was Nature which developed it, who is to say?

The most important episodes in the life of a man or woman are those which have to do with marriage and the relations arising out of that marriage. Surely it would be better to fail in everything else and succeed in this, than to succeed in everything else and fail in this. If this is true—and it must be left to the reader to decide—it is rather surprising that information on this subject should be so frequently suppressed. . . .

The relations that exist between a husband and wife, who are deeply in love with each other, are good and clean and pure. . . . It is impossible to suppose that the source of all life is unclean or indecent. Therefore, *sex is good.* It is clean unless dragged in the dirt. Even then, usually it can be made clean again if the persons concerned are willing to get themselves out of the gutter and into a decent way of living.— *Thurman Rice, M.D., in Sex, Marriage, and Family.*

The great variety of individual opinions about sexual matters reflects the restless uncertainty, most intense among marriageable women and young bachelors, as to whether their current conduct will lead them to get the most out of their natural sexual instincts. It must be abundantly clear, however, to any thinking person that managing one's sexual drives cannot be divorced from the overall, continuing problem of living with one's whole armory of emotions.

Personal decisions concerning sexual conduct are and must always be intimate, individual decisions, unique in time, place, and personalities involved. In making your own decisions, however, it is always helpful to have a long perspective and wide range point of view on the possible outcomes of the actions you propose to take. The information presented here is for the purpose of helping you to appreciate the long view for yourself.

Marriage itself does not automatically solve all sex problems; the evidence is all to the contrary.

On the other hand, for *most* people, sex life in marriage represents the ideal way of handling the great, beautiful, and potentially dangerous sex drive of the individual.

It must be pointed out, however, that sex adjustment before marriage will inevitably have an effect upon sex life in marriage. This is an exceedingly complex topic with scanty scientific information on the subject. To what extent the use, nonuse, or abuse of one or more varieties of sexual outlet before marriage will affect the personalities involved and their interaction with one another in "building a marriage" is a question to which there is no single answer.

It has sometimes been suggested that early marriage is the solution for the common problem of sexual adjustment before marriage. However no one has seriously suggested lowering the legal age for marriage down to that of puberty or biological readiness for reproduction. Experience shows that very early marriage too often results in either unhappiness or divorce. There is a trend toward earlier marriage in the United States, but no one can pretend that this has eliminated the problem of premarital sexual adjustment.

It should also be pointed out that for *some* men and women sexual adjustment never was, is, or will be a problem. Of these some are secure in their moral tenets; others have a comparatively weak sex drive. For still others, the problem of sexual adjustment will not appear as a problem or be recognized as such. For some of this group, hidden and diverted sexual energy may operate capriciously in the unconscious mind.

How Physiological Factors Influence Sex Attitudes. Physiological factors also influence an individual's attitudes toward sex matters and the conduct stemming from such attitudes or feelings. This implies more than the drives associated with increase of sex hormones at the time of puberty. It relates also to the acceleration of growth in all dimensions that the present generation of young people have enjoyed. Young men and women today are 3 to 4 inches taller than their immediate and remote ancestors. This acceleration in growth begins early; indeed, by the end of the first year of life babies are about $1\frac{1}{2}$ inches taller than were year-old infants a century ago.

This early maturation and larger size of children and young men and women today (teenagers can literally "look down on" their parents) has widespread social and medical significance. As Dr. Harry Bakwin, of New York, put it in 1962:

The frustrating period between the time when drives for self-expression, social dominance, sex experience, economic independence appear and the time when these drives and desires can be satisfied is prolonged. Attitudes must be re-evaluated regarding the length of compulsory education, the proper age for military service, the age for marriage, the time to choose a career, the age of responsibility for criminal acts, inheritance laws and child labor.

That the problem is serious may be further attested by the fact that in the 1960's somewhere between 100,000 and 120,000 illegitimate births to teenage mothers were expected annually.

Biological Bases of Feeling. The intensity of sexual feeling and interest varies enormously with age, sex, condition of health, and other factors. A kind of imitative "puppy love" is occasionally observed between childhood sweethearts in elementary school, but sexual feelings—in the more specific and narrow sense of the term—do not really arise until biological readiness for reproduction occurs at puberty. This is accompanied, by significant changes in the endocrine gland secretions within the body ("leaping hormones" is the popular term) and is outwardly evident in the development of secondary sex characteristics—growth of pubic hair, change in body contours, menstruation (in women), change of voice (in men), and other changes. The physical factors underpin the psychological feelings and the social conduct. There is what we might call a biological rudder steering the course of life. Disease sometimes twists the rudder.

In addition to the obvious anatomical differences between male and female, it is also important to recognize that the biological patterns of sexual development differ between the sexes. In boys the physical changes of adolescence come on more or less abruptly, usually somewhere between the ages of 11 and 15. Their active sex interest begins at that time and is soon stepped up to the point where most males reach their maximum rate of sexual outlet in their middle teens.

It is also generally true that sexual feelings in men are more volatile; they are more quickly aroused and more speedily satisfied. Furthermore, men are often involuntarily subject to evident physical response to sexual stimuli of almost any kind, for example, the mere presence or picture of a woman.

In the human female, even after the onset of menstruation, sexual development occurs more gradually. Women generally reach their peak of sexual outlet a good many years later than men.

Sexual feelings are reflex reactions of the human organism. Given adequate stimulus, a normal man or women cannot help having some sexual feelings any more than he or she can avoid feeling hungry, thirsty, or angry under the appropriate circumstances. The feeling itself cannot be wiped out, but the action based upon the feeling can be controlled and modified.

We must distinguish between the normal sexual reaction and more complex behavior patterns of which it is only a part, for example—lust, love, romance, and infatuation. Lust is an *excess* of feeling, often leading to selfish or violent action; its goal is as often power or money as sexual license. Love in its fullest sense is an emotion that pervades all of life. It need not be directed solely to sexual objects; nor should mere sexual desires be masked or disguised as love. Infatuation may be described as the temporary delusion that "love conquers all."

Self-Direction of Sexual Desires by a Guiding Philosophy. There is no harm in suppressing one's sexual desires. In fact, throughout life, they must be suppressed most of the time by the responsible individual. This suppression represents willing obedience to a personal code of ethics which stems from or includes the more formal religious, ethical, and moral codes.

Control of one's sexual feelings is possible and to a great extent inevitable; it is also desirable and valuable. The emotions centering in sexual desire are intertwined with all the other powerful emotions that energize and motivate the individual—love, hate, jealousy, anger, and fear. These too must be controlled, if one is to achieve a happy, well-balanced life.

Experience in self-control is not *denial* of oneself or one's demands and needs; it is *direction* of these desires and needs toward fulfilling the greater goals of the total personality. In this self-direction toward life goals, control of admitted sexual feelings has an important place.

The "trick" in controlling sexual desires is to accept them for what they are but not to overemphasize them either by indulgence or denial. Act need not follow feeling. An attitude may properly interpose between the stimulus and the response.

Sex-Releasing versus Sex-Stimulating Practices. In practice, this means thinking out a philosophy of sex for yourself in advance of possibly dangerous encounters with it. This may prevent many embarrassing situations. Sometimes it may mean deliberately choosing courses of action which are sex-releasing rather than sex-stimulating. Take social dancing, for example. You can dance for fun, attending to the rhythm of the music, the grace and conviviality of your dancing partner, and the whole pattern of social gaiety at the dance you are attending. On the other hand, you can concentrate exclusively on the physical contact and intimacy of the dancing posture. In the first case your activity is sex-releasing without being sex-denying. In the second instance it is sex-stimulating.

Reading as an avocation also plays this dual role. You can read the same book for the sexual stimulation you get out of its carnal passages, or you can read to achieve understanding of human personality under the stress of passion. The primary difference between sex-stimulating and sex-releasing activities is in the attitude with which you approach them.

The Conspiracy of Silence. The evidence is now overwhelming that the *problem* aspect of sexual adjustment in American society is being solved in large part by the conspiracy of silence,

or, as Hollingshead has described it, *the clandestine complex.* In a brilliant study of the impact of social classes on adolescent behavior (*Elmtown's Youth*), he wrote:

Young people . . . must repress their sexual desires or violate the mores. This perennial problem has been solved, in a way, in our culture by the development of a clandestine complex that enables individuals to release sex tensions secretly and simultaneously to maintain their "good name" and dignity publicly, but not without compromising the mores and creating serious personal and social problems. As a result, an adolescent who breaks the sex taboos does not talk about his "vices" even to his closest friends, for so long as the mores are adhered to outwardly no public embarrassment is experienced by youngsters who profess one thing and do another. It is only when accident or ill fortune brings secret violations into the open, and persons other than the participants in the experience learn what has happened, that delinquents are compromised by their conduct and condemned severely by the community. . . .

The strongest moral judgments in the culture are applied to the violations of the sex mores. Perhaps the clandestine complex has developed as a reaction to the severity of these judgments. . . . [It is] a conspiracy of silence.

The publication of the "Kinsey reports" on sexual behavior in the United States put numbers on the open secret of the conspiracy of silence. The shock of these reports arose more from surprise that the unofficial secrets of the conspiracy should be openly published than from the statistical facts they revealed. These well-known reports have limitations, admitted by the scientist-authors themselves and generously pointed out by their critics. Nevertheless the findings of these reports offer the largest and most significant statistical samples of sexual behavior in the United States. The Kinsey reports do not presume to tell what such behavior *should* be; they simply reveal what it is.

The following comments from a distinguished college president, Dr. Sarah Gibson Blanding, president of Vassar College, on the occasion of the publication of the third Kinsey report (1958), underline the importance of these reports from the standpoint of the college community:

The late Dr. Kinsey, and now his collaborators, have engaged in studies which are sincere, objective, and determined explorations into an area of human behavior which is manifestly important to educators. [These] volumes are a concise, sober, factual presentation of an aspect of life which is emotionally charged and which has not previously been regarded as within the province of the scientist. . . .

Like all new discoveries, these findings must be subjected to further scientific research to confirm or disprove the conclusions drawn from the available data. The three published studies indicate that sexual behavior and reproductive experience are at variance with the official moral code and traditional beliefs and values. Most of us find it hard to think of sexual behavior in purely objective terms. We defend ourselves against unwelcome truths by passionate denial. We try to interpret the facts in accordance with our own understanding of moral behavior. We protest the data not because it may be untrue but because of its social and moral significance. In our society sex is a dramatically exploited commodity. . . .

If the facts are what they seem to be on the basis of the studies to date, the problems of duplicity they imply cannot be solved by indignation or ostrichlike denial. Sensational exploitation can only exaggerate the discrepancy between what people do and what society sanctimoniously thinks they do or should do. Parents and educators, ministers and doctors, psychologists and sociologists are challenged to straightforward, openminded, courageous thinking. Concepts, beliefs, values and goals must be constantly re-examined in the light of scientific truth and intellectual honesty and with deep concern for human dignity and the integrity of society.

Some Premarital Adjustment Problems

Expectation and anticipation of marriage is very high among college men and women. Their basic sexual interest, therefore, lies in choosing (or refusing) a mate through the accepted processes of dating, "falling in love," courtship, engagement, and finally marriage. But this is often a turbulent course and may require along the way a fuller understanding of other problems of premarital sexual adjustment, which, if not properly understood and managed, might upset the more fundamental goals. The problems lie in the areas of premarital intercourse, petting, autosexuality (masturbation) and homosexuality.

The Risks of Premarital Intercourse. The risks of premarital intercourse are well-known: venereal disease (discussed on pp. 100–103), unwanted pregnancy, illegitimate children, social stigma, psychic trauma, loss of self-respect, and others. Why, then, are so many found willing to run these risks? Some explanation is in order.

The risks are relative, what the military strategist calls "calculated risks." Those who take the risks are buoyed up by a false sense of optimism, fatalism, or, more rarely, responsibility. The optimists say, "Nothing can happen to *me*"; the fatalists, "Whatever happens, happens"; those who are responsible, "Whatever happens, I can take care of it."

Many who know the risks are temporarily blinded to them by love, hate, and other emotions, or by drugs like alcohol.

We need not stress the difficulties that those who gamble with premarital sexual intercourse sometimes encounter—for example, the boy trapped into marriage with a wife who will be a stone around his neck.

Fiction has made much of these tragedies. On the other hand, it must be admitted that these results are not the inevitable outcome of all sexual adventures.

While the sex drive is strong, it is not relentless. It does not begin as an overwhelming force; it has its rhythms. The motive which prompts sexual adventures in youth is not always love. Among the other common motives are to feel "grown up," search for adventure or romance, gang spirit, fear of not being "normal," rebellion against parents and other authority, and virtual seduction by older persons.

Young men take the risks of premarital intercourse generally for fear of "missing something"; young women often for fear of "losing someone."

Yet to divorce sex relationships from the total social context in which they take place is to denigrate their essential value. A few moments of sexual embrace in the back seat of an automobile or a night in a shady motel does not qualify as a sexual experience. The sense of "conquest" and the release of sexual tensions, if any, are only temporary and offer no positive, enduring satisfactions. To some degree such experience always engenders feelings of guilt or shame, overpowering and damaging to many people although lightly passed off in others.

There is a normal and natural tendency in any sex-tinged relationship to overvalue one's personal feelings. However, the lasting satisfactions to be derived from sexual experience depend upon social approval. Personal feelings are not entirely personal; they derive from the feelings of other people.

For some young people premarital intercourse has a negative value rather than a positive one. It is a symbol of rebellion and emancipation from parental control. The unconscious motives for doing something that parents have long forbidden are masked and unrecognized feelings of anger or hate against them, their ideas, and their guidance. Hence casual love affairs are often an expression of hate against one's parents rather than love for one's partner.

Petting. "Petting," a word that has many synonyms, describes a wide variety of bodily contacts and explorations undertaken both for the stimulation and satisfaction of sexual impulses. It represents a kind of sex play engaged in by many lower animals as well as human beings. Sometimes it is carried to climax.

The incidence of petting appears to have increased in recent years. The evidence seems to be that petting has become more accepted as a substitute for premarital intercourse, especially on the higher educational levels. There is little or no reason to suspect that petting *per se* causes any direct physical harm to those who engage in it. The psychological effects and social implications are something else again. Expert opinion is divided as to whether petting promotes or impedes later marital adjustment.

Certainly petting can invoke feelings of guilt, shame, disgust, and other uncomfortable emotions in young men and women who find a sharp conflict between what they are doing and what they think they ought to do. On the other hand it would be abnormal in modern society rigidly to refuse all physical contact with a person of the opposite sex, especially under conditions of a growing love relationship.

Some of the questions worth asking about the practice of petting are: "Is this getting me more deeply involved with someone than I want to be?" "Do I feel differently about the aftermath of this experience than I expected to feel?" "Am I getting a reputation for petting?" The question of "how far" one goes in petting is often a less important question than the question of under what circumstances one pets at all.

Petting and promiscuity are not the same thing. There are no good arguments in favor of promiscuity, which debases potentially valuable feelings to the level of a "cheap thrill." The Don Juan types, whether male or female, are basically unhappy people who sadly enhance their own feelings of insecurity by flitting from one person to another. They never really find the satisfactions they presumably seek.

Other Adjustment Problems. *Nocturnal Emissions.* Nocturnal or seminal emissions are spontaneous ejaculations of semen during sleep. They are often, but not necessarily, accompanied by dreams in which erotic fantasies occur. Over 99% of the men who enter college report nocturnal emissions at some time during their lives. Some individuals have many nocturnal emissions; others, very few. More imaginative individuals may have more erotic dreams, but these are not necessarily accompanied by ejaculations.

The incidence of nocturnal emissions is highest in the teens and gradually falls to very low levels. Very little is actually known about the physiological or psychological mechanisms involved. The semen ejected is, of course, exactly the same type of fluid released in all other types of ejaculations. No harm arises from nocturnal emissions, even when they are frequent, and most young men today simply accept them as a normal male experience.

Masturbation. Since very high percentages of both men and women report engaging, or having engaged in autoerotic practices (autosexuality, masturbation), the practice cannot be called abnormal. In the past great harm was done to emotional lives of young men and women by the false preachment that autosexuality had seriously damaging physical effects. Everything from pimples to insanity was blamed on it. There is *no* scientific evidence that any harmful physical effects result from autosexuality. The practice normally (and statistically) diminishes steadily with increasing age.

Homosexuality. In the normal course of psychosexual development, every individual goes through a stage of orientation to his own sex. This is the period of "gangs" and "crushes." However this is something quite different from overt homosexuality as an adult sex practice (in women referred to as Lesbianism). Any student who is genuinely bothered by homosexual feelings and longings is strongly advised to seek professional help for his problem. Attention should also be called to the fact that there are sophisticated and experienced homosexuals of both sexes who deliberately prey upon inexperienced young men and women.

A good marriage, conceived in affection and observed with fidelity, offers the best opportunity for successful resolution of problems of sexual adjustment. In the next chapter we shall discuss the factors involved in making a good marriage, particularly those concerned with choice of a mate.

Venereal Disease

Venereal diseases are so designated because they are usually the outcome of venery, a word whose origin goes back to Venus, the Roman goddess of love. The five commonly recognized venereal diseases are syphilis, gonorrhea, chancroid, lymphogranuloma venereum, and granuloma inguinale. The last two mentioned are comparatively rare and chiefly tropical diseases.

The principal venereal diseases are syphilis and gonorrhea, two quite different infections but occasionally acquired at the same time. Untreated syphilis is a long-range, sometimes fatal disease. Untreated gonorrhea is a shorter, some-

times crippling disease. Chancroid describes a soft chancre or ulcer on the genital organs.

When a "hush-hush" attitude toward venereal disease pervaded society, the venereal diseases altogether were politely called "social diseases." Then it was both conscientiously believed and vindictively taught that venereal diseases were "the wages of sin." With all that is known about them today they might more properly be described as "the wages of ignorance." Intelligent community health organization, better treatment (antibiotics), and public education have all helped to change community attitudes toward venereal disease.

The extreme fear in which these dieases have been held was undoubtedly more justified in earlier generations than in our own. Like other communicable diseases, their etiologic agents were then shrouded in mystery, and there was no effective treatment for them.

Unquestionably, moral and social issues such as promiscuity, prostitution, and personal sex conduct are associated with the spread of venereal disease. However, since we have previously dealt with these problems, we shall limit our discussion here to venereal diseases as communicable diseases that fall into the province of the physician and the public health officer and his staff. With the introduction in the 1940's of penicillin and other antibiotics for the treatment of venereal diseases, the incidence of these diseases fell sharply. However, in the mid-fifties the incidence of the venereal disease began to rise again.

Syphilis. The antiquity and origins of syphilis are still disputed by scholars. According to some it originated in the Western Hemisphere and was imported from America to Europe by the sailors of Columbus. At any rate the disease first came to serious public attention in France and Italy shortly after the discovery of America. It followed the Armies of Charles VIII at Naples in 1495— and it has been following armies ever since.

Syphilis has been called by many names: historically, the French pox, the English pox; scientifically and politely, lues (for which the adjective is luetic); vulgarly, "bad blood," "the dog," and other names. In the late 1800's Sir William Osler gave it the nickname of "the great imitator," for in its final stages syphilis can produce signs and symptoms which mimic almost every known disease.

The specific causative agent of syphilis is the corkscrew-shaped microorganism called *Treponema pallidum,* formerly *Spirochaeta pallida.* It is capable of invading all tissues of the human body and does not, as some believe, stay only in the blood stream. It is an eager parasite on a human host, but outside the human body it is relatively delicate and fragile. Dried up, it dies. Exposed for any length of time to temperatures as high as those of an extremely hot bath, it perishes.

The source of infection in syphilis is always another infected human being. The sphirochete travels to its new victim in discharges from his or her obvious or concealed lesions on the skin or mucous membranes. Spirochetes can also be discharged in semen and in blood. Direct contact with infected persons is the chief means of transmission of syphilis.

How Syphilis Is Spread. In well over 90% of all cases this direct contact is by sexual intercourse. It is occasionally contracted by professional workers in the course of their duties— through dental, surgical, or technical accidents.

Indirect contacts are responsible for the transmission of syphilis only in the rarest of instances. Articles freshly soiled with discharges or blood containing the spirochete might transmit the disease if the second person touched them within just a few minutes after they left the infected individual and they were still moist. Towels, toilet articles and articles held in the mouth, such as pipe stems or some musical instruments, are, practically speaking, about the only objects on which a viable spirochete might be conveyed.

The fear of contracting syphilis "innocently" by touching doorknobs or coming in contact with bathtubs, eating utensils, or toilet seats is *unwarranted.*

The only other way of getting syphilis is congenitally—through the placenta during intrauterine life from an infected mother. However, the protection of the unborn infant by treating the mother is very effective. Even if treatment is begin as late as the fourth or fifth month of pregnancy, the chances of preventing congenital syphilis in the child are 90% or better.

The individual who has syphilis is not always capable of transmitting it. The disease is communicable during its primary and secondary stages. Infrequently the skin lesions of secondary syphilis later reappear, within a year usually, and these too may be infectious. Technically these lesions are designated as mucocutaneous relapses. The most important period of communicability is during the first few months or year or two of infection. Yet inadequately treated patients *may* transmit the infection through sexual intercourse for a period up to approximately five years.

Like many other communicable diseases, syphilis is carried along through a chain of infected individuals. A single infected prostitute might give the disease to 100 men. There is no such thing as a "safe" prostitute or call girl even though they receive periodic medical inspections.

The Stages of Syphilis. If untreated, syphilis runs a long course and goes through the following stages: primary, secondary, latent, and tertiary.

Primary Stage. This is marked by a sore at the site where the spirochetes entered the body. It is usually found on the sex organs, but occasionally in the mouth. This sore, called a chancre (pronounced shanker), is generally hard and painless. It may look like a small pimple or ulcer, ranging from pinhead size to an inch or more. It is often concealed and may pass unnoticed.

The chancre appears anywhere from 10 days to about 3 months after exposure, but on the average in about 3 weeks. By this time the spirochetes have spread through the body, but there are no general symptoms of disease. Treatment of syphilis should begin promptly whenever a chancre is discovered, for this is the best time to drive out the spirochetes. The disease is highly communicable while the chancre is present.

Secondary Stage. Even without treatment, the chancre disappears in about 3 to 6 weeks. The secondary stage of syphilis begins as the chancre is disappearing; at this time the spirochetes diffuse themselves throughout the body, and can be found in the circulating blood. The secondary stage lasts for a variable period of time, usually a few months but sometimes for several years. The disease is still readily curable in the secondary stage.

Latent Stage. The signs and symptoms of secondary syphilis gradually pass away although no treatment be given. This disease then lapses into a latent or quiescent stage, which usually lasts from 5 to 20 years but may range from 2 to 50 years. There are no symptoms in the latent stage, but the spirochetes are still present in the body and can be discovered by serologic ("blood") tests.

Tertiary (third) Stage. In this final stage of syphilis, the untreated disease often comes to a hideous flower and imitates many other diseases. It may attack the brain and spinal cord (neurosyphilis), the heart and blood vessels (particularly the aorta), the bones, and the skin.

The effects of late syphilis on the nervous system go under such names as paresis, general paralysis of the insane, dementia paralytica, locomotor ataxia and tabes dorsalis. Late syphilis can be treated—but not so effectively as the earlier stages of the disease.

Diagnosis and Treatment. The diagnosis of syphilis requires laboratory confirmation. In the primary stage it is confirmed by examining fluids from the chancre under a dark-field microscope and actually seeing the pale, wriggly spirochetes. In the subsequent stages the diagnosis is made by serologic tests, (*blood tests*). Spinal fluid is also used. The best-known of these laboratory tests for syphilis is the Wassermann test, but there are a great many others also named after the laboratory men who developed them—for example, the Kahn, Kline, Kolmer, Hinton, and Eagle tests. A four-plus Wassermann signifies a completely positive reaction on the test.

Syphilis at all stages is now effectively treated and usually cured with penicillin and other antibiotics. The treatment period is *short,* and the injections can be given easily and painlessly in any doctor's office. A series of four or five injec-

tions of penicillin in the course of a week can change a positive Wassermann to a negative Wassermann in that time. Relapses are few, although reinfection can occur.

Gonorrhea. Gonorrhea is both the most common and the most readily curable venereal disease. Its incidence is about five times higher than syphilis. It is an acute, communicable disease, specifically caused by infection with the gonococcus microbe (*Neisseria gonorrheae*). Untreated gonorrhea may have a chronic, serious, and crippling aftermath, resulting in sterility, arthritis, or blindness.

The only source of gonorrheal infection is discharges from lesions of the mucous membranes or lymph nodes of persons currently afflicted. Hence the disease is almost always transmitted by sexual contact or direct personal contact with the discharges. In rare instances articles freshly soiled with discharges—wash cloths, towels, and other bathroom accessories—may transmit the disease. Little girls under 6 are especially susceptible to vaginal infection with such discharges, and epidemics of vulvovaginitis sometimes occur in girls' schools. These are the principal instances in which gonorrhea is innocently acquired.

Symptoms. The symptoms of gonorrhea appear from 1 day to 2 or 3 weeks (usually 3 to 5 days) after exposure. In the male the symptoms of the early and acute disease include pain—stinging or burning—when urinating, some slight swelling and discomfort in the urinary region, and the discharge of a few drops of pus from the tip of the penis. These symptoms grow worse as the infection of the mucous membranes of the urinary system and adjacent organs progresses.

In women the early symptoms are likely to be less acute. In addition to pain on urination (which is less acute because the female urinary tract is shorter than the male), the early symptoms may include a yellowish vaginal discharge and a painful swelling or abscess of the glands (Bartholin's glands) at the mouth of the vulva.

Even without treatment, the acute, painful symptoms of gonorrhea gradually fade away. But there is no absolutely positive way of knowing that the gonococcus has completely disappeared from the body. Chronic or recurrent inflammation with discharge is a common occurrence in untreated gonorrhea even after the initial, acute stage has passed. So long as the gonococcus persists, the infected individual can transmit the disease.

The mucous membranes of the eye are particularly susceptible to gonorrheal infection. Newborn babies were once frequently infected during the process of birth. "Babies' sore eyes"—gonorrheal ophthalmia—was once a common cause of blindness. This condition has been practically eliminated by laws requiring silver nitrate or other equally effective gonococcus-killing drugs to be instilled in infants' eyes immediately after birth.

Treatment. Present-day treatment of gonorrhea is swift and sure. Cure rates approaching almost 100% have been reported. Any doctor can give the treatment. Most cases can be cleared up in a day or two by a single injection of delayed-action penicillin or administration by mouth of some other antibiotic drugs.

Control of Venereal Disease. Syphilis case rates in the United States and other parts of the world fell precipitously to new low levels when penicillin and other antibiotics highly effective in the treatment of venereal diseases were first introduced in the 1940's. The effectiveness of these drugs has not diminished, but their consistent application apparently has. For a variety of reasons the rate of reported syphilis has been increasing in the United States since 1957.

About 60,000 *new* cases of syphilis are now reported yearly; and there are about 2 million cases still needing treatment. There are about 1 million *new* cases of gonorrhea in the United States every year. Very few of them—perhaps 10%—are reported by private physicians to public health authorities.

The control of venereal disease has many ramifications—moral, legal, social, educational, medical, and personal. Guided by knowledge and by moral and common sense any alert individual can guarantee himself freedom from contracting venereal disease or suffering its consequences. This is more than can be promised for almost any other class or type of disease. The rules for freedom from venereal disease, or perhaps more properly the precautions against them, can be summed up simply as follows:

Precautions Against Venereal Disease. Avoid exposure to venereal diseases and to the circumstances inviting them, especially alcoholic indulgence.

If exposed, take prompt prophylactic measures.

Watch out for the danger signals of infection—the chancre of syphilis, the pain and pus of gonorrhea.

Seek treatment promptly from a reliable physician.

Continue treatment until pronounced cured.

Have a blood test taken as part of a medical examination.

Prophylaxis may be mechanical (the rubber sheath), chemical (ointments and solutions for application to the genitals), or chemotherapeutic (antibiotics). As one of several methods of control of syphilis and gonorrhea the American Public Health Association's official *Control of Communicable Diseases in Man* recommends: "teaching methods of personal prophylaxis applicable before, during, and after exposure."

Theoretically—if every person with venereal disease was immediately put under adequate treatment—it would be possible to eliminate these diseases entirely. In Sweden, where the police power of the state has been invoked for this purpose, this goal is nearly attained.

In the United States, public health authorities have not thought it wise to press for such drastic power. Legal action is confined to setting up free clinic programs, repressing commercial prostitution, forbidding sale of liquor to minors, requiring premarital and prenatal blood tests (which some authorities believe are no longer worth the cost and effort), and regulating the conduct of taverns.

Unfortunately, with respect to many other communicable diseases, such as the cold, there are no laws which can possibly wipe them out.

SUMMARY REVIEW QUESTIONS

1. What are the functions of the family? Elaborate.
2. What do you consider to be the trends in family life in the United States today? How does this help create and how is this reflected in the total population pattern of the United States?
3. How do you interpret the statement: "Marriage is the normative pattern of sexual behavior"? Elaborate.
4. What is the historical background for the present American ideal of marriage?
5. How are private and personal attitudes toward sex formed? Why do you think they sometimes differ so greatly from person to person?
6. Do you think it is important to have a guiding personal philosophy for the management of sexual instincts? Why or why not? What is your personal philosophy of sexual behavior? Has it changed much in recent years? Why or why not?
7. What is the "conspiracy of silence" in the United States? How does it operate? What do you conceive to be its purpose? Its results?
8. What are the risks of premarital intercourse? Why do some young men and women take these risks?
9. Are the following statements sense or nonsense? Why? *The population of the United States will exceed 250,000,000 by 1980. . . . Love conquers all. . . . Early marriage is the best answer to all problems of sexual adjustment. . . . Men attain real sexual maturity years ahead of women. . . . The girl who will pet/Is a poor marriage bet.*
10. What do the following terms mean to you: matriarchy, birth rate, polygamy, polyandry, fertility cult, lust, infatuation, promiscuity, autosexuality, homosexuality?
11. What measures for the control of venereal disease do you *personally* advocate? What measures—briefly—do you think you would emphasize if you were: A police chief? A public health officer? A physician? A clergyman? A parent of teenage boys or girls? An army officer? A high-school principal? The proprietor of a public dancehall?
12. What are the early and evident signs of syphilis? How is the disease spread? What are the stages of the disease?
13. How does gonorrhea differ from syphilis? What are the presenting symptoms of gonorrhea? In what way, if any, is the treatment of the two diseases different?

Worth Looking Into: *Elmtown's Youth: The Impact of Social Classes on Adolescents* by August B. Hollingshead. *Love against Hate* by Karl Menninger. *Male and Female* by Margaret Mead. *Human Sex and Education: Perspectives and Problems* by W. R. Johnson.

8

PREPARING FOR MARRIAGE

THE TRANSITION FROM CHILDHOOD TO MAN-
hood in modern American culture often
seems to be particularly turbulent. One paradoxical reason for this is the comparatively high
degree of independence enjoyed by young people,
since parental authority wanes early. The formal
landmarks of growing up have been erased; there
are no traditional initiation ceremonies to mark
acceptance into adult status. In youth the underlying theme of conduct is independence and
the goal is maturity.

In early adolescence the physical changes
wrought by new hormone patterns and differ-
ential growth rates of different body parts create
problems of adjustment; adolescent awkwardness
must be mastered. In the late teens and into
college years the need for making new kinds of
social and emotional adjustments becomes more
intense. The relationship of college students with
their parents and other members of their family
changes and sometimes becomes strained.

More important, the need for establishing new
kinds of attitudes and relationships with members of the opposite sex becomes paramount. A
feeling for adventure is gradually modified by
a desire for permanence in man-woman relationships. The drive toward growing up is slowly
integrated with the feeling for settling down in
marriage. But interposed and imposed on these
feelings is the demand for love, that is, the need
to love and be loved by a particular mate. The
choice of a marriage partner becomes an expedi-
tion for discovering the sensation of "falling in
love." This predominantly American way of ar-
ranging for marriage has both its advantages

and disadvantages, its successes and its failures.

In this chapter we shall give particular consideration to the factors in choosing or refusing
a mate that enhance the chances of success in
marriage and minimize its risks. We shall also
discuss briefly the social processes of dating,
courtship, and engagement through which marriages in the United States occur.

Taboos on Choice of Mate

Prohibitions and taboos on one or another
kind of sexual conduct are as universal as marriage itself. Most elaborate and complicated rules
exist among many primitive tribes to say whom
a man or woman may or may not marry. Most
of these rules prescribe *exogamy*, that is, selection
of a mate outside one's own family, tribe, clan,
"totem," or village. More rarely, but with equal
insistence, they demand *endogamy*, which means
that the marriage partner must be found within
a particular group.

Endogamy is generally practiced, if not enforced, among higher social class and caste
groups and sometimes along religious lines, for
the preservation of that particular social group
within the larger social structure. The peak of
endogamy was reached among the Pharaohs of
ancient Egypt and the Incas of Peru, where
brother-sister marriages were prescribed. But endogamy is still subtly enforced in old, upper-class
society in the United States. Utmost family and
social pressure, sometimes including the threat
of disinheritance, is brought against many a socially elite young man or woman who proposes

to contract a marriage with a mate of dissimilar background. Fiction has made much of this dilemma; *Kitty Foyle* by Christopher Morley and *Back Street* by Fannie Hurst are good examples.

Exogamy is fundamentally a bar to marriage rather than a ban on sexual relationships. As observed in primitive tribes and enforced by its social and religious taboos, the practice of exogamy forbids marriage between members of the same "clan" or "totem." This does not, however, exclude marriages between rather close blood relatives. Indeed, in some tribes cross-cousins are the preferred marriage partners; this means that it is considered an exceptionally good match if a young man marries his mother's brother's or his father's sister's daughter. This comes close to the practice of *homogamy,* or like marrying like. Homogamy is actually the practice in most modern civilized societies. Contrary to the opinion that "opposites attract," they do not often marry; most individuals choose and marry someone with a background very much like their own.

Universal Incest Taboo. The taboo on primary incest is almost absolutely universal. Primary incest may be defined as sexual congress or marriage between mother and son, father and daughter, brother and sister. Among thousands of societies studied by anthropologists, none —even the most primitive and culturally backward—fails to impose the strongest kind of prohibitions and punishments on incest. Primitive people explain their system of exogamy as an extension of incest taboo; their extensive kinship acknowledgements therefore provide for different "degrees" of incest which must be prohibited. In some places the risk of incest is held to be so great, and regarded with such awe, that no contact between brother and sister is permitted from infancy onward. In extreme cases all the children of one or the other sex are removed to different households for rearing.

A completely satisfactory explanation for the incest taboo has not yet been formulated. Malinowski and others hold the opinion that incest taboos are rigidly enforced and universally accepted because of their high social utility in keeping family and clan together. Without them, the family might too easily be torn apart by sexual rivalries and jealousies, and hence fail to fulfill its other functions. The so-called eugenic argument for prohibitions on incest has never been proved; "first-cousin" marriages do not commonly engender defective children.

Whatever their origin, incest taboos have a great social usefulness in safeguarding the family. They are rooted in the deepest folk wisdom of the human race. Even if there is no agreement on a rational basis for them, any scientific study of society would warn against relaxing them.

Taboos on Adultery. Almost as universal as incest taboos are those against adultery. In a world-wide study of 250 societies, Yale anthropologist Murdock found only five, a mere 2% in which adultery was socially condoned. Social utility again is probably the reason for this stricture. Extramarital affairs generally threaten the stability and function of the family. Scientific study does not justify the position that fidelity in marriage is an "outmoded superstition." Indeed, it is just the contrary.

The definition of adultery, however, is more flexible than that of incest. In most primitive tribes adultery means only sexual intercourse with a married woman. This was the Biblical definition of the word on which the Seventh Commandment rests. In some societies adultery is considered a theft. The property rights of the husband have been infringed, and his recourse is against the offender.

Adultery on the part of the husband has almost universally been more lightly regarded than on the part of the wife. In some tribes, for example, it is frequently expected when the wife is under a taboo of sexual continence—as when she is still nursing an infant.

In many societies the taboos against adultery have been circumvented by other legally permissible customs, for example concubinage and polygamy. In our culture "serial polygamy," frequent divorce and remarriage, has been attempted as a solution to the taboos on extramarital affairs.

Few Primitive Taboos on Sexual Experimen-

tation. In contrast to their strong and almost universal taboos against incest and adultery (and also against rape and child seduction) most primitive societies are more permissive than our own about premarital sexual experience. Murdock found that 70% (of 250 societies) permitted varying degrees of sexual experimentation before marriage. In the remaining 30%, the taboos were directed mainly against females. Premarital pregnancy is often severely castigated, though sometimes it is considered desirable. The basic premise seems to be concern for the status of the child without a "legal" father. Who will be responsible for it?

Dating and Courtship

Where do you find the person you marry? Practically all studies made on this subject by sociologists show that most people find their marriage partners within a few blocks of their own homes, and the nearer they live, the more likely they are to marry. Young people tend to choose mates whose backgrounds are substantially like their own. In some communities, however, the number of marriageable men or women may be smaller than the number of persons of the opposite sex seeking marriage. The moral is plain: if you seek marriage, go where the sex ratio is favorable.

A unique factor in the American social scene is the amount of casual contact between young men and women before marriage. "Dates" and "dating" as practiced in the United States are not characteristically found in other cultures. Dating is certainly a preliminary to courtship and always includes the possibility of "falling in love," but it has other values. It is a social experience, of which young people today may acquire more in a few years than their grandparents did in a lifetime.

On every college campus we know that there is a "dating and rating" pattern whose object is not necessarily matrimony. The crucial point here is that a good "date" is not necessarily a good mate. The relationship of dating to marriage is very indirect, even though each individual meets or gets to know the person eventually married on some sort of dating or social occasion.

The social process leading toward marriage, a pattern which American young people have evolved for themselves in the past few decades, usually moves in the following sequence: group dating (parties), double dating, single dating, going steady, courtship, engagement, and marriage.

The values of courtship are not the same as the values of marriage. During courtship individuals tend to be on their best behavior toward their prospective spouses and often wittingly, or unwittingly, conceal their true personalities and mask their flaws from each other.

Courtship is a time of psychological exploration. Couples already in love, or on the verge of it, may properly raise questions about the suitability of a particular marriage and the probable compatibility of a particular partner.

Engagement. Engagement is a trial period in which the engaged couple has the time and freedom to discover each other. It is not and should not be mock marriage. It is a time when many subjects previously avoided, such as sex, children, money, and relatives, can be realistically discussed. It is a time when fundamental character and emotional reactions can be carefully scrutinized and evaluated.

How long should an engagement be? Long enough to begin to learn much about one's intended marriage partner, but not so long as to put both man and woman under needless stress. There are no figures in weeks or months that apply to all cases. Every couple must decide this for themselves.

Love

In the 1950's around 1,700,000 weddings a year took place in the United States. By the mid-sixties this number had decreased somewhat but a higher marriage rate was forecast. The vast majority of these marriages, it may be assumed, were conceived in romantic love.

Marriage for love is the accepted American pattern of mating; romantic, monogamous marriage is both the ideal and the norm. Yet it is necessary to draw a sharp distinction between romantic love and other manifestations of this "profound and complicated sentiment."

The poet Shelley has given as scientific a definition of love as you are likely to find, thus: "That profound and complicated sentiment which we call love is the universal thirst for a communion not merely of the senses, but of our whole nature, intellectual, imaginative and sensitive. . . . The sexual impulse, which is only one, and often a small part of those claims, serves, from its obvious and external nature, as a kind of type of expression of the rest, a common basis, an acknowledged and visible link."

There persists among young people a zealous but naive curiosity for the answer to the question, "How can you tell you're in love?" The only sensible answer that can be given is the standard one: "When you are, you'll know it yourself and you will stop asking how you can tell." You may also encounter some cynical answers, such as Voltaire's. "If one were to judge love solely by its effects, it would seem a great deal more like hate than like friendship."

The phenomenon of love at first sight does occur. More commonly there is a gradual intensification of interest in and feeling for another person which, when it reaches a certain pitch, can be dignified with the name of love. There are three simple tests that can be applied: the test of time, the test of absence, and the test of companionship. If your interest in and feeling for the other person rapidly pass away, are easily diverted, quickly submerged, or casually overridden by other interests, don't dream that you are in love. If reasonable absence or separation makes your heart grow emptier not fonder, if you find yourself more and more forgetting the person you suspected you might be in love with, drop the suspicion. If you are increasingly bored with your companion, you are not likely to be in love with that person.

Psychologically speaking, a human being has no greater single need than that of giving and receiving love. We must "love or perish." But there is no law which says that all valid love must be romantic love.

The great fallacies in the American pursuit of romantic love are the beliefs that it will "last forever," that with it everything can be conquered, and that without it nothing else counts much. This is nonsense; there are many kinds of love beyond the romantic that yield superb life satisfactions. Romantic love may spark a wedding, but unless it ripens into a deeper conjugal love, it may later burn itself out. It is easier to fall in love than to stay there.

The gospel of the supreme value of romantic love has left far too many people so busy being "in love with love" that they cannot establish firm and genuine love relationships with other people; others who spend their whole adult lives trying to recapture the rapture of their first romantic love.

This emphasis and overvaluation of romantic love on the American scene may be viewed as the outcome of a number of factors, some long in the making, for example, urbanization, social mobility, economic emancipation of women, and global war. Against the casual impersonality of the big city, or the threat of atomic annihilation, romantic love shines as a protest and a last opportunity for happiness. Progress in transportation has brought about greater mobility and the automobile has supplanted the family parlor as the scene of courtship. Since women have won a high degree of economic emancipation, they do not have to accept marriage as their only road to economic security. Against the "soulless organization" for which one works and the stark objectivity of modern science, romantic love often stands out as a bright (and therefore presumably valuable) personal possession.

The ancient Greeks thought of romantic love as a kind of madness visited upon men and women by the caprice or malevolence of the gods. Certainly the socially acceptable conduct of many eager young lovers is such as would be considered symptomatic of mental illness in other people. Yet we accept the fact that people in love should "go around in a trance"; lose appetite and weight; suffer from illusions, delusions, compulsions, and the alternating heights of joy and depths of despair that mark a manic-depressive cycle.

Romantic love has had the effect of bulwarking the American ideal of monogamous marriage. The reason is simply that romantic love demands an *exclusive possession* of the beloved, and this is the essense of monogamy. The token of the engagement ring should be understood in this connection. When the young man places it on his sweetheart's finger, he is not only saying to her, "I love you." He is also jealously asserting to all other men, "She's mine. Stay away."

Romantic love probably will govern American marriage practices throughout the foreseeable future. Yet it is wise to understand it for what it really is—the prelude, not the whole feast of marriage.

Marriage

If marriages are "made in heaven," they nevertheless have to be lived out on earth. The simple determination to make a marriage succeed is one of the most important factors in its success. There are no marriages completely without crises, just as there are no lives without problems. The words of the wedding ceremony are full of truth: "for better or worse, in sickness and in health. . . ."

Children who have had the advantage of observing "good marriages" in their own homes often enjoy a greater chance of success in their own marital adventure. They have had the benefit of seeing how "normal" marital quarrels and difficulties can be compromised and happily resolved.

Nature of Marriage. Marriage provides an opportunity for two people in love to live, work, play, and worship together. Living together obviously requires readjustments in personal habits on the part both of man and wife, and demands emotional realignments. Because of serious flaws in their own personality structures some individuals cannot properly adjust to the needs and demands of their mates. This is the real source of marital unhappiness.

Marriage may in many ways be regarded as a *sublimation,* in which primitive emotional energies, including sexual drives, are directed to higher social ends. A certain amount of immediate renunciation of self is required to discover a greater self. In a happy marriage one no longer thinks in terms of "What am I doing for *you*" but rather "What can I do for *us.*" The marriage becomes a third entity, above and beyond the partners to it—a deep well from which the whole family, mother, father, and children, draw strength, sustenance, and love.

Divorce. One in every three or four marriages in the United States ends in divorce. In addition, probably another one in six ends in annulment, informal separation, or desertion ("the poor man's divorce"). This situation, though distressing, is probably not so socially alarming as it is sometimes depicted. The general pattern is early marriage and early divorce, with a high rate of remarriage. Because so many people whose marriages are broken by divorce or annulment tend to remarry, the number of "broken homes" actually existing in the United States is nowhere near so great as the number of divorces on the statistical records.

Despite so-called "legal grounds" for divorce, the real source of wrecked marriages lies in incompatibility of temperament (immaturity usually) of the partners. Sexual maladjustment, though often mentioned, is not really a very common cause of divorce.

In possibly 50 to 75% of current American divorces, no children are involved. A sensitive discussion of "children of divorce," of whom there are about 1.5 million under eighteen, has been provided by Dr. J. Louise Despert. It is her opinion that children are more likely to suffer when "emotional divorce" between parents is *not* followed by legal divorce.

Marriage on the Campus. Marriage has been woven pretty firmly into the fabric of campus life since World War II. Undergraduate marriage is taboo today only in very few collegiate institutions—primarily the armed service academies. In the graduating classes of June 1964, almost one-fourth of all graduates were already married and a high percentage already had children. Approximately 38% of this "class of '64" were women; they received 40% of the 490,000 bachelor's and first-professional degrees and one-third of the 90,000 master's degrees.

Within 20 years, since 1949, the number of women graduating from college nearly doubled, increasing from 117,000 to 224,000. Within this same time, as for 35 years earlier, there has also been a decline in the average age at marriage in the United States. In the present decade the modal age at marriage—the most frequent age at which women get married—is 18. The modal age for men is 21. However, it is 2 to 3 years lower for women who did not attend high school, and it averages 4 years higher—age 22—for women college graduates.

Why girls who attend college tend to marry considerably later than those who do not, is a subject for speculation. It may seem paradoxical that college education delays marriage for a girl since she is constantly in contact with boys her own age. It may be imagined that familiarity with many young men may evoke a more critical and choosey attitude. Furthermore, while a good many young men marry while they are still in college, the majority do not.

Many married coeds manage to continue their studies on a part-time basis: 44% of all part-time coeds are married. In 3% of all American families, both husbands and wives have college degrees. However, four out of every ten men graduates choose wives who have had no college training.

There have been variations in the overall marriage rates in the United States in the past few decades. For instance, in 1950, when the population was 151 million, the marriage rate was 11.0 per thousand; and there were 1.7 million marriages that year. In 1963 the marriage rate was only 8.8 per thousand and only 1.65 million marriages took place. In 1964 the rate was between 9 and 9.5 per thousand, producing slightly more marriages than in immediately previous years.

It may come as a surprise that brides and grooms in the United States are younger and closer in age at first marriage than are those in any other major urban-industrial country in the world. Indeed the American age-at-marriage pattern is now closer to the Asian than the European.

Choosing or Refusing a Mate

We all speak glibly about selecting a mate. The real question is *on what grounds to reject as a mate*—before marriage—an individual of the opposite sex toward whom you have feelings that already are or may unmistakably become classified as love. This is a difficult decision for the simple reason that few, if any, unmarried young people really know what to expect of marriage or of each other in marriage.

Young men and women in the United States enjoy exceptionally free choice of marriage partners. In far too many cases, however, they do not really exercise this choice. They plunge, jump, fall, leap, drift, stumble, rebound, march, or amble into a particular marriage partly because of outside pressures from family or friends or sometimes because of inner fears or drives.

Some young women, approach the grave responsibility of marriage as if it were a game of musical chairs in which the sole object is not to be left out. Some bachelors stalk wives as if they considered a wife a trophy of the chase, like a stuffed moosehead. Many accept husband or wife because they are weary, afraid, or ashamed to look further. Some couples marry hastily because, as they put it, "We're in love and that's all that matters." Some are eventually nagged into apparently unattractive marriages by family pressure or conversation, including one or another variation of that most infuriating remark: "Such a nice girl! Why isn't she married?"

A very high percentage of marriages contracted on trivial grounds nevertheless turn out remarkably well. On the other hand, even the most plausible matches fail. The attempt to select a mate on completely reasonable grounds is ludicrous. Marriages made by computers which attempt to match mutual compatibilities and traits are among the most foolish of all. A wedding is a commencement, not a termination. It is also a gamble, never a sure bet.

Let us review briefly the areas in which questions about the suitability of a particular marriage partner commonly fall.

What probable effect on the outcome of a

marriage shall we assess for each of the following factors?

Physical Attractiveness? This factor is often overrated. It may be enough to get a marriage started, but not enough to hold it together.

Physical Size? Matching for size is a trivial consideration. Incompatibility on account of disproportions in physical size can be considered negligible.

Age? There are two questions here. Are the parties individually too young to be married (no one is ever really too old) and is the discrepancy in their ages so great as to suggest difficulties?

Mature, well-adjusted adults are more likely to make a success of marriage than adolescents. Society acknowledges this by laws establishing minimum ages for marriage. In about three-fifths of the states in the United States the age is 21 years for men, 18 for women, without parental consent; 18 years and 16 years, respectively, with consent. Biological readiness for reproduction, of course, occurs much earlier.

Marriages with great discrepancies in age between husband and wife are comparatively rare, about one marriage in twenty. The much older husband usually assumes a predominantly father role toward his wife, the older wife a strong mother role toward her spouse. If the psychological demands of *both* parties to the marriage are thus fulfilled, who can object?

Health? A medical certificate of physical fitness for marriage is required in three-fourths of the states of the United States before a marriage license is issued. In too many cases this requirement is purely perfunctory and means only that the applicants have passed a laboratory test which certifies them to be free of syphilis. A complete premarital physical examination by a physician is an excellent idea for both men and women. Such examinations should not be approached with the fear of finding something wrong, or as a bar to marriage, but rather as an opportunity for discussing and preventing specific health problems that might later complicate the marriage.

Heredity? When a person contemplating marriage knows for certain that one of the rare diseases (e.g. hemophilia or "bleeder's disease," or Huntington's chorea) transmitted by defective genes runs in his family, he should surely reveal this fact to his intended partner. Other worries about heredity should be discussed frankly with a physician.

Religious Faith? All organized religions frown on intermarriage, but all permit it under specific conditions and provisions. The circumstances surrounding a given or proposed intermarriage are always unique and highly individualized. Some succeed, some fail completely; many are maintained at uncertain medium levels of happiness. Young men and women contemplating intermarriage may well inquire into *all* their psychological motives at such a time and ask themselves such questions as: How strong are my deepest religious convictions? Do I secretly resent and *want* to hurt my parents and family by marrying out of their faith? Am I doing this because I want to be different and thus attract attention, concern, and even sympathy to myself? Have I the maturity and strength of character to make this marriage work? Will I feel truly at home in the new household I am helping to create?

Intelligence? The ability to think clearly is an asset in any human undertaking. What passes for intelligence (or the lack of it) is often only a reflection of different interests and motivations. A wife does not have to understand the intricacies of her husband's business or profession. She only has to be intelligent enough to appreciate him.

Education? The mere possession of an academic degree per se has no bearing on suitability for marriage or on the outcome of marriage. Insofar as degrees reflect intelligence, the promise of professional competence, a record of personal development, and opportunity for employment and advancement they do have value on the marriage market.

The present generation of college students in the United States is not quite so troubled by the dilemmas that acutely plagued their parents and grandparents. They often had to choose sharply between college or marriage, between marriage or a career. Since World War II, and the GI Bill, which provided educational benefits for veterans, the choice between going to college or getting married is no longer an either/or proposition. Young people today can have both, provided they have the strength and courage to accept both challenges. Married students do as well academically as unmarried students, often better.

Personal Abilities? This is a factor that can be grossly overrated. You don't marry a man because he is a good dancer or a woman because she is a good bridge player. You don't dismiss potential marriage partners on such trivial grounds as not liking the way they dress or comb their hair. Extreme fanaticism in any direction, however, may be a warning signal.

Money? The relationship of money to marriage has more ramifications than we can deal with here. Historically the relationship of wealth to marriage was more important than the relationship of love to marriage. For centuries marriages were arranged by families, and the marriage contract was a legal document that dealt largely with exchanges of property. Wives were chattels.

The question, "Can we afford to get married?" does not bother the present generation of young people so much or as often as it bothered earlier generations. One reason for this is the simple calculation that if both husband and wife work full or part time, they can make enough money together to support a small apartment or household. Prejudice against the working wife, once strong, has largely disappeared. The modern young woman does not expect her husband to support her immediately in the style to which she was or would like to have been accustomed. She frequently wants to share the financial responsibility of establishing and maintaining a household.

Any young couple insistent on marriage can scrape up enough money to get married and "get by" on what they make for some length of time. They are buoyed up, and properly, by hope for the future. But when financial hopes are disappointed, when family expenses rise, when the wife has to stop working to stay home with the children, crisis and test of the marriage occur. This is when strength of character and compatibility of temperament become important, when wise choice of a mate becomes more clearly apparent, when the power of personal love and true understanding of the meaning of marriage is revealed.

Millions of married couples weather their money troubles and build firmer, happier marriages out of their times of financial and other crises.

Money has many meanings to different people. It is not just a simple commodity or means of exchange. Attitudes toward money and the handling of money reflect some of our deepest psychological needs and basic philosophical outlooks on life. Money values reflect life values, and these change with age. When married, engaged, or even "dating" couples disagree about money, it is usually symptomatic of significant cultural and psychological differences in their total views of life.

Compatibility? The ability of two people to get along with each other is not a predictable factor and can be tested only by the experience of marriage itself. Strong youthful differences of opinion on political issues of the day are not an indication of incompatibility for marriage. A practical test is the ability to disagree on questions or problems, then compromise and agree on solutions.

Personality Structure in Marriage. Each man and woman brings to marriage the personality structures that they have developed through all their previous life experiences from infancy onward. Though marriage itself exerts a strong stabilizing influence on later personality development, it cannot undo traits and characteristics already ingrained. These normal emotional reactions are firmly established long before the individual is thinking of marriage.

The greater insight you have into the personality structure of another person, the better you can get along with him or her. Nowhere does this obvious rule of trying to understand one another apply with greater force than between mates, actual or intended. During a period of courtship, engagement, or "going steady," you should, if possible, observe the *emotional reaction* of your intended husband or wife to a variety of life problems.

The things to watch out for are overreaction, excessive reaction, rigid reactions, and "clang reactions" (like a firehorse at the clang of a firebell). Such reactions will give you quite valuable clues to the underlying personality of your intended.

Sex and Religion

The ancient religious codes are still the prime sources of the attitudes, the ideas, the ideals, and the rationalizations by which most individuals pattern their sexual lives. The apparent conflicts between the religious codes and the patterns of sexual behavior may lead one to overlook the religious origins of the social patterns.

The author of this forthright statement is the late Dr. Alfred C. Kinsey, professor of zoology at Indiana University, presenting a scientific study of sexual behavior in the United States. He says further: "For the individual who is particularly concerned with the moral values of sexual behavior, none of these scientific issues are, of course, of any moment. For such individuals, moral issues are a very real part of life. . . . They should not be overlooked by the scientist who attempts to make an objective measure of the outcome of [sexual practices, such as] premarital intercourse."

In discussing the social and psychological aspects of sexual adjustment, especially as it affects the lives of young men and women in American colleges, we have chosen to examine the moral and religious issues in depth and detail.

"Why have religions generally failed to help the individual with his life problems by not admitting the force of the sex drive?" is a question commonly asked by college students during discussions of the religious and moral point of view toward sexual adjustment. Other common questions are: "Why have organized religions placed so much emphasis on wedding ceremonies and so little on personal adjustment in marriage?" "Dare I have premarital intercourse with a clear conscience?" and "Are there religions which today condone premarital intercourse?" These questions demand information, discussion, and decision on the part of every student who poses them out loud or to himself. They are central to American college life today, and they cannot be ignored.

The questions themselves betray an ignorance, not by any means limited to college students, about the present and true interest of the great modern religions in sex behavior and their authoritative statements on the subject. There is a widely held, flippant, and cynical attitude that this interest is limited to enforcing the Seventh Commandment: "Thou shalt not commit adultery." There is an appalling lack of knowledge concerning the stress placed today by all the major religions of Western culture on the positive and happy aspects of sex and marriage relationships. It seems to be generally overlooked that organized religions stemming from the Judaeo-Christian tradition take their primary warrant for concern with the sexual life of mankind from the first words of God to man. As anyone who opens the Bible to the first chapter of Genesis can rediscover, these words (in English) are, "Be fruitful and multiply."

Organized religion in all societies has taken this Biblical commandment most seriously and attempted only to stipulate conditions, coordinate with the rest of the culture, under which it can be most effectively carried out. In American society, the right to accept or deny these codes remains an individual right and responsibility. Obedience cannot be commanded, but the consequences of disobedience, however light or grave, cannot be avoided. Choice is free, but ignorance is no excuse for a poor choice.

Fundamental to any personal decision or to any real understanding of the social and psychological aspects of sexual adjustment in modern American society is an awareness of what religions actually have to say on the subject. We are fortunate in being able to present verbatim quotations from official documents and authorized statements emanating from the three major religious denominations in the United States.

In presenting this material we have sought for the common ground in these three points of view; but we have not neglected to point out significant differences where they occur. We have not and we do not imply any criticism, nor do we concern ourselves with any of the properly theological questions on which these statements ultimately rely. Space limitations prevent giving the statements in full, and some students may wish recourse to the complete texts.

The Protestant Point of View

The following statements are direct quotations from the document *Christian Marriage*, issued in 1952 by the National Council of Churches of Christ in the United States of America:

This is an attempt to state unofficially the Christian view of marriage as generally held by the great body of Christians constituting the National Council of the Churches of Christ in the United States of America. These include a majority of non-Roman [Catholic] Christians in North America. While these bodies represent a wide range of opinion on many debated points, they hold strongly to the ideal of chastity, of reverence for personality, and the sacredness of family ties. . . .

While there have been times when the efforts of the church seemed more defensive than constructive, in the long run great progress has been made. Gradually the inherent democracy of the Gospel has helped to emancipate women from the disabilities and handicaps of patriarchal culture, and young people have been defended in their rights to select marriage partners according to their own ideals and preferences.

On the Christian Conception of Marriage. Stated by Christ Himself in beautiful and sensitive words, He speaks of how "He who made them from the beginning made them male and female," and quotes the words, "for this reason shall a man leave his father and mother, and be joined to his wife." The man and woman in marriage become one flesh, that is to say, the union is organic, and it is God who unites them, which means that it is a profound biological-spiritual experience which comes out of the depths of life. The union is permanent: "What therefore God hath joined together, let no man put asunder." The Mosaic law which permitted a man to divorce his wife with no recourse for her is abrogated. . . .

In this sort of marriage the two become not merely "one flesh" but one in spirit, for the highest values of marriage are in the realms of personality. In Christian marriage the meeting of all the needs of personality and the enhancement of delicate mutual regard must be sought. At the same time the welfare of society must be loyally promoted through the home. . . .

On Freedom of Personality. The home calls for a fine combination of responsibility and freedom. The fullest freedom is not gained in isolation but in a set of well-chosen loyalties. . . . Yet a certain amount of restlessness in the home and of irritation between husbands and wives is due to unnecessary limitations of freedom. . . . Differences may be handled successfully . . . if each through kindly interest in activities and tastes which are different from his own gives encouragement to the full self-expression of the other.

But beyond this there is also great reward in transforming as many one-sided interests as possible into common interests mutually shared. In fact this process of the sharing of life is the very essence of marriage on its inner side.

On Tensions in Marriage. A measure of tension in making adjustments in marriage is almost inevitable. . . . The romantic emotions of the early period must grow into something hardier and more discerning. . . . Success results from meeting these difficulties with patience, with resourcefulness, and especially with great mutual consideration. People must win their happiness and sometimes wrest it from hard conditions.

On Love. Love, however, has an incalculable power to transmute life. Married people by continuing as lovers can create a home atmosphere in which the little difficulties can be absorbed and all obstacles to full success can be put in a setting of endeavor to reach the higher levels of personal fellowship. . . .

On Children. Although a man comes of age at twenty-one, he becomes more fully a citizen when he is married. When his first child is born he enters more consciously into relationships which are universal and eternal. . . . The high calling of parenthood is one of the supreme fulfillments of personality at the same time that it enables the parents to make their contributions to the future as well as to the present life of the church and the community. . . .

On Rearing Children. Parents should be encouraged to give full personal attention to children and to share sympathetically in their daily lives. Other persons, capable as their service may be, can never take the place of mother and father. . . . The home needs much of the presence of the father as well as of the mother. . . . Children need the contribution which their father is in a position to make to their training. . . .

On Economic Resources Adjusted to Family Needs. [A nation] must be concerned to give every family its fair access to economic opportunity and to its share of national production. . . .

Abnormal deferring of marriage on economic grounds is a serious problem for some young people and their families. This fact challenges society to create an order more favorable to family life. For the young people concerned it requires emphasis on the fact that a home may be begun on a modest basis. . . .

On Attitudes toward Sex. Mistaken attitudes make sex a serious problem. . . . Christianity regards sex as God-given in its origin and purpose, not to be disdained but rather to be fitted into a Christian way of life. Sex union, however, when it occurs outside of marriage is a menace to the welfare of the individual, the family, and society.

Sex desire, if no more than desire, passes with satisfaction. Therefore this desire must always be in subjection to a plan of living which safeguards all the values of the personality. It can never be put first and expressed irresponsibly. To do so

is to degrade not only the mind but sex itself.

Sex experience is elevating and wholesome to body and mind only when it is under moral control and when it is transmuted into a spiritual experience by love and devotion. Love includes but transforms desire and lifts it to a spiritual plane.

The Christian ideal of marriage can therefore make no compromise with laxity in sex relations. No matter how great the compassion of the church, or how swift its sympathy and its redemptive action, it must always speak to sex delinquents as did Christ to the woman whom He refused to condemn to a shocking death, but to whom He said, "Go, and sin no more."

What people need is purposeful restraint, not greater freedom in the form of sex indulgence. . . . Young people are in the difficult situation. . . . The problem of sexual self-control often becomes aggravated under such circumstances. Moreover, the situation is affected by the widespread and increasing knowledge of the use of contraceptives. However, the solution is in the correction of the social and economic maladjustments and not in the violation of our sex ethics. The convictions of religion based on long experience and the findings of modern research studies agree in indicating that the forward path is not in the direction of laxity.

On Divorce. Differences of conviction as to divorce, and freedom of divorced persons to marry again, must be recognized. Civil divorce and remarriage are now provided in all nations, even in those predominantly Catholic. The state exercises wider latitude as to permissible grounds of divorce than the church, as a teacher of ideals, can allow itself to recognize. All churches, however, either recognize divorce and remarriage on one or more grounds, or, as in the Roman Catholic Church, grant annulment of marriage. . . .

The most beautiful and satisfying experiences are for those who, having chosen wisely their life partners, achieve a life-long marriage with ever deepening love and loyalty. . . . [However] divorce or separation may seem preferable to the enforced continuance of a relation which has no true basis in mutual respect and affection as far as the two individuals concerned are involved; but the effect on the children, the family, and society must never be ignored or minimized. Moreover, it is evidence of failure, always to be deplored, and to be avoided if by any means success can be achieved even over what may appear insurmountable obstacles.[1]

On Family Planning. Marriage should provide for the fullest development of personality, and at the same time homes should carry on and continually reinvigorate all traditions which aid fine family living. . . . [Under such circumstance] family planning takes greater prominence, both in respect to size of the family and to the genuine quality of family life.

*   *   *

The likenesses between the Protestant, Roman Catholic, and Jewish points of view on marriage and family life deserve to be emphasized. Despite some traditional and historic differences, they all point to the same goal. These statements which present the Roman Catholic and Jewish attitudes toward sex, marriage, home, and children, may be profitably compared with the Protestant attitudes already delineated.

The Roman Catholic View

The following statements are direct quotations from the Encyclical Letter on Chaste Wedlock (*Casti Connubii*) given at Rome, in St. Peter's, on December 31, 1930, by Pope Pius XI:

How great is the dignity of chaste wedlock, Venerable Brethren, may be judged best from this—that Christ . . . not only ordained it in an especial manner as the principle and foundation of domestic society and therefore of all human intercourse, but also raised it to the rank of a truly and great sacrament of the New Law, restored it to the original purity of its divine insti-

[1] This paragraph is from *Social Ideals of the Churches,* published by the Federal Council of the Churches of Christ in America.

tution, and accordingly entrusted all its discipline and care to His spouse the Church. . . .

On the Divine Institution of Matrimony. Let it be repeated as an immutable and inviolable fundamental doctrine that matrimony was not instituted or restored by man but by God; not by man were the laws made to strengthen and confirm and elevate it, but by God. . . . Hence these laws cannot be subject to any human decrees or to any contrary pact even of the spouses themselves. . . .

On the Nature of the Marriage Contract. Yet, although matrimony is of its very nature of divine institution, the human will, too, enters into it and performs a most noble part. For each individual marriage, inasmuch as it is a conjugal union of a particular man and woman, arises only from the free consent of each of the spouses; and this free act of the will, by which each party hands over and accepts those rights proper to the state of marriage, is so necessary to constitute true marriage that it cannot be supplied by any human power. This freedom, however, regards only the question whether the contracting parties really wish to enter upon matrimony or to marry this particular person; but the nature of matrimony is entirely independent of the free will of man, so that if one has once contracted matrimony, he is thereby subject to its divinely made laws and its essential properties. . . .

By matrimony, therefore, the souls of the contracting parties are joined and knit together more directly and more intimately than are their bodies, and that not by any passing affection of sense or spirit, but by a deliberate and firm act of the will; and from this union of souls by God's decree, a sacred and inviolable bond arises. Hence the nature of this contract . . . makes it entirely different both from the union of animals . . . and also from the haphazard unions of men, which are far removed from all true and honorable unions of will and enjoy none of the rights of family life. . . . The sacred partnership of true marriage is constituted both by the will of God and the will of man. . . .

On the Blessings of Matrimony. "These," says St. Augustine, "are all the blessings of matrimony on account of which matrimony is itself a blessing; offspring, conjugal faith, and the sacrament." And how under these three heads is contained a splendid summary of the whole doctrine of Christian marriage. . . .

On Children. Amongst the blessings of marriage, the child holds first place. . . . The blessing of offspring, however, is not completed by the mere begetting of them, but something else must be added, namely the proper education of the offspring. . . . This is also expressed succinctly in the Code of Canon Law: "The primary end of marriage is the procreation and the education of children." . . .

On Conjugal Fidelity. Nor did Christ our Lord wish only to condemn any form of polygamy or polyandry, as they are called, whether successive or simultaneous, and every other external dishonorable act, but, in order that the sacred bonds of marriage may be guarded absolutely inviolate, He forbade also even willful thoughts and desires of such like things: "But I say to you, that whosoever shall look on a women to lust after her hath already committed adultery with her in his heart." . . .

On Mutual Love. This conjugal faith, which is most aptly called by St. Augustine the "faith of chastity," blooms more freely, more beautifully, and more nobly when it is rooted in that more excellent soil, the love of husband and wife. . . . For if man is the head, woman is the heart, and as he occupies the chief place in ruling, so she may and ought to claim for herself the chief place in love. . . . If the husband neglect his duty, it falls to the wife to take his place in directing the family. . . .

On Marriage as a Sacrament. Since the valid matrimonial consent among the faithful was constituted by Christ as a sign of grace, the sacramental nature is so intimately bound up with Christian wedlock that there can be no true marriage between baptized persons "without it being by that very fact a sacrament" . . . from which they draw supernatural power. . . .

On Modern Fallacies. When we consider the great excellence of chaste wedlock, Venerable Brethren, it appears all the more regrettable that particu-

larly in our day we should witness this divine institution often scorned and on every side degraded.

For now, alas, not secretly nor under cover, but openly, with all sense of shame put aside, now by word, again by writings, by theatrical productions of every kind, by romantic fiction, by amorous and frivolous novels, by cinematographs portraying in vivid scene, in addresses broadcast by radio telephony, in short by all the inventions of modern science, the sanctity of marriage is trampled upon and derided; divorce, adultery, all the basest vices either are extolled or at least are depicted in such colors as to appear to be free of all reproach and infamy. . . .

Not all the sponsors of these new doctrines are carried to the extremes of unbridled lust; there are those who, striving as it were to ride a middle course, believe nevertheless that something should be conceded to our times as regards certain precepts of the divine and natural law. But these likewise, more or less wittingly, are emissaries of the great enemy who is ever seeking to sow cockle among the wheat. . . .

To begin at the very source of these evils, their basic principle lies in this: that matrimony is repeatedly declared to be . . . invented by man. Some confidently assert that they have found no evidence for the existence of matrimony in nature or in her laws, but regard it merely as the means of producing life and of gratifying in one way or another a vehement impulse. . . . How grievously all these err! . . .

On Family Planning. First consideration is due to the offspring, which many have the boldness to call the disagreeable burden of matrimony. . . . But no reason, however grave, may be put forward by which anything intrinsically against nature may become conformable to nature and morally good. Since, therefore, the conjugal act is destined primarily by nature for the begetting of children, those who in exercising it deliberately frustrate its natural power and purpose sin against nature. . . . Holy Mother Church very well understands and clearly appreciates all that is said regarding the health of the mother and the danger to her life. And who would not grieve to think of these things? . . . Holy Church knows well that not infrequently one of the parties is sinned against rather than sinning. . . .

Secondary Ends of Matrimony. In matrimony . . . there are also secondary ends, such as mutual aid, the cultivating of mutual love, and the quieting of concupiscence, which husband and wife are not forbidden to consider so long as they are subordinated to the primary end. . . .

On Mixed Marriages. The maternal love and providence of the Church dissuades her children. . . . [from] mixed marriages. This attitude is . . . summed up in the Code of Canon Law. . . .

On Divorce. The advocates of neopaganism . . . continue by legislation to attack the indissolubility of the marriage bond. . . . Opposed to all these reckless opinions, Venerable Brethren, stands the unalterable law of God, fully confirmed by Christ, a law that can never be deprived of its force by decrees of men, the ideas of a people or the will of any legislator: "What God hath joined, let no man put asunder." . . .

If, therefore, the Church has not erred and does not err in teaching this, and consequently it is certain that the bond of marriage cannot be loosed even on account of the sin of adultery, it is evident that all the other weaker excuses that can be, and usually are, brought forward are of no value whatsoever. . . .

In certain circumstances the imperfect separation of the parties is allowed, the bond not being severed. This separation, which the Church herself permits . . . removes all the alleged inconveniences and dangers. . . .

On Due Preparation for Marriage. The basis of a happy wedlock, and the ruin of an unhappy one, is prepared and set . . . during childhood and adolescence. There is the danger that those who before marriage sought in all things what is theirs, who indulged even their impure desires, will be in the married state what they were before, that they will reap that which they have sown. . . . Worst of all, such parties will find themselves left alone with their own unconquered passions. . . . For the preservation of the moral order . . . religious authority must enter in to enlighten the mind, to direct the will, and to strengthen human frailty by the assistance of divine grace.

The Roman Catholic View on Moral Questions Affecting Married Life. The following statements are direct quotations from a discourse by Pope Pius XII delivered on October 29, 1951, under the title of "The Apostolate of the Midwife—Moral Questions Affecting Married Life," and these statements may be regarded as further explanation of the text set forth by Pope Pius XI, his predecessor, already quoted:

Nature puts at man's disposal the whole chain of causes giving rise to new human life. . . . Once man has performed his part and put into motion this wondrous evolution of life, his duty is to respect its progress religiously, and this is a duty that forbids his halting the work of nature or hindering its natural development.

The child formed in the womb of its mother is a gift of God, Who entrusts it to the parents. . . . Unfortunately there are many cases where speaking, even cautiously, of children as a "blessing" is sufficient to provoke contradiction or even derision. Very often the idea and remarks about the great "burden" of children dominate. . . .

On Acceptance of Motherhood. It is one of the fundamental demands of the right moral order that sincere inner acceptance of the office and duties of motherhood corresponds to the use of conjugal rights. . . .

Unfortunately, it is not always thus. Often the child is not wanted. Worse, it is feared. Under such conditions, how can people be ready to carry out their duty? . . .

On Periods of Natural Sterility. There is the serious question today as to whether and how far the obligation of ready disposition to serve motherhood can be reconciled with the ever more widely diffused recourse to periods of natural sterility (the so-called agenetic periods of the woman) which seems to be a clear expression of the will contrary to that disposition. . . . The medical point of view about this theory and of the progress that is likely to be made in it . . . [should be] founded on scientific objectivity and the authoritative judgment of specialists in medicine and biology. It is the office [of the obstetric professions, e.g., physicians, midwives], not that of the priest, to instruct married people, either when they come for private consultations or through serious publication, on the biological and technical aspects of the theory. . . .

[But on] the norms of morality to which the application of this theory is subordinated, here it is the Church that is the competent judge. . . .

There are serious motives, such as those often mentioned in the so-called medical, eugenic, economic, and social "indications," that can exempt for a long time, perhaps even the whole duration of the marriage, from the positive and obligatory carrying out of the [conjugal] act. From this it follows that observing the non-fertile periods alone can be lawful only under a moral aspect. . . .

If, according to a rational and just judgment, there are no similar grave reasons of a personal nature or deriving from external circumstances, then the determination habitually to avoid the fecundity of the union, while at the same time to continue fully satisfying their sensuality, can be derived only from a false appreciation of life and from reasons having nothing to do with proper ethical laws. . . .

On Attitudes toward Sexual Pleasure. The Creator, Who, in His goodness and wisdom, has willed to conserve and propagate the human race through the instrumentality of man and woman by uniting them in marriage, has ordained also that, in performing this function, husband and wife should experience pleasure and happiness both in body and soul.

In seeking and enjoying this pleasure, therefore, couples do nothing wrong. They accept what the Creator has given them. Nevertheless, even here, couples must know how to contain themselves within the limits of moderation. As in eating and drinking, so in the sexual act, they must not abandon themselves without restraint to the impulse of the senses. The right norm, therefore, is this:

The use of the natural inclination to generate is lawful only in matrimony, in the service of and according to the ends of matrimony.

Transgression of this rule is as old as original sin. But in our times there is risk of losing sight of the basic principle. . . . At present it is the custom to maintain in word and writing (and some Catholics do it too) the necessary autonomy, the proper end and the proper value of sexuality and its performance independently of the object of procreation. . . .

If nature had aimed exclusively or even primarily at a mutual gift and mutual possession of couples for pleasure, if it had ordained that act solely to make their personal experience happy in the highest degree and not to stimulate them in the service of life, then the Creator would have adopted another plan in the formation and constitution of the natural act. . . .

A Further Statement on Family Planning. The following passages are excerpts directly quoted from an address to the Cardinals of the Roman Catholic Church given in Rome on July 23, 1964, by Pope Paul VI. These remarks may be considered as an extension of the affirmations on this subject made by his predecessors in the papal office:

Thus our speech takes us from looking at the present and the past to the future. And here also we face a wide panorama, full of formidable problems and great events for us.

We will talk, in conclusion, about only one of these problems, and about only one of the events which the future prepares for us. The problem [which], everyone talks about, is that of birth control, as it is called; namely, of population increases on one hand and family morality on the other.

It is an extremely grave problem. It touches on the mainsprings of human life. It touches on the feelings and interests most close to the experience of man and woman. It is an extremely complex and delicate problem.

The Church recognizes the multiple aspects of

it; that is to say, the multiple competences, among which certainly are in the forefront those of married people, [including considerations] of their freedom, of their conscience, of their love, of their duty.

But the Church must also affirm her own [competence]; namely, that of God's law, by her interpreted, taught, favored, and defended. And the Church will have to proclaim this law of God in the light of the scientific, social, and psychological truths which in these times have undergone new and very ample study and documentation. . . .

The question [of birth control] is being subjected to study, as wide and profound as possible, as grave and honest as it must be on a subject of such importance. It is under study which, we may say, we hope will soon be concluded with the cooperation of many and outstanding experts. We will, therefore, soon give the conclusions of [this study] in the form which will be considered most adapted to the subject and to the aim to be achieved.

But, in the meantime, we say frankly that up to now we do not have sufficient motive to consider out of date, and therefore not binding, the norms given by Pope Pius XII in this regard. These must, therefore, be considered valid, at least until we feel obliged in conscience to change them.

In a matter of such gravity it seems well that Catholics should wish to follow one law—that which the Church authoritatively puts forward— and . . . that no one, for the present, takes it on himself to make pronouncements in terms different from the prevailing norms.

Jewish Attitudes

The Jewish ideal of marriage and family life is reflected in many of the already stated Christian ideals of marriage stemming from the same Old Testament tradition. The following statements are direct quotations from materials issued over the signature of the Synagogue Council of America, an organization representative of the three major divisions of American Judaism:

Reform [Liberal], Conservative, and Orthodox:

Judaism has always looked upon the home as the posit of religious life and sought to manifest religious teachings in family relationships. . . . Jews have always been aware of the unique value of the family, not only for the development of human personality but also for the survival of the individual within the framework of the group. Judaism has nourished the family by traditions and customs . . . rites and institutions. . . .

The Jewish family has a special function. The Jewish people owe their survival in large part to three institutions: the school, the synagogue, and the family. Of the three the family is the most important. ("One may even sell a scroll of the Torah [the Law] if he needs money for the purpose of getting married.")

The Jewish family becomes through the cultivation of its own genius a sacred circle in which members are bound together in a spirit of common understanding, mutual sympathy, and unremitting sacrifice. . . . Judaism has always stressed the integrity of the family . . . [and with it] such values as love, sanctity, purity, stability, responsibility of parents and children, companionship, familial happiness. . . .

At the present time the family is passing into a new stage of development . . . reorganizing itself under the spell of the spirit of our age, the spirit of democracy. . . . The failure to recognize this change that is taking place results in many conflicts. An autocratic form of family organization can never train men and women for a democratic social order. . . . It is necessary, therefore, to combine every possible skill to deal with the complexities that go into the process of marriage, the rearing of children, the creating of a home, the conserving of a family.

The following statements are direct quotations from the pamphlet, *Judaism and Marriage,* by Felix Levy, Ph.D., issued by the Commission on Information about Judaism, representing the Reform [Liberal] position:

On Monogamy. Monogamy was probably the prevailing mode even in earliest Biblical times.

That this was the Jewish ideal can be inferred from the creation legend, where one human couple are parents to the race. Though polygamy occurred among the ancient Hebrews from Adam onward, and was sanctioned, this can hardly be said to have been the norm. Moses and Job have each one wife; the prophets take for granted single partnership as the proper state; the spiritual relationship between God and Israel is conceived as an ideal marriage between the one divine husband and the single people Israel.

On the Position of Women. Proverbs and Ecclesiastes exalt the character and the position of the wife in the home and in society. ("Her children rise up and call her blessed,/Her husband also, and he praiseth her"—Proverbs 31. . . . "The joy of the heart is a wife"—Ecclesiastes 10:7). . . . The very part that women played throughout Jewish history takes the edge off the assertion that woman was man's property to dispose of at his will. . . . Even though admittedly woman was not man's equal before the law, the teachers assert that the unmarried man's existence is incomplete. . . .

On the Marriage State. Marriage is the most exalted state in the eyes of the Jew, and if the wife is good and virtuous, the greatest blessing has come to the home. The idea that marriage is more than a union of the flesh or nature's arrangement for insuring the continuity of the race lies behind the Hebrew term for marriage, "Kiddushin" ("Consecration"). . . . For the Jew it meant holiness and was symbolic of the sacred relationship between husband and wife, of a hallowed state in which they were to live. They were to be one flesh, but more, one spirit.

Marriage for the Jew never became a sacrament, with its mystery, or a concession merely to the weakness of the flesh; for the Jew believed in the satisfaction of all legitimate appetites as a duty, the condition imposed being that desire, including that of sex, should be directed into proper channels for the good of the person and the group. Hence marriage became obligatory, so that a man might build a home, rear a family, and grow in personality thereby.

On Children. Man became creator when he begat children, and the intimate physical relation between man and woman was only for the sake of founding a family. Celibacy was unnatural, and hence abhorrent, particularly in those of marriageable age. . . .

On Family Life. The family life of the Jew with its wifely purity and its husbandly fidelity, the counsel of prenuptial chastity for both sexes, are more eloquent testimony to the Jewish idea and ideal of marriage than all the codes and decisions of [its] courts. The beautiful service in the home that welcomes the Sabbath, itself poetically conceived as a bride, . . . reflects actualities.

On Attitudes toward Sex. A considerable body of statute and lore is discoverable in Jewish literature which attempts to protect the group against physical or moral taint—by insisting on sexual purity for man and woman before and after marriage, by discountenancing any union except in marriage, by advising early matings . . . by regulation of intercourse to safeguard the woman and the possible child, by the high esteem in which parenthood, especially motherhood, is held . . . by insistence on caring for bodily health, even to the extent of regulation of diet. . . .

[Judaism teaches that the expression of sexual love is the exclusive right of husband and wife— for whom it is altogether normal, wholesome, and desirable. Such expression for any couples not joined in marriage is immeasurably damaging to them, is sinful before God, and is antisocial in the eyes of man. Judaism expects the daughters of Israel to remain virgins until their marriage and Jewish men to be chaste and continent until they are wed.][2]

On Marriage Laws. Reform [Liberal] Judaism . . . has recognized the right of the state to supervise and control marriage . . . and though it does not encourage civil ceremonies, it does, unlike orthodoxy, recognize their validity. . . . In short, Reform Judaism looks upon marriage as a purely religious act, the contractual part involving prop-

[2]From *Wife of Thy Youth*, by Stanley R. Brav, Chairman, Committee on Marriage, the Family, and the Home of the Central Conference of American Rabbis. Published by the Union of American Hebrew Congregations, 1946 (Reform Judaism).

erty and dower rights governed by the civil regulations of the state, while orthodoxy still acts in the double capacity of "state and religion." Reform Judaism . . . waives the right to perform the old contractual marriage as documented in the "Ketubah" ("marriage contract") with its property stipulations.[3] . . .

On Mixed Marriages. Mixed marriages, or unions between Jews and non-Jews, are discouraged by Judaism, the chief reasons being that differing religious views in the household are not conducive to the peace and harmony, love and understanding, that an intimate relationship such as marriage must foster. . . . Judaism is the religion of a small minority, which can ill afford to weaken itself by loss of any of its members. . . . If, however, the stranger embraces Judaism wholeheartedly and willingly joins the Jewish people, he or she is made welcome and an intermarriage may take place. [Cf. The Book of Ruth.]

On Divorce. Divorce has a history as old as

---

[3] In understanding Jewish marriage law, two facts should be kept in mind: (1) from the time of Abraham until less than a century ago almost all Jewish marriages were arranged by parents with the help of a professional matchmaker or marriage broker ("shadchon"); and (2) marriages were made when couples were still in their teens.

marriage, though less is known about its beginnings. In the Bible we find the simplest procedure, viz., that a man could send his wife away at will. . . . Rabbinic legislation . . . made it increasingly difficult for the husband to get rid of his wife, by safeguarding her dower rights, far more so than did the Bible. . . .

Chief among the grounds for divorce was adultery . . . [which] then meant something else from what it did in the New Testament or does now. It was unfaithfulness on the part of a wife, and the guilty parties were punished by death. A married man who erred with an unmarried woman was a sinner but not an adulterer. . . .

Modern Jews try to follow the spirit of the Jewish law even though they may not agree with all its prescriptions. Reform Jews have yielded to the state as possessing exclusive rights in the question of divorce . . . and no Reform rabbi grants the "Get" ("divorce") or recognizes one other than that issued by the courts of the country. . . .

Religion then must reluctantly recognize the need of divorce and bewail it whenever it occurs. . . . Divorce is a remedy of last resort . . . and the means to lessen it must be those which invest marriage, as does religion, with sacredness and solemnity.

SUMMARY REVIEW QUESTIONS

1. What is the normal social process or pattern leading to marriage among young people in the United States? How does this differ from the patterns in other nations and cultures?
2. Where do you usually find the person you marry? Why should this be so?
3. What taboos on choice of mate are commonly found within primitive cultures? What are two almost universal taboos with regard to marriage practices?
4. What are the values of "dating" as practiced in the United States? What is the fundamental rule for behavior on a date?
5. How do you interpret the statement, "The values of courtship are not the same as the values of marriage"? What is the function of engagement?
6. How would you define love? How many different kinds of love can you think of?
7. What is romantic love? Why does it often carry the seeds of its own destruction? In what ways does it support the American ideal of romantic, monogamous marriage?
8. What do you expect of marriage? What personal attitudes toward marriage on the part of husband and wife can help to make it more successful?
9. What significant changes in attitudes toward marriage among college students have occurred since World War II? Why?
10. How would you personally assess each one of the following factors in accepting or rejecting

a prospective marriage partner: physical attractiveness, physical size, age, health, heredity, religious faith, race, intelligence, education, social status, personal habits, wealth, compatibility? Which factors do you consider more important? Which least important?

11. How would you attempt to determine before marriage whether a particular person was a good marriage risk for you? What kind of questions about him (or her) would you ask yourself?

12. What is the relationship of love to marriage? Expound.

13. Are the following statements sense or nonsense? Why? *A good date makes a good mate. . . . Marriages are made in heaven. . . . When poverty comes in the door, love flies out the window. . . . College spoils a girl's chances of getting married. . . . When you're in love, you'll know it. . . . Every marriage is a gamble.*

14. On the basis of the texts presented in abridged form in this chapter, and any other documented information you may have, what would you say was the "common ground" of present-day Protestantism, Roman Catholicism, and Reform (Liberal) Judaism on the following points:
    a. The conditions that make for a happy marriage.
    b. The role of parents toward their children.
    c. Religious symbolism drawn from family life.
    d. Attitude toward sex in marriage.
    e. Attitude toward sexual relationships outside of marriage.
    f. The relationship of love and marriage.
    g. Monogamy.
    h. On the *value* of permanence in marriage relationships.
    i. Intermarriage.
    j. The *desirability* of parenthood.

15. In what ways, if any, have these official statements of present-day attitudes toward sex, marriage, and the family on the part of Protestant, Jewish, and Catholic faiths changed or corrected the ideas and beliefs that you formerly held?

16. Why should a discussion of moral and religious values be given a place of primary consideration in any presentation of the topic of "sex education"?

17. Do you think that the goals and aims of marriage, as defined in the official statements in this chapter, would be significantly different in cultures and societies not so strongly influenced as the United States by Judaeo-Christian traditions? If so, why? If not, why not?

18. Discuss the implications of the statement: "Children are a gift of God."

19. What do the following terms mean to you: endogamy, monogamy, homogamy, "falling in love," engagement ring, "poor man's divorce," "going steady," sublimination, compatibility, overreaction, chastity, celibacy, adultery, divorce, annulment, prenuptial, canon law, Judaeo-Christian tradition, *Kiddushin, Casti Connubii?*

Worth Looking At: *Love: A Garland of Prose and Poetry Woven Together* by Walter de la Mare. *Facts of Love and Marriage for Young People* edited by Aron Krich. *How To Understand the Opposite Sex* by William C. Menninger and others. *Marriage* by Herman R. Lantz and Eloise C. Snyder. *Christian Marriage* by the National Council of Churches of Christ in the United States of America. *Casti Connubii: Encyclical Letter on Christian Marriage* by Pope Pius XI. *Judaism and Marriage* by Felix A. Levy, from the Union of American Hebrew (Reform) Congregations.

9

HUMAN REPRODUCTION

THE URGE OR NECESSITY TO REPRODUCE one's kind is the mark, and one of the fundamental mysteries, of life itself. On the shadowy borderline between animate and inanimate objects, in the field of virus research, the ability to reproduce (or replicate) remains the basic test for classifying a *living* virus as against an inert chemical.

Among many living species reproduction appears to be the aim of life. Salmon swim upstream, leaping impossible falls, to return to their spawning grounds. Eels at maturity swim downstream to go back to their own place of birth in the black depths of the ocean, reproduce a new crop of elvers, and disappear. Among higher animals, the dog and the horse, for example, the instinct for reproduction is equally powerful, and involuntary. It is controlled by seasons of "heat" or "rut," which can be correlated with the activity of endocrine glands, especially in the female.

The human reproductive process has different rhythms of its own. After puberty, the time of attaining biological maturity, human beings are capable of reproduction at any time of the year. In fact, however, this capacity is physiologically limited in the female to certain times of the month and is controlled over the years by powerful social pressures.

It is profitless to ask why mankind desires to reproduce itself. Or why the overtones of the reproductive process, sexual pleasure, sound so sweet to the human race. It has proved equally futile to debate the question of bisexuality, to ask why in the course of evolution the union of male and female elements became necessary to initiate new life.

We may profitably consider, however, the observable processes by which a "gleam in the eye" may eventually become a full-fledged living infant which itself grows up to repeat the cycle of human reproduction. We shall deal here with the biological facts of human reproduction since we have already dealt with their social and psychological implications. Such information is properly described as education for family living, because it is for the sake of creating a happy family of one's own that one seeks fuller knowledge of the phenomenon of human reproduction along with perspective on risks and opportunities surrounding it.

No intelligent man or woman can afford to play ostrich with the facts about and surrounding human reproduction. The most elementary activities of our daily lives and our most fundamental feelings and attitudes are largely controlled by these facts. We are educated for and in family living, as male or female, from infancy onward. The attempts on the part of some individuals and groups to veil the facts of life behind prudish attitudes are responsible for much needless human doubt, guilt, suffering, and misery. "Nice-Nellyism" is out of key with our modern, science-oriented civilization.

The Reproductive Process

A human life begins with the penetration at the proper time and place of a single, ripe human ovum (egg) by a single, viable human sperm.

HUMAN SPERM CELL. Here are two diagrammatic views of a human sperm cell, magnified approximately 2000 times actual life size. A. Side view (profile). B. Top view (looking down).

This is the critical moment of conception, but it is in fact a "microscopically small and unfelt event." It occurs, normally, in one uterine tube of the female some hours after the deposit of semen in the vagina. The ovum arrives at this rendezvous by maturing and bursting out of a follicle in the nearby ovary. The sperm originates in the male testis, but the whole reproductive apparatus of the male, and some of that of the female, is required to get the sperm to the place of conception.

Sperm. Sperm[1] are microscopically small, measuring only 50 to 60 microns (thousandths of a millimeter) in length. You could pick up on the head of a pin all the sperm necessary to sire the next generation in North America.

Each normal human sperm can be seen in profile to have a spear-shaped head, a neck, and a threadlike tail. The tail is about ten times as long as the head and gives the sperm a whiplike power of locomotion. As observed under the microscope, it wriggles along by lashing its tail. Sperm move ahead, or "swim," at the rate of about an inch in twenty minutes. Comparatively speaking, this is roughly the speed of a good human swimmer. Sperm moving at approximately this rate, and normally shaped and proportioned, are considered *viable,* that is, living and capable of fertilizing a human ovum.

Sperm leave the male body in an ejaculate of

[1] The singular form of the word sperm is sometimes written as spermatozoon; the plural, spermatozoa.

semen, a white, viscous fluid, whose function appears to be exactly that of serving as a vehicle for the sperm. A normal ejaculate contains from 2 to 5 cubic centimeters of semen, each cubic centimeter carrying on the average about 100 million spermatozoa. When an ejaculate of semen is deposited in the female vagina, its huge swarm of sperm, numbering perhaps from 200 million to 500 million, begin to move under their own power toward that site in the female genital tract where a mature ovum is likely to be encountered. If encountered, however, one and only one sperm cell actually punctures, penetrates, and fertilizes the egg.

The sperm which do not fertilize the egg simply perish, like any seeds scattered on barren ground. Some of the sperm deposited in the female genitalia appear to remain viable up to seventy-two hours if they have entered the uterus. Most of those left in the vagina perish within an hour or two. Under controlled laboratory conditions the hardiest of ejaculated sperm can be kept alive in a test tube for one or two days. At least they retain some motility.

Beginning at puberty and continuing to old age, though at a slower rate in later years, the normal human male produces literally billions of sperm in the course of his lifetime. There is not ground for the belief that, if men "waste" their sperm early in life, the supply will run out. Nature's prodigality with sperm perhaps reflects the high degree of hazard that any single one will succeed in reaching a mature egg cell.

Ovum. Timing is a crucial factor in human conception. The mature or ripened human ovum has a comparatively short life span, probably not more than forty-eight hours and possibly less. Unless fertilized in the uterine tube during these crucial hours, the egg dies, disintegrates, and is discharged from the body in the course of menstruation.

A ripe (mature) human egg cell is about $\frac{1}{100}$ of an inch in diameter, just about visible to the naked eye.

The two female ovaries contain altogether about 50,000 egg cells, but these are immature cells laid down during embryonic life. These egg cells do not ripen or become mature until puberty. Then, with the onset of menstruation and ovulation, a small number of the ova eventually mature at about the rate of one a month. The outside limit would be about 500 in a lifetime. Each egg cell matures in its own pocket, called a *Graafian follicle*. This process continues until the menopause, which usually comes in the late forties.

Twins. On some occasions more than one mature ovum may happen to be released from the ovaries at about the same time. The proof that this occurs is the birth of so-called *fraternal twins* or triplets. Each separate egg cell is under these circumstances fertilized by a different sperm cell. Fraternal twins, therefore, are no more alike than any other brothers and sisters. *Identical twins,* however, come from the same egg and sperm cell; the egg splits after being fertilized. Identical twins are always of the same sex; they usually look almost exactly alike. About one pair of twins in every four is made up of identical twins.

Twins are born about once in every 80 pregnancies; triplets, once in every 6000 to 7000—roughly 80 times 80; quadruplets, once in approximately a half-million—roughly 80 times 80 times 80. Quintuplets occur once in about 50 million to 60 million pregnancies. There is some evidence that the tendency to multiple births runs in families.

The Male Reproductive System

The purpose and design of the male reproductive system is to deliver viable sperm for the impregnation of the ovum. Its essential anatomical apparatus includes the testes, also called male gonads; a series of sperm ducts, the prostate gland and seminal vesicles for elaborating and storing semen; and the penis, urethra, and accessory glands.

Testes. Two testes, or testicles, each about the size of a walnut, are enclosed in a sac of skin, called the scrotum, suspended from the groin.

INSIDE THE OVARY. An ovary cut across looks like this. The Graafian follicles, in which the ova mature, are shown in various stages of development. Note also the corpus luteum, containing the old follicles whose eggs have been discharged. The egg cell itself is about as big as the period at the end of this sentence.

Hanging outside the body, between the legs, the scrotum has a temperature slightly lower than the rest of the body; this appears to be an essential condition for production of sperm. The testes normally descend from the abdomen into the cooler scrotum just before or shortly after birth. If they fail to descend (undescended testes, cryptorchidism), medical or surgical treatment may be needed.

The first important function of the testes is to manufacture sperm. This takes place, so far as is known, in a series of little twisted (convoluted) tubules, where the sperm develop from immature sex cells laid down in these membranes early in the life of the embryo. Mature sperm, capable of fertilizing an ovum, do not appear until puberty. The testes may continue producing sperm well into old age, as is evidenced by the not infrequent birth of children to aged fathers. From collecting tubes in the testes, the sperm move on to a series of ducts, beginning with the epididymes, through which they are eventually conveyed outside the body.

The second important task of the testes is to manufacture the male sex hormone, *testosterone,* which brings about development of secondary sex characteristics at puberty: growth of beard and pubic hair, deeper voice, comparatively rapid increase in size of the male sex organs, and general muscular development. The male sex hormone is produced in a set of specialized cells located in the tissues that support the tubules making sperm; a lesser amount is elaborated by the *adrenal glands.* Testes are part of the *endocrine* system.

Epididymes. These are coiled-up tubes, several feet long but looking like a twisted ball of string, attached like a hood or pouch to the outer surface of each testicle. They collect and store sperm. In them the sperm become mature and motile, that is, capable of moving under their own power. However, they do not do this until they are discharged from the body. They are propelled through spermatic ducts by contractions of the tubes and tubules.

Spermatic cords, or ducts, convey sperm from the epididymes up to the seminal vesicles. They are winding tubes, about a foot long, including the *vas deferens* and other structures. The spermatic cords, one from each testicle, issue from the scrotum into the abdomen by way of the inguinal canal. Spermatic cords can be felt where they pass over the pubic bone near the base of the penis. Cutting the cords near this point is the simplest operation for *sterilization* of the male.

Seminal vesicles are the upper outlets of the spermatic cord. They are two small pouches or sacs located in the abdomen just behind the bladder. They secrete a large part of the thick, white, alkaline fluid, *semen,* in which the sperm float. Like the rubber bulb on an eye dropper, they can contract vigorously and spurt or squirt semen out into the *urethra,* the mucus-lined tube that traverses the penis and carries urine as well as semen. Because some of the same bodily organs are used for the discharge of urine as well as semen, the entire system is sometimes called *genito-urinary.*

Ejaculation of semen from the seminal vesicles is a nerve-reflex act, associated with the sensation called *orgasm.* The motor nerves that control orgasm respond to both physiological and psychic stimuli. The stimulating impulses usually arise in the head (glans) of the penis. The distention of the seminal vesicles with an accumulation of semen may also prompt the discharge of semen as a nocturnal emission.

The prostate gland, normally about the size and shape of a chestnut, is situated just below the bladder and seminal vesicles and surrounds the urethra where it emerges from the bladder. It is involved with secreting fluids which make up part of the semen. Anatomically it is the homologue of the uterus in women: its function as a genital organ, however, is still poorly understood.

Accessory glands among the male sex organs include a pair called *Cowper's glands.* They are about the size of a pea, are located near the base of the penis, and open into the urethra. They secrete a clear, oily lubricating fluid. A few drops of this fluid may come out of the penis following sexual excitation not carried to the point of orgasm.

The *penis,* a cylindrical organ suspended from

ureter

bladder

seminal vesicle

prostate gland

Cowper's gland

penis

scrotum

vas deferens

spermatic cord

epididymis

testis

urethra

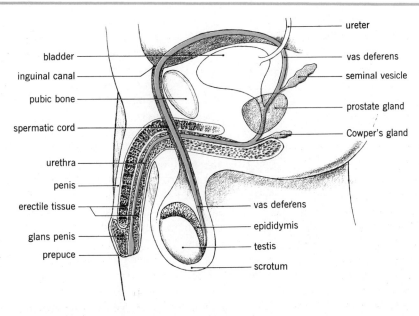

ureter

bladder

inguinal canal

pubic bone

spermatic cord

urethra

penis

erectile tissue

glans penis

prepuce

vas deferens

seminal vesicle

prostate gland

Cowper's gland

vas deferens

epididymis

testis

scrotum

THE MALE REPRODUCTIVE SYSTEM. The upper diagram is a straight front view. The lower diagram is a side view shown as if a section had been made a little to one side of the center of the body, from front to back.

the front and sides of the groin, is the male organ of intercourse, designed for delivery of semen into the vagina. Enlargement, or erection, of the penis is normally necessary for this function. This occurs when the usually retracted and flaccid organ becomes engorged with blood. The shaft and head of the penis are composed of a spongy, cavernous, erectile tissue, traversed by many blood channels. When stimulated, these channels become filled with blood, whose immediate return to the rest of the circulation is temporarily cut off by constriction of the veins leading away from the penis. Under conditions of adequate sexual excitation, erection of the penis is a normal and natural reaction of the male animal—part of nature's design to assure perpetuation of the species.[2]

Circumcision. The penis is covered with loose folds of skin, allowing for enlargement. The extra skin at the tip, or glans, is called the *foreskin* or *prepuce.* The operation for its removal is known as circumcision. Among Jews, Mohammedans, and some other peoples, the operation is performed as a ritualistic measure. Among Orthodox Jews it is always performed on the eighth day of life. In the Bible it is stated that the "tribe of Abraham" is to affirm its "covenant" (*bris*) with the Lord by this measure.

---

[2] At puberty the size of the penis usually increases markedly. The length of the organ is sometimes falsely taken as a measure of manliness. This is nonsense. Except in rare individuals in whom the sex organs fail to develop normally, usually as a result of some disease requiring definite medical attention, the size of the penis has no relationship to fertility, or marital adjustment. Despite the bawdy jokes that are brought to bear on the topic, fears on the part of the male that he will be unable to give or receive satisfaction in the marital act because of the size of his penis are completely unwarranted. The psychological satisfactions surrounding the act, the tenderness, warmth, affection, and love brought to it, are of far greater moment than the physiological mechanics. Furthermore, the innervation of the female genital tract—the comparative paucity of nerve endings in the distensible vaginal tissue itself—is such that actual penile dimensions are of insignificant import in the totality of sensations and satisfactions involved. To think otherwise is to retreat to a level of phallic worship found in primitive tribes. (The male organ and representations of it in model or symbol are designated by the word phallus.)

The origin of circumcision is lost in the history of antiquity. In modern times it is performed for both its ritualistic and sanitary values. It keeps "cheesy" secretions (smegma) of the foreskin from accumulating and irritating the penis, and it prevents cancer of the penis. Circumcision does not alter sexual satisfaction.

The Female Reproductive System

The female reproductive system consists of a pair of *ovaries,* a pair of tubes, the uterus or womb, the vagina, external genitals, and some accessory glands. The mammary glands (breasts) are sometimes considered part of this system.

All the important female sex organs are located inside the body. The whole system is greatly influenced at all times by hormones produced both in the ovaries and in other endcrine glands.

The female sex organs have at least three functions: to produce and yield mature ova for union with viable sperm, to shelter and nourish the fertilized egg cell until it has developed into a newborn baby, and to elaborate female sex hormones.

Ovaries. The ovaries, or female gonads, are two small glands, each about the size and shape of an almond, set in the pelvic cavity (lower abdomen). One is about 3 inches to the right and the other the same distance to the left of the midline of the body. The ovaries do two jobs: they bring ova to a point of readiness for impregnation and they secrete hormones.

The hormones released by the ovaries have several functions. They help to govern the monthly rhythm of ovulation and menstruation. They do this partially by their effect on other endocrine glands. Furthermore, these hormones spur the development and maintenance of secondary sex characteristics, for example, deposition of fat under the skin to give the characteristic feminine curves, enlargement of the breasts, growth of pubic hair.

Fallopian Tubes. When the matured egg cell escapes from its follicle, it is caught or picked up by one or the other of the two uterine tubes, or oviducts. Each of the two uterine tubes is about

body of uterus

oviduct

ureter

fimbria

ovary

bladder

neck of uterus

urethra

vagina

Bartholin's gland

labium minus

labium majus

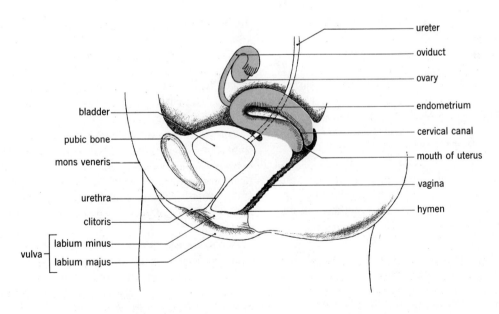

ureter

oviduct

ovary

bladder

endometrium

pubic bone

cervical canal

mons veneris

mouth of uterus

urethra

vagina

clitoris

hymen

vulva

labium minus

labium majus

THE FEMALE REPRODUCTIVE SYSTEM. The upper diagram is a straight front view. The lower diagram is a front-to-back section through the center of the body.

3 to 5 inches long. Its lower end clearly opens into the uterus. Its trumpet-shaped far end, however, is not really attached to the ovary. It just lies close to it and holds out fingerlike projections (called fimbria) toward it, reaching for the ripened egg.

The upper, inner lining of the tubes has little hairlike organs, called *cilia,* which by waving back and forth carry the egg down the tube. This action is essential because the egg itself has no power of locomotion. The journey down the tubes takes 3 to 6 days. This is the time and place at which the egg must meet and be penetrated by a viable sperm if pregnancy is to occur.

The fertilized egg normally completes its journey to the uterus. About once in 500 times, however, it implants itself in the tube, causing a *tubal,* or *ectopic, pregnancy.* This usually becomes a serious emergency, demanding surgery.

If both uterine tubes are blocked, usually as a result of inflammatory disease, pregnancy cannot occur. A common test to tell whether the tubes are open (patent) is to blow carbon dioxide gas into them with a special apparatus for this purpose.

The uterus, or womb, is the central organ of the female reproductive system. Non-pregnant, it lies just above and slightly behind the urinary bladder, in the center of the pelvic cavity. Enlarged with pregnancy, the womb fills a large part of the lower abdomen, displacing other organs as it rises.

The non-pregnant womb is a hollow, pear-shaped pouch of muscle, about 3 inches long and 2 inches wide. The stem of the pear points down. This narrower, lower end is called the *cervix,* or neck, of the womb. The upper, round portion, where the embryo actually grows, is called the body, or fundus, of the womb. The uterus is held in place, loosely, by a number of ligaments. This looseness of attachment is essential because it permits the changes in shape, size, and position of the womb that occur during pregnancy.

The uterine muscle is one of the strongest in the body. It has to be to expel a full-grown, newborn infant when the time of labor comes.

The inner lining (endometrium) of the womb is one of the most unusual tissues in the body. A soft, velvety tissue, greatly influenced by hormones, heavily interlaced with blood vessels, it grows and disintegrates in the monthly cycle of ovulation and menstruation.

The lower end of the cervix, called its os or mouth, extends into the upper vault of the vagina. A short cervical canal passes through the cervix. Male sperm must get through this canal to reach the uterus and the uterine tubes above it. If this canal is plugged with mucus, or otherwise blocked, conception cannot occur.

The vagina serves both as the female organ of intercourse and the birth canal through which the newborn infant enters the world. It is a tubular cavity about 3 or 4 inches long, extending from the cleft of the legs to and beyond the mouth of the womb. It is set at an angle of about 45 degrees to the front of the abdomen, and just below the bladder. The muscles that make up the vaginal tube can be greatly stretched without harm. The inner lining is soft membrane.

Accessory glands secrete some fluids during sexual excitation, which lubricate the vagina. These are *Bartholin's glands,* two small oval glands located on each side of the vagina, near its external opening, and *Skene's glands,* multiple small secreting glands located near the opening of the urethra into the vaginal vestibule.

The external genitalia of the female, found adjacent to the vaginal orifice, are the vulva and clitoris. The vulva consists of two pairs of "lips": the *labia majora,* elongated folds of skin covered with hair in the adult woman, and, underneath these, the *labia minora,* thinner folds of tissue covered with mucoid membrane. The clitoris appears at the far forward fold of the labia minora. It is a small, rudimentary structure, consisting, like the penis, of erectile tissue responding to stimulation.

Across the opening of the vagina appears the thin, perforated mucous membrane called the *hymen* (or maidenhead). This structure, whose biological purpose is not known, varies greatly in size, thickness, and extent. In many women it is merely rudimentary. Its absence is of no significance. It is usually broken by the first sexual intercourse, but may otherwise be reft. Being perforate, it does not block menstrual flow. Superstition notwithstanding, its presence is not an absolute sign of virginity, nor is its absence proof to the contrary.

Above the external genitalia, in front of the pubic bone in the area covered by pubic hair, is often found a thick mound of subcutaneous fatty tissue—the *mons Veneris* (hill of Venus).

Menstruation

Menstruation is a characteristic bodily function common to all healthy, adult, nonpregnant women. A menstrual period need not interfere with a woman's regular schedule of activities.

Myth, mystery, and superstition have long enveloped the facts about menstruation, the periodic issuance of blood from the female genital tract "at the waxing or waning of the moon." To the ancient Hebrews, Greeks, Romans, and early Christians the menstruating woman was "unclean." The American Indians, believing the moon to be the First Woman, saw in her waning the periodic "sickness" of the female. The Koran forbade the menstruating woman to pray or enter a mosque. Practically the only fact in the great cluster of erroneous superstitions was that menstruation occurred in cycles corresponding approximately with lunar months. The lunar (moon) calendar has 13 months of 28 days each. The word menstruation derives from the Latin word *mens,* meaning month.

Myths and Misconceptions about Menstruation. While we, fortified by scientific knowledge, tend to laugh at primitive myths about menstruation, nevertheless certain modern misconceptions of the hygiene of menstruation continue to crop up. Mark down as myths and misconceptions, entirely incorrect, such statements as the following:

"Don't take a bath or a shower—don't go swimming or wash your hair when you are menstruating." "Menstruation is a sickness—it's naturally painful." "Any exercise during a menstrual period is harmful—the best policy is to stay in bed." "Your hair won't take a curl or a wave when you are menstruating." "If you have your teeth filled at this time, the fillings will fall out." Nonsense!

The hygiene of menstruation can be summed up in one phrase, "Take it in your stride." Extremes, of course, are wisely avoided. Although some physicians would still interdict it, there are many others who accept evidence[3] that even such an activity as swimming, except in very cold water, can be safely permitted during the menstrual period. (Internal protection—a tampon—is worn.)

There is no objection whatsoever to ordinary bathing, showering, or shampooing or setting of the hair during the menstrual period. Going to bed when a menstrual period arrives is sometimes evidence of an unhealthy attitude not only toward the menstrual function itself, but also toward normal sexuality. Mild exercise will probably tend to relieve rather than promote menstrual discomfort.

Some women nourish the myth that they are as "regular as clockwork" in their menstrual function. This is rarely, if ever, so, as carefully kept calendar records for large groups of women reveal. A few days' so-called irregularity is perfectly normal. Extreme irregularities may be considered signals for a medical check-up. It is to be remembered, however, that many severe diseases, such as pneumonia, and even some mild ones, like a common cold, can upset the regularity of the menstrual cycle. So too can sudden change of altitude or climate, physical shock or emotional excitement, like an airplane trip, an auto accident, or an engagement. Irregularities are also to be expected at the beginning and toward the close of the childbearing years.

On the *average,* the length of the menstrual cycle is twenty-eight days. But every woman has her own rhythmic cycle of ovulatory and therefore menstrual function. For some women cyclic periods of twenty-one or thirty-five days, and occasionally even longer or shorter periods, if reasonably regular, are quite normal.

[3]Grace Thwing, "Swimming during the Menstrual Period," *Journal of Health and Physical Education,* (March 1943).

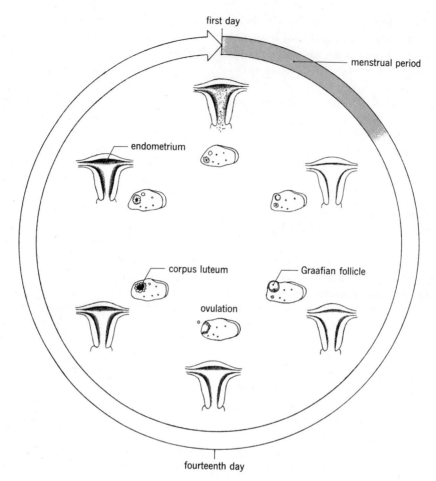

first day

menstrual period

endometrium

corpus luteum

Graafian follicle

ovulation

fourteenth day

THE MENSTRUAL OR OVULATORY CYCLE. This diagram of the menstrual or ovulatory cycle is based on an average (theoretical) 28-day cycle in the human female.

The total amount of blood lost in a normal menstrual period is usually only about three ounces and is quickly regenerated by the blood-forming organs (bone marrow).

A checkup is indicated for the woman who finds herself staining between regular periods, who skips one or more periods, who finds her periods extremely painful, or whose menstrual flow continues much more than a week. The *average* menstrual period is three to five days, but two to seven days are within normal range.

It is not to be denied that painful menstruation (dysmenorrhea) occurs. Yet this is far more commonly—by a ratio of at least 4 to 1 among normal college women—the exception rather than the rule. As Boynton has pointed out, this condi-

tion can often be relieved and prevented by a change in attitude toward the menstrual process.[4] Self-imposed invalidism or unconscious resentment can magnify slight cramps into apparently intolerable pain. When indicated, the physician can prescribe medication for relief of menstrual pain and tension.

The Menstrual or Ovulatory Cycle. Though we commonly speak of the menstrual cycle, dating from the first day of menstrual flow, we can also designate it as the ovulatory cycle, guided and controlled primarily by the time of ovulation. There is no completely accurate way of

[4] Ruth Boynton, "A Study of the Menstrual Histories of 2282 University Students," *American Journal of Obstetrics and Gynecology,* **23**:516 (April 1932).

determining the day of ovulation, although there is evidence that there occurs at this time a slight decrease, by fractions of a degree, in body temperature, following which a relatively sharp rise occurs.

Ovulation occurs at about the midpoint of the menstrual cycle. This is the time when a ripened egg cell bursts out of the tiny sac, or Graafian follicle, in which it has been maturing. This follicle manufactures ovarian hormones; it is a kind of "temporary endocrine gland." Most amazing, it makes one kind of hormone before the egg erupts, another kind afterward. The emptied follicle is called *corpus luteum* (literally, yellow body). Its hormone influences the endometrial lining to disintegrate. But it also influences the pituitary gland to issue hormones that speed another egg cell to maturity and another Graafian follicle to open up, thus starting the whole cycle of events over again.

The menstrual or ovulatory cycle is a complex process that involves the uterus, ovaries, and endocrine glands. However, the most evident changes during the cycle occur in the inner lining (endometrium) of the uterus.

During the menstrual flow this lining is being shed, torn away from the underlying uterine tissues to which it is attached. Small blood vessels (capillaries) are broken as this takes place, and this is the source of the menstrual blood. But even as this old lining is being shed, a new lining is commencing to grow. It gets thicker and thicker, soft and velvety, and enlaced with blood vessels, for the next 3 weeks.

The function of this lining is to receive a fertilized ovum, if one should appear. If none appears, which is usually the case, the lining is again shed, with bleeding, and still another begins to grow. If a fertilized ovum *is* present to embed itself in endometrium, the menstrual cycle comes to an abrupt halt, to resume after childbirth.

The Menopause

The menopause, sometimes called the "climacteric" or "change of life," marks the end of the potential child-bearing period that begins with the onset of menstruation (menarche). The menopause usually comes anywhere from the early forties to the late fifties, occuring on the average at about forty-seven. Just as the onset of the menses was marked with a sudden increase in ovarian hormones, so the menopause occurs when there is a gradual decrease in these hormones. The elaboration of ovarian hormones (by the ovaries) finally ceases. No more ova are matured. The menstrual flow becomes scanty and irregular or stops abruptly. That is all there need be to the menopause, and in about 85 out of 100 cases there are no other changes. Childbearing is no longer possible, but sexual feeling is not necessarily decreased (in some women it is heightened).

The outward physical symptoms of the change of life are usually mild and transient, if they occur at all: a few "hot flashes," lasting a minute or two; a feeling of fatigue at times; an occasional pain in the joints. It should be noted that many of the symptoms often associated with the menopause are today amenable to much relief with hormone and psychological treatment.

Some attempts have been made to define a "male climacteric," similar to the menopause. It may occur in a few men, but the cessation of function of the male sex hormones usually tapers off so gradually that no well-defined symptoms can be definitely associated with it.

Contraception

Despite the marvel of human reproduction, it must be admitted that there are millions of married couples (and others) who do not want to run the risk of pregnancy occurring with every incident of sexual intercourse. These people are more interested in contraception than in conception. Contraception is known by other names: birth control, birth prevention, family planning, child spacing, and planned parenthood.

A number of methods of contraception are now available, some more reliable than others, some very new, others very ancient. With one exception—surgical sterilization in the male—they are all reversible. That is to say, conception can be expected to occur when the particular technique(s) of contraception are no longer employed. Among the popular methods of contraception now employed are (1) "the pill," (2) intrauterine devices, abbreviated to IUD's, (3) rubber diaphragm with or without spermicidal creams or jellies, (4) the rubber condom or male sheath, and (5) "the rhythm" or "safe period" system.

As one expert in this field has pointed out,[5]

The knowledge of the so-called new birth control methods has been shared with the public with a haste that seems almost unparalleled in medical history. The daily press, the weekly news periodicals, the romantic magazines of the newsstands, even staid financial journals have published articles in their own particular styles or from their own particular points of view. . . .

The new methods of birth control have brought with them special problems of application, of acceptability, of reliability, and sometimes of unwanted side effects. Much work on evaluation remains to be done and much research is required for the perfection of technics which are perhaps still in the early stages of their development.

Here is a brief rundown of the principle current contraceptive methods.

"The Pill." The ovulation-suppressing pill is a hormonal stimulant and depressant, whose basic ingredients are related to the female sex hormones. The pill, taken orally, contains some synthetic progesterone and a little estrogen. These hormones suppress the follicle-stimulating hormone of the anterior pituitary gland. As a result, the ripening of an ovum in the ovary fails to occur. Without the presence of a ripe ovum in the uterine tubes or cavity, pregnancy cannot occur.

The woman who wishes to avoid pregnancy takes one pill a day for about 20 or 21 days, beginning on the fourth or fifth day after the start of her menstrual period. Properly used, the pill can offer close to 100% protection against pregnancy. When discontinued for a month or two, normal pregnancy can be expected to occur following intercourse. In fact, it must be taken regularly, for even if one day is missed, ovulation and pregnancy might occur. Furthermore, investigations now under way indicate possible relationships between thromboembolism and other diseases and the taking of the pill. The risk, however, appears to be within permissible limits.

. . . It was to be expected that the method would have to defend itself against numerous apprehensive allegations. This it seems to have accomplished successfully. It was at first feared that fertility, after long use of the progestins, might be permanently impaired, but it has been shown that conception will occur within one or two cycles after discontinuation of the medication, and indeed there is some evidence for even a temporarily heightened fertility. The specter of a carcinogenetic effect has of course also been raised and apparently been excluded, at least so far as the cervix of the uterus is concerned, by the finding of an actually smaller number of positive Papanicolaou smears among the users of this method than was to be expected. Because the progestins are said to produce a physiologic state somewhat resembling that of pregnancy, and since thrombophlebitis is of slightly increased frequency in pregnancy, the observation of a few cases of thrombo-embolic disease among women taking Norethynodrel led to new anxiety. A careful study by an ad hoc committee of the Food and Drug Administration led, however, to the conclusion that no significant increase in the risk of thrombo-embolic deaths had been demonstrated.

At the moment, then, there are no well-founded accusations pending against the progestins as health hazards. They have now been in use for [over a decade] and reservations are still held by some as to the possible results of 20 years of use. Such concern, taking the form of worry about effects on any subsequently conceived offspring, or about possible carcinogenic effects on breast and endometrium, especially from the estrogen usually combined in the "pill," is largely theoretical. It is troublesome in that it cannot possibly be excluded completely until another decade has come and gone.

There remain a certain number of so-called "side effects," annoying symptoms, which cause a certain number of women to discard the method. These consist in nausea, some intermenstrual, so-called "breakthrough," bleeding, and gain in weight due principally to the retention of electrolytes and water.

[5]This quotation, and those that follow in this section, are from Howard C. Taylor, Jr., M.D., "Evaluation of Developments in Contraceptive Technology," *American Journal of Public Health* (January 1966 supplement).

Consequently, a small number of users, possibly 5 or 10 percent, abandon the method for reasons other than the decision to have another child.

Nearly ideal as this method appears to be, there are a number of improvements that are needed before it can be considered perfect. The price is still high, about $2.50 a month, if the 21 tablets are purchased at retail, and this, though far less than the cost of maintaining an average cigarette habit, is still out of the financial or psychological reach of a large segment of the world's population. Further, the taking of even one tablet a day may be hard to remember, and research is under way to produce longer-acting compounds which might require only a single dose for a whole cycle.

Intrauterine Devices—IUD's. These are usually made of a flexible plastic in the shape of loops, rings, spirals, "butterflies," etc. and can be folded down to small size for insertion through the narrow cervical canal of the uterus. Once inserted, they snap back to their original expanded state. This method has the advantages of low cost and relative permanence. Under the best conditions, it is from 97 to 98.9% effective in preventing unwanted pregnancies. The method has some disadvantages. In some women the device causes extreme menstrual flow and uterine cramps. In perhaps one woman in seven there is a tendency toward spontaneous expulsion of the device. It must then be replaced with a different shape or size.

First of all it is clear that the effectiveness of the intrauterine device is very high, the cumulative pregnancy rate during the first year after insertion, for all devices combined, being 2.6 per 100 patients. For certain forms and sizes of the device the figure was as low as 1.1 or 1.3 per 100 patients. An additional small figure must be added for pregnancies occurring after spontaneous expulsion of the ring when this occurrence is unnoticed by the patient. Even with this addition the protection offered is substantially better than that from the traditional methods of birth control when used by the average clinic patient. If the undetected expulsions can be eliminated, the degree of security would approach, although perhaps never quite reach, the perfect safety afforded by the pharmacological technic.

The point of superiority of the intrauterine device is of course its relative permanence, since only a single decision is required. Once the device is inserted, there is no need for further responsible action. This feature, coupled with the low cost, has given the device great promise for use by the less educated, less motivated, and less self-controlled.

Certain disadvantages of the intrauterine devices must still be faced. In a proportion of women wearing the ring, menorrhagia and uterine cramps develop, requiring removal of the device in about seven percent. The tendency to spontaneous expulsion of the device is a further problem. In perhaps 13.8 percent, the figure varying considerably with the shape of the device, the first one tried is expelled and must be replaced, or a new type or size tried. Finally, there is the possibility that the ring predisposes to infection. The old Gräfenberg ring was held responsible for pelvic inflammatory disease and instances of such inflammation have certainly occurred among the women in the present investigation. However, an incidence of 1.7 cases per 100 women using the device for 12 months is perhaps not very different from that to be found among a similar group of women not using the device.

Future work with the intrauterine device must still be somewhat concerned with health hazards. The possibility of slight predisposition to pelvic inflammatory disease needs to be somewhat further considered. The hazard of carcinogenic action from a long retained foreign body has of course been thought of, and although this effect seems improbable, the question can finally be answered only by the passage of time. Studies of changes in the cervical epithelium, as measured by successive Papanicolaou tests, have been inconclusive. . . .

The technical developments that are needed include the development of shapes and sizes that will not be expelled, and, hopefully, such that will cause a minimum of cramps and bleeding. The need of a simple method by which the continued presence of the device in the uterus can be detected has given rise to some electronic thinking leading to some interesting and some frivolous proposals. In summary, the intrauterine device like the pharmacological method, given the proper means of public information and application, could also solve the problem of overpopulation.

Diaphragm with or without Spermicidal Creams or Jellies. Until recent years this was the form of contraceptive most commonly recommended by physicians and birth control centers. The diaphragm is a rubber cap, shaped like a shallow dish, with a flexible metal spring or coil forming its outer edge. The diaphragm is fitted over the mouth of the uterus, and prevents viable sperm from entering. The diaphragm has to be anchored firmly between the back of the vagina and, in front, the pubic bone. This distance varies from woman to woman. Hence the diaphragm has first to be fitted precisely by a physician skilled in this work. It must be inserted by the woman each time sexual intercourse is anticipated. There has been some complaint that this method takes too much of the spontaneity out of sexual intercourse. However, it is a highly reliable method, especially when used as recommended with a spermicidal cream or jelly, which provides a chemical barrier to the diaphragm's mechanical barrier between sperm and egg.

Newlywed couples may have to use some other form of contraception (e.g., the condom) on their honeymoon because it is not easy, and sometimes not possible, to fit a diaphragm to a woman with an intact maidenhead (hymen).

Condom (male sheath). The condom is a thin rubber sheath, shaped like the finger of a glove, which rolls down to fit over the erect penis. It is probably the most popular form of contraceptive and has the added advantage of helping to guard against the risk of venereal disease. It is freely sold in drugstores as a "prophylactic."

"The Rhythm" or "Safe Period" System. This method depends upon the fact that there exists in most women of child-bearing age a reasonably regular menstrual or ovulatory cycle. Menstruation and ovulation are generally about halfway apart in the cycle. Pregnancy can occur only in the ovulatory phase of the cycle, that is, the time when a ripened ovum is present in the uterine tube. Hence the days that surround the menstrual period are "safe" from pregnancy, while those immediately before and immediately following the time of ovulation are the "fertile" period. In a woman with a regular menstrual cycle, the tenth to the eighteenth days following the onset of menstruation are the time when the fertile period occurs. A viable sperm may re-

main in the female genital tract for three days (72 hours) or possibly longer. The life span of the unfertilized ovum is less than one day (24 hours).

To prevent conception the couple must practice abstinence during the fertile period of the menstrual cycle. Illness, shock, emotional storms, and other events may influence the time of ovulation and throw the menstrual cycle out of kilter. The difficulty with the method lies in knowing exactly when ovulation occurs. A daily temperature record can help to determine this. If taken daily, the first thing in the morning, the body temperature will tend to rise a half to a whole degree about the day that ovulation occurs. The Roman Catholic Church has permitted birth control by the rhythm method (also by prolonged abstinence and celibacy).

The effectiveness of the "rhythm" method, that of abstinence during the days when ovulation is expected to occur, remains somewhat of a mystery. Physiologists swear that it should be a success; statisticians doubt somewhat that it has been.

The resolution of this apparent contradiction is to be found, of course, in the number of days a month abstinence must be practiced if "safety" is to be assured [since] even the most regular menstrual pattern has a variability of three days, these authors conclude that with the Ogino formula the days of abstinence must be 11 each month. For women with less regular cycles this figure may increase to as much as 15 or 18 days a month. Yet they point out that the observation of the rules implied by this theoretical model should give a 90 percent chance of avoiding pregnancy for five to ten years.

Data derived from actual use of the method are not numerous but that which exists indicates a high failure rate, apparently several times that cited for the usual traditional methods. The conclusion seems inevitable that the use of the rhythm method gives only relative protection unless there is strict adherence to the Spartan regime required for real effectiveness.

Yet the physiological facts seem sound and the method is potentially an effective one. Success might be attained by a fundamental revision of current concepts of sexual behavior in marriage and, indeed, the standard frequencies of intercourse may be related more to fashion and custom than to physiological necessity. Alternately, the method must apparently await the discovery of a test, easily applied, which would indicate when ovulation was about to occur, or a simple medication which would precipitate ovulation on a convenient date. Such possibilities are indeed being worked upon in a number of laboratories and are quite within the realm of possible development.

Among other contraceptive methods are douching, withdrawal, and surgical sterilization.

Douche. This is a common but highly unsatisfactory method of contraception. It calls for cleansing the vaginal tract with water (sometimes with something added) immediately after sexual intercourse. Speed is the key to practicing this method. Within 90 seconds after intercourse some sperm are already within the uterine cervix, where they cannot be reached by the douche fluid.

Withdrawal. The essence of this method is that the male withdraws the penis from the vagina just before he reaches his climax or orgasm. However, there may be a leakage of semen into the vaginal tract even before orgasm. Though it has the advantage of requiring no apparatus, it cannot be depended upon for safety against the risk of pregnancy.

Surgical Sterilization. Sterilization in the female is accomplished by tying off the uterine tubes; in the male, by cutting through the spermatic cord as it emerges under the skin at the groin. In women, at any rate, the procedure is reversible and tubal potency can be reestablished by surgery. About 5% to 6% of white U.S. couples with three or more children have undergone the simple operation of surgical sterilization for contraceptive purposes.

. . . Since this procedure is rarely undertaken until after there are three or more children in the family, its effect on birth rates may not be considerable. Nevertheless, the frequency with which sterilization is now carried out makes it a factor to be noted. [Indeed], some 200,000 operations preventing pregnancy were performed in the United States annually from 1955 to 1960 and of these 110,000 were contraceptive in intent.

The majority of contraceptive sterilizations in women consist in a tubal ligation carried out during the first week after delivery. . . . The frequency of this procedure among 177,433 live births . . . proved to be 3.2 percent of all deliveries.

Puerperal sterilization is an almost completely safe procedure and requires so small an incision that little discomfort follows it and the patient's postpartum hospital stay is scarcely prolonged. Psychological and even physiological disturbances have been alleged to follow it, but these have not been proved or checked against unsterilized controls. A small percentage, perhaps half of one percent, of failures to prevent pregnancy have been reported. A very few sterilized women regret their decision, but here there is evidence that the surgical reestablishment of tubal continuity will be successful in a considerable percentage of patients. The freedom from concern and the absence of need for any continuously applied method of contraception are the great assets of this method.

The obstacles to the still wider application of surgical sterilization are two. One is the nagging fear in each case that the operation once done will be regretted. The other is the prevailing feeling in the medical profession, not at all limited to those of the Catholic faith, that the operation of sterilization is a special one, interfering with a provision of nature and not to be lightly undertaken.

There is still objection to birth control—on moral, religious, political, and other grounds. However, with the rapidly increasing population of the globe, some effective form of birth control will be necessary to curb the population explosion.

Conditions seem to be rapidly changing in the United States and it appears that in a few years some consideration of family planning will be as integral a part of pre- and post-partum care as is the detection of physical illness. In such a program, the subject of birth control should certainly be introduced during the mother's classes in the antepartum period. Reference to the subject and a stress on the importance of the postpartum visit should be given at the bedside while the patient is still in the hospital. Finally, at the postpartum visit birth control should again be discussed and the patient given a chance to select a method satisfactory to her taste and conscience.

SUMMARY REVIEW QUESTIONS

1. Why should an educated man or woman know the facts about human reproduction? Why do some supposedly mature adults fail to get the facts straight?
2. What is "conception"? Where does it occur? What are the crucial factors that make it possible? What sharp contrasts can you point out between human sperm and human ova with relation to size, shape, number, life span and mode of travel?
3. What is the difference between fraternal and identical twins? Approximately how often do multiple births occur?
4. What are the essential parts and functions of the male reproductive system?
5. What are the essential parts and functions of the female reproductive apparatus?
6. What myths and misconceptions, ancient and modern, about menstruation can you cite? How could you combat such misconceptions?
7. What is the menstrual cycle? The ovulatory cycle? How are they interrelated and how are they regulated?
8. What are the most effective means of contraception now employed? What are the objections to contraception?
9. Are the following statements sense or nonsense? Why? *Barrenness is always a woman's fault. . . . The menopause is usually a painful process. . . . Never wash your hair when you are menstruating. . . . If a man "wastes" his sperm when he is young, the supply will soon run out. . . . Shocking experiences during pregnancy can put marks on the unborn child.*
10. What do the following terms mean to you: bisexuality, Graafian follicle, Fallopian tube, circumcision, dysmenorrhea, ovulation, ectopic pregnancy, seminal vesicles, IUD, "The pill," diaphragm, accessory glands?

Worth Looking At: *Sex Anatomy* by Robert L. Dickinson. *Essentials of Human Reproduction* by Velardo. *Sex in Marriage* by Baruch and Miller. *Planning Your Family* by Alan F. Guttmacher.

10

BIRTH OF A BABY

CHILDBIRTH HAS LONG BEEN SHROUDED IN secrecy, as a reaction to the pain and risk it entailed in earlier generations. Scientific progress in medicine, obstetrics, surgery, and anesthesiology has now reduced these hazards to the barest minimum. Women today can have their babies safely and relatively easily if they take advantage of the modern safeguards of adequate prenatal care and hospital delivery. In the United States today better than 3099 out of 3100 mothers come through childbirth safely.

Twentieth-century changes in the social and economic relationships between the sexes have also operated to make present-day attitudes toward pregnancy and childbirth quite different from those of our Victorian grandparents. Proper Victorians never "talked obstetrics." To the present day "organization man" and his wife, living in suburbia and exurbia, obstetrics is the grist of everyday conversation.

Modern fathers are no more directly engaged in childbearing than was Prince Albert, the consort of Queen Victoria. But it is the rare father today, among educated people, who can or wants to escape the responsibilities of child-rearing. He will be concerned with his children and children-to-be from the very moment that a diagnosis of pregnancy is established in his wife. Pregnancy is a family affair.

The gist of the modern enlightened attitudes toward pregnancy and childbirth is that these are normal, *natural* events of human life; there is no need to conceal them. The risks, as always, lie in ignorance and suppression of the facts.

Life Before Birth (Embryology)

When you were one month old, you were one-quarter of an inch long; at two months, an inch long; at three months, three inches long; at six months, a little over a foot long; and at nine months, when you were actually born, about twenty inches long. We are counting, of course, from the date of conception, not the date of birth.

Your weight increased as astonishingly as your length. The human embryo, growing in its mother's womb, weighs less than an ounce until the end of its first three months of life. At four months, on the average, it weighs six ounces; at five months, one pound; at six months nearly two pounds; at term, after nine months of intra-uterine life, about seven and a half pounds, more or less.

These facts are known to us through the science of embryology, characterized by Margaret Shea Gilbert, as writing "the biography of the unborn." Scientific inferences about human growth are based in part on microscopic examination of the embryological development of other mammals, for example, the monkey, the rabbit, and the cat.

From Egg to Embryo. Conception of the new individual occurs at the moment when sperm and ovum unite in the uterine tubes, leading from the uterus to the ovaries. The fertilized egg cell (zygote) quickly divides into two cells, the two into four, the four into eight, and so on. This process is called subdivision or cleavage. It continues while the zygote makes its way down the

LIFE BEFORE BIRTH
DEVELOPMENT OF HUMAN EMBRYO—COMPARATIVE SIZES

AT
CONCEPTION

human ovum
impregnated

amniotic sac
yolk sac
ectoderm
endoderm
mesoderm
embryonic disc

ONE-TWO
MONTHS

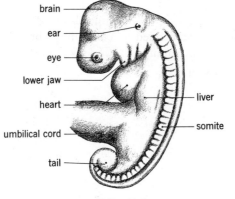

brain
ear
eye
lower jaw
heart
umbilical cord
tail
liver
somite

¾″

28-Day Embryo
(the human tadpole)

8½-Week Embryo

AT
FOUR MONTHS

4½″

4-Month Fetus

uterine tube, about a three-day journey, and while it floats, so to speak, for a week to ten days in the cavity of the uterus. During this period is uses up the food substances contained in the human egg itself. Then it attaches or embeds itself in the uterine wall prepared for its reception. By this time the subdivision of cells has advanced to a point where the single fertilized egg cell has become a hollow ball with several layers of cells. At this point it is called a morula, from the Latin word for mulberry.

Not all the cells in the morula become the embryo out of which the individual develops. Some of them are in a sense shunted off to become accessory structures necessary to the growth and development of the embryo, for example, the placenta, the umbilical cord, and the amniotic sac ("bag of waters"). The placenta, embedded in the uterus, and the umbilical cord, running from the placenta to the developing embryo, function primarily as food supply lines, for the human embryo, a true parasite on its mother, must get from her body all the nourishment it requires. The amniotic sac forms in effect an elastic bottle of fluid within which intra-uterine growth of the embryo actually takes place.

The *placenta,* called the *afterbirth* following delivery of the child, is a flat disc of tissue by which the infant is attached to the mother's womb and through which it is nourished. It grows along with the embryo and fetus. At term it is a pancake-shaped tissue, an inch or two thick, 6 to 9 inches in diameter.

The placenta interlocks with the tissues of the uterus. The nourishment for the growing child in the womb seeps through the membranes of the placenta from the maternal blood stream. These membranes filter out many things that might harm the infant. But some things, like the spirochete of syphilis, certain viruses (like that of German measles), blood elements like the Rh factor, and some drugs (including anesthetics), can get through this membrane. The growing fetus has its own blood supply and circulatory system. The mother's blood does not circulate through the infant in the womb.

The *umbilical cord* runs from the middle of the placenta to the navel (umbilicus) of the developing infant. The cord increases in size as the placenta and the infant grow. At birth the cord is usually about 2 feet long, $\frac{1}{2}$ to 1 inch in diameter. It is usually twisted, and on rare occasion a loop of it may snare the neck or limbs of the fetus.

The *amniotic sac* or "bag of waters," is a kind of elastic bottle in which the growing infant develops, floating in amniotic fluid. This fluid is secreted by the inner lining of the bag of waters (amnion). It protects the child from pressures on the mother's body and helps regulate the infant's temperature. Just before the bag of waters breaks at term, it carries between 1 and 2 pints of fluid.

The embryo proper arises from a spot on the inner layer of cells of the morula. This spot is called the embryonic disc. The disc comprises two tiny layers of cells. In very crude terms, you can imagine the shape of the disc as that of two round pancakes rolled up. For the sake of convenience we call the outside layer of cells the ectoderm and the inside layer the endoderm. Almost immediately another layer of cells begins to form between these two. This middle layer is called the mesoderm. These events occur not only in human but in all embryos. The ectoderm layer, for example, always turns out to form the outer covering—skin, scales, or feathers—as well as the nervous system and sensory organs of the creature-to-be.

We shall now trace the growth of the strictly human embryo.

The First Month of Life. The human body, as we know, is made up of a myriad of cells. The first specialized cells to appear in the embryo are young blood cells. They are found in the mesoderm layer in patches called "blood islands," and show up about seventeen days after conception. With their appearance begins the formation of the body's blood and circulatory systems. Soon thereafter, the young blood cells take predictable shape. Tiny tubules, that is, blood vessels which are forerunners of the veins and arteries, begin to form, and the blood flows through them to initiate a kind of circulation. These tiny blood vessels gradually fuse to form a "heart tube." On about the twenty-fifth day after conception this tiny heart tube, precursor of the human heart, begins pulsating or beating. It will continue beating until the creature dies. The embryo heart beats much faster than the adult's or even the child's heart.

The human nervous system takes its origin in the embryo just about the same time that the heart tube is forming. The first step in the development of the nervous system is the appearance of a "neural plate" on the ectoderm layer of tissue. This plate then "rolls up" to form a "neural tube." This tube takes position right straight down the middle of what will later take shape as the human backbone or spinal column. The front end of the neural tube eventually becomes the human brain; the tail end becomes the spinal cord.

Heart and brain begun, the embryo next goes about forming its food (alimentary) canal. In its earliest stage this structure is called the "embryonic gut." It has two parts: a foregut and a hindgut. At the head end of the foregut, tissues from the ectoderm join it to form what will be the human mouth and lips.

The Human Tadpole. A month after conception the fertilized egg cell has grown into something that resembles a tadpole. It is a soft creature, about one-quarter of an inch long; and it has a head and a tail, but scarcely a face. Yet most of the essential human organs are already in the process of formation.

The head end of the "human tadpole" is approximately one-third its total length. Its heart is so large that it bulges out against the wall of the chest-to-be. Its lungs are scarcely more than little sacs.

At four "corners" of the embryo, where arms and legs will later appear, are to be found four little nubbins of flesh described as "arm buds" and "leg buds." Along the back of the tiny human tadpole are to be discovered 38 little bundles of tissue, called "somites," from which the strong muscles of the human frame will eventually take shape.

The Second Month of Life. In the second month of life, dating here always from conception, the "tadpole" that was changes into something that can be identified as being human. We may summarize the changes during the second month of intrauterine existence by saying that it begins with a tail and ends with a face. The human tail at its longest measures only 1 to 2 millimeters; it reaches its maximum length during the fifth week of life. Then it disappears. On very rare occasions the tail fails to regress and an infant may be born with a tail.

By the end of the second month the embryo has a face, queer looking to be sure; a neck supporting a large head that is mostly brain; four limbs, the arms budding faster than the legs; five digits already in the process of formation on each limb; a trunk that houses the internal organs; some muscles; the beginnings of many bones; and internal sex organs which can often be identified as male or female.

The face is gradually put together around the head end of the foregut, where the preliminary structures of the mouth appear. The eyes, originally placed on the sides of the head, like those of a bird, converge toward their proper forward-looking position above the mouth and nose. Skin, that is, ectoderm, tissue above the eyes forms eyelids which seal the eyes shut for at least the next three months. The chin, mostly bony tissue, remains small.

The skeletal system, including bones and connective tissue, get properly under way during the second month. The "tadpole's" somites commence to swell out and form all the typical human muscles, which gradually insert themselves between the skin and the internal organs. The pattern of the bones-to-be is first laid down in a softer kind of connective tissue which we call cartilage (or "gristle"). The cartilage forms models for the bones in somewhat the same way that a sculptor forms in soft clay what he will later cast in harder stone or metal.

The process of exchanging cartilage for bone is called "ossification." The harder bone tissue contains minerals like calcium and phosphorus.

The bones of the skull and the face are an exception to the general rule for the ossification of ribs, backbone, long bones of the legs and arms, and other bones. The skull and face bones, some seventeen in all, are not first modeled in cartilage. They do not become completely and finally fused into one another to form a solid skull until the embryo has grown into an adult. The newborn infant normally has certain soft spots, called fontanelles, on his skull where the bones have not yet fused.

Beginning of Sex Differentiation. The sex of the person-to-be, is determined at the time of conception. During the second month of life those embryonic organs which will eventually be parts of the finished sexual apparatus of the adult man or woman begin to develop. By the end of the seventh week of life the internal sex organs of the embryo can usually be identified by an embryologist as either male or female.

The first internal sex organs developed in the embryo are the same for both sexes. Later they differentiate.

The sex-organs-to-be take their origin and make their first appearance on the embryo's middle kidney. There during the second month of life appears a little ridge of flesh, which embryologists call either a "genital" or a "sexual" ridge. Within it develop the individual's first "primitive" sex organs.

On the surface of the ridge are to be found growing little cords of cells, called "genital cords." The cords push or infiltrate their way down below the surface of the ridge. They make a place for themselves in the interior of the ridge which is then properly described as a sex gland or gonad.

If the embryo is to be a male, the genital cords continue growing as they started. They become the tubules of the testicles (seminiferous tubules), where the male in part manufactures his sperm.

However, if the embryo is to be a female, the genital cords stop growing and a new process takes place. Now from the surface, not the interior, of the tiny gonad (later to be a true ovary) a new set of cells start to grow. These surface cells are the forerunners of what will later be the female's egg cells.

The remarkable thing to be observed here is

that inside every female ovary there is the undeveloped (embryonic) testis of the male.

The external sex organs in the male or female embryo do not become visible and apparent until the third month of life, though they start out in the same way during the second month. At this earlier time just in front of the "human tadpole's" tail can be located a little protuberance which the embryologists describe as the "genital tubercle." It appears the same in both sexes. Later it will develop into the penis in the male and its homologue (similar structure), the clitoris, in the female.

The Third Month of Life. By the time the embryo begins its third month of life, its internal organs have been pretty well laid down. We have now the recognizable sketch of a human being. It is all out of proportion, like a child's crude drawing of the human figure. Here are some of the important details in the development of the living creature that are filled in during the third month of life:

Sex emerges, more rapidly evident in the male than in the female. The teeth begin to sprout, though they will not become visible above the gum margins for years. Arms, legs, hands, and feet become more fully formed. Fingernails and toenails appear. The ears are formed. Liver, stomach, and kidneys commence functioning.

The stomach begins tentatively to pour out mucus; and other parts of the alimentary tract stir vaguely toward functioning. The liver starts its life-long job of manufacturing bile and takes on the temporary task of making red blood cells. The manufacture of mature red blood cells is eventually taken over by the bone marrow.

Mouth and jaws, nose and throat, including vocal cords, become more fully fashioned during this third month. On the rudimentary framework of the upper and lower jaws-to-be there now appears a dental ridge. Beneath it are soon to be found small cones of cells which turn out to be the "tooth buds" for the child's first set of baby (deciduous) teeth. There are normally ten sockets for baby teeth in each jaw. The dental ridge then sinks deeper into the jawbone, where it sets out buds for the thirty-two adult (permanent) teeth that will make their appearance above the gums anywhere from six to twenty years later.

After the third month the embryo is usually called a fetus. This change in name is a purely arbitrary matter, for which there is no special reason.

Fourth, Fifth, and Sixth Months of Life. During the fourth, fifth, and sixth months of life, the normal fetus makes rapid strides toward physiological maturity. As it leaps in weight from an ounce at the end of the third month to about two pounds at the end of the sixth, its presence generally becomes evident to the outside world in the rounding contour of its mother's abdomen.

The fourth month usually marks the time when the mother first feels a "quickening in the womb." This means that the fetus has grown to a stage where it can begin to move about.

Another interesting development in the fourth month is the increase in the volume and intensity of the fetal heart beat. With the use of a stethoscope, which conducts sound, the physician can often hear this minuscule heart beating through the mother's abdomen.

The forging of the human brain also makes significant progress at this time. The growth of the brain, which commenced in the "neural groove," is gradual. At first the hindbrain is most conspicuous. The midbrain appears less important. Most slowly developed of all is the forebrain. This is the part of the brain which gives rise to the large cerebral hemispheres of the adult where, it is commonly held, the real "thinking" part of the brain is located.

During the fourth month convolutions ("wrinkles") appear in the cerebral hemispheres of the fetus. From then on the brain develops with astonishing rapidity. Soon it outruns every other mammal's brain in complexity and capacity for ideation.

Beginning in the fourth month many changes occur in the external appearance of the fetus. The external sex organs for both sexes become more specifically delineated. Eyebrows and eyelashes may appear. A fine, soft, down-like hair, called "lanugo," covers the gnome-like body. Often it is especially prominent on the face. The dark-wine color of the skin, which is produced by the blood vessels showing through it, becomes slightly less pronounced as the skin adds a few layers of thickness. The whorls and ridges on the skin of the toes and fingers are more or less fully patterned at this time; the four-month-old fetus already has the fingerprints by which he can be identified for the rest of his life.

In the fifth month real hair, something more than lanugo, shows up on the head of the fetus. Fingernails and toenails are also to be found, growing out beyond the tips of fingers and toes. Sweat glands and sebaceous (oil-secreting) glands come into being.

By the fifth month the internal organs are all present but they have not yet assumed the size, position, and function that they will have at birth. Heart and liver, for example, are still comparatively large and high up in the body framework. As the fetus continues to grow, its back straightens, its trunk lengthens, and its internal organs settle into their proper places.

During the sixth month of intrauterine life the fetus begins to open its eyes, previously sealed shut. The eyes at birth usually appear an indeterminate gray-blue color.

The Final Months of Intrauterine Life. During the seventh, eighth, and ninth months of normal intrauterine life the fetus fills out and develops in many ways. It gains much weight and strength. It waxes fat; its skin loses its wrinkles and improves in color. In the male an especially important event normally occurs during the seventh month, namely, the testes descend from their place of origin in the abdomen to the scrotal sac appended outside the body trunk.

During its sojourn in the uterus, the human fetus can theoretically assume any position and it certainly does move around. However, it rarely assumes strange or abnormal positions. About 95% of the time it grows head down.

The normal gestation period of the human infant is about forty weeks or nine months. Some infants, born prematurely[1], are not fully enough

[1] Technically speaking, any newborn infant weighing less than 2500 grams ($5\frac{1}{2}$ pounds) is considered premature.

developed to withstand the shock of birth and of facing survival outside their intrauterine homes. The less the premature infant weighs at birth, the lower are his chances of survival, yet many can be saved and continue their development to full maturity.

Pregnancy

Pregnancy begins with conception and ends with childbirth (labor) or abortion (miscarriage).

In the very early stages of pregnancy even the wisest doctor may find it difficult to make a positive diagnosis. False pregnancies, with many of the classic symptoms of pregnancy, are sometimes discovered in women who have an overwhelming fear or desire of having a child. Tumors sometimes mimic pregnancy.

A delayed or missed menstrual period may raise a *suspicion* of pregnancy, but it should not be taken as a certainty that pregnancy has occurred. If *two* periods are missed, the woman should consult her doctor.

Starting about two weeks after a missed period, the condition of pregnancy can usually be confirmed by a laboratory test, the "mouse" or "rabbit test." These tests are about 98% accurate, but they do give a few false positives and false

PLACENTA includes:

(1) blood sinuses (mothers blood)

(2) fingerlike projections of the chorion

(3) blood vessels leading to and from the embryo

umbilical cord

muscle layer of uterine wall

lining of uterus (endometrium)

chorion

amnion

amniotic cavity filled with amniotic fluid

uterine cavity

mucous secretion

vagina (birth canal)

THE UTERUS IN PREGNANCY. This is a diagrammatic cross section of the uterus containing a fetus about three months old. The cross section of the placenta is very much simplified.

THE FIGURE IN PREGNANCY. A. This is a diagrammatic cross section of the mother's body at the beginning of pregnancy. B. This is the same figure at full term, just before the child is to be born. The figure returns to normal shortly after childbirth. Many women have better figures after bearing one or more (but not an excessive number of) children.

negatives. In the rabbit (Friedman) test, a sample of the woman's urine is injected into the ear of a virgin rabbit. If the woman is pregnant, changes in the rabbit's ovaries can be detected within 24 to 48 hours.

The rabbit and mouse tests, and all others depending on reactions in test animals (for example, toads and fish), are based on this fact: when pregnancy occurs, there is a drastic change in the hormone and endocrine balance of the body. This, incidentally, explains in part why many women feel different during pregnancy. Some may feel wonderful, others melancholy.

In particular, large quantities of gonad-stimulating hormones are made and released into the blood stream in early pregnancy. The kidneys extract hormones from the blood stream and release them into the urine. It is these hormones that stimulate the changes in the sex organs of the test animals, such as the virgin rabbit.

Timetable of Pregnancy. The following timetable suggests what a woman going through a normal, uneventful pregnancy may anticipate although, needless to say, not all women have the same experience.

1st Month. Within 2 to 3 weeks after conception, the suspicion of missing a period must arise.

Some of the early symptoms of pregnancy, described below, may appear at this time, but they usually come on somewhat later.

2nd Month. Morning sickness—nausea and vomiting—may develop; it is not inevitable. Easy fatigue, extreme sleepiness, full and sensitive breasts, frequent urination often appear—but not all these symptoms in all women.

3rd Month. The breasts begin to enlarge; the ring around the nipples may darken. The abdomen is not yet noticeably extended, but the uterus can be felt either as a small hard ball or softening and enlarging. The feeling of fatigue may be tremendous. An appetite for "strange foods" may begin. Neither symptom is essential.

4th Month. The pregnancy usually begins to show on the abdomen, unless concealed by obesity or artful dressing. Gain in weight commences. This usually continues at the rate of about *3 pounds a month,* with considerable variation in different women.

5th and 6th Months. The quickening of the baby is definitely felt by the mother; these at first are light, fluttery movements. Later they can be felt as definite kicks against the wall of the enlarged abdomen. The baby's rapid heartbeat can be definitely heard by the doctor.

7th and 8th Months. The rapidly growing baby kicks vigorously against the still-enlarging abdomen, on which striations, or stretch marks, usually appear. Skin color on the abdomen and face may darken slightly, but not permanently. A few drops of fluid—colostrum, a precursor of mother's milk—may begin to flow from the breasts. Weight gain continues.

9th Month. The abdomen no longer enlarges. The fetal movements are felt less often, less vigorously. This is nothing to worry about. The enlarged uterus may cause pressure symptoms on other abdominal organs and on the veins, giving symptoms of temporarily enlarged veins in the legs. The need for frequent urination is common. However, the expectant mother is often filled with unusual energy at this time. She cleans house, buys clothes, gets ready for the baby.

About 2 weeks before childbirth, the infant's head may begin to sink into the pelvic cavity and the uterus correspondingly descends with it. This is the "lightening." The woman usually feels more comfortable.

At last, somewhere around 280 days after conception, labor begins and the baby is born.

The Date of Birth. When will the baby be born? In round numbers, 280 days, 40 weeks, or 9 months after the day of conception. But there is no way of foretelling this *exactly,* because no one yet knows what sets off the trigger mechanism of normal labor. Unless the labor is artificially induced or Caesarean section done, the exact date of birth cannot be assured. A common method of predicting birth date (Naegle's rule) is to add 7 days to the date of the first day of the last menstruation and then count back 3 months. Only 1 in 10 babies is born on this calculated calendar date. But 75% are born within 2 weeks of this time.

Prenatal Care

Pregnancy is a natural, normal physiological process. The hazards of pregnancy are today comparatively few, and the discomforts are more often determined by the woman's own psychological attitude toward her particular pregnancy than by anything else.

Some women are depressed by their pregnancies, especially if they have had any trouble before or have borne many children. Other women find their health improved during pregnancy (relief from arthritis or migraine, for example, often occurs).

Nulliparas (women who have not been pregnant nor had a child before) are likely to be overenthusiastic, overmeticulous, and overfearful. Such anxiety in the presence of what is, after all, a profoundly important experience is natural and to be anticipated.

From the standpoint of the patient, prenatal care looks deceptively simple. From the doctor's standpoint it often requires consummate skill to keep the patient and her human freight out of trouble.

Personal hygiene during pregnancy is the same as good health care at any other time, magnified by the responsibility for the life and health of two (or more) lives instead of one.

A patient receiving adequate prenatal care from a private physician or a clinic is expected to:

1. See the doctor regularly—once a month during the early months of pregnancy, twice a month or oftener in the later stages.

2. Bring urine samples when requested.

3. Do what her doctor tells her and not listen to old wives' tales, the misinformation peddled by well-meaning friends, sensational magazine articles, or half-baked books.

4. Report promptly to the doctor any unusual signs or symptoms of disease or any sudden changes in her condition.

Repeated urinalyses are performed because the kidneys are under special strain in pregnancy; the waste products from the fetal circulation are passed back into the mother's blood stream by way of the placenta, and these wastes are removed from the maternal blood by the kidneys.

Childbirth

Pregnancy normally terminates in labor, that is to say, in the spontaneous delivery of a healthy, well-developed, full-term infant.

Labor. *Labor* is well named. The uterine and

other muscles work hard. The mother sweats, sometimes losing several pints of fluid. A normal fatigue usually follows labor. Women accustomed to hard physical labor every day may be less affected by childbirth.

Labor is normally divided into three stages. The *first* stage extends from the beginning of labor pains to the time of full dilation (opening) of the mouth or neck of the womb. It is the longest stage, lasting perhaps 10 to 16 hours with the first baby. The *second* stage extends from the time of the dilation of the cervix until the actual birth of the baby. It may take anywhere up to 2 hours. The *third* stage extends from the birth of the baby to the expulsion of the afterbirth (placenta). It may be completed in 2 or 3, but usually 5 to 10 minutes.

The length of labor varies in different women and in the same women in different pregnancies. Rarely it may be over in less time than it takes for a taxicab to get to a hospital. On the average, a woman bearing her first child will be in labor for about 18 hours; if she has already had a child, about 12 hours.

NORMAL SPONTANEOUS DELIVERY I. At term, as the first stage of labor begins. This illustration shows the position of the fetus in the uterus at the beginning of labor. The cervix has not begun to dilate (open up).

NORMAL SPONTANEOUS DELIVERY II. At the end of the first and the beginning of the second stage of labor. The rupture of the membranes ("bag of waters") usually occurs at the end of the first stage of labor. The cervix of the uterus is now completely dilated.

Labor pains usually begin in the small of the back and progress to the abdomen. True labor pains are always associated with contractions of the uterus. Between pains (contractions) there is usually no discomfort. The first contractions may occur every quarter or half hour and last a quarter to half a minute. The pains gradually begin to last longer, to become more frequent and intense, and to come at more regular intervals. As soon as they become *regular* it is time to call a doctor and, on his advice, to be off to the hospital. *False* labor pains often occur, frequently about a month before the baby is born. The

diagnosis here is a problem for the doctor. False labor pains are usually irregular.

Delivery. Most women are admitted to the hospital while still in the first stage of labor. The woman is immediately put to bed and prepared by nurses for an aseptic delivery. Pubic hair is shaved, an enema usually given. Members of the hospital house-staff of physicians may look in and perhaps examine the patient. Her pains are timed by an attendant. If necessary, one or more drugs may be injected to help relieve pain or discomfort.

When examination reveals that the cervix is

NORMAL SPONTANEOUS DELIVERY III. The second stage of labor, when the child is actually born. The infant's head is impelled into the birth canal (vagina), now greatly enlarged, by the force of uterine contractions. The top of the infant's head appears here at the vaginal orifice.

NORMAL SPONTANEOUS DELIVERY IV. The moment of birth, the end of the second stage of labor. The physician gently grasps the head of the infant and prepares to help the rest of his body into the world.

fully dilated—it has a temporary diameter of about 4 inches—the mother-soon-to-be is taken into the delivery room, usually on a wheel table, and placed on the delivery table. It has elevated leg rests, or stirrups, on two corners.

The woman lies on her back, her feet elevated by the leg rests. Her body is draped with sheets.

About this time the bag of waters breaks, and amniotic fluid pours out of the vagina. This sometimes happens early in the first stage of labor, causing a so-called *dry labor*. In other cases, the doctor has to puncture a thick amniotic membrane.

The rhythmic contractions of the uterus continue, exerting a powerful force squeezing the child out into the world. The contractions or pains cannot be voluntarily controlled by the mother. She can, however, "bear down" by using abdominal muscles to help along the contractions. Or she can relax and let the uterus work.

At length, in about 95 out of 100 cases, the top of the baby's head appears at the vaginal orifice. It recedes somewhat as the contraction that brought it down subsides. With each new contraction, the baby's head comes out farther and farther—and finally does not recede between pains.

At this point the doctor grasps the child under the chin. He turns the head gently to one side and then the other as he releases the shoulder. The rest of the child can be easily lifted out of the birth canal. The infant is still attached to his mother by the umbilical cord.

While waiting for the third stage of labor to be concluded (delivery of the afterbirth), the doctor immediately swabs out the baby's mouth and waits for the first cry. Most infants cry lustily as soon as they are born (a few, even, just before). If regular breathing is not quickly established, the doctor may hold the baby upside down, give him a few gentle slaps on the buttocks, or if necessary, apply a tiny oxygen mask. Breathing air is the first of the many new experiences that await the baby. Rapid changes occur in his lungs and heart while he is getting used to it.

After a final surge of blood from the placenta, the umbilical cord is tied off, about 3 inches above the navel, and cut. The cord stump is covered with a sterile dressing and placed over the abdomen. Infection must be avoided.

Drops of silver nitrate or other acceptable antiseptic (e.g., penicillin) are immediately put into the baby's eyes to protect against possible blindness from gonorrheal infection. The baby is cleaned off as much as necessary, wrapped in a blanket, weighed, footprinted, encircled with an identification bracelet (so that babies can't possibly get mixed up), and placed in a warm crib.

When the afterbirth is expelled, the physician examines it to be sure that it is all out. Immediately after the child has been expelled, the uterus begins to contract. In so doing it squeezes off the blood vessels that were broken when the placenta was torn off. To speed this process and prevent needless bleeding, the doctor may give drugs (ergot and pituitrin), which are called *oxytocics*. Only $\frac{1}{4}$ to $\frac{1}{2}$ pint of blood is usually lost. If more, it can be promptly replaced by transfusion.

Following delivery the new mother usually sleeps. Doctors now make every effort to get the mother back on her feet as soon as possible after childbirth—anywhere from the first day on. A few days' to a week's convalescence in the hospital is usually enough—if there are no complications. Many women are anxious to leave earlier. The maternity ward is usually the gayest one in the hospital. A gradually increasing schedule of activity and social life is desirable. Visitors with colds or other communicable infections should not be welcomed. It takes about six weeks for the mother's body to return to the size and shape it had before pregnancy.

Complications of Childbirth. These do occur, but most of them are prevented by adequate prenatal care. Approximately 95% of all babies present themselves to the world head first and go through the normal spontaneous delivery just described. In about 4% the buttocks show first (breech presentation). In the other 1% a shoulder, leg or arm may first present. All these presentations can be handled by appropriate obstetric maneuvers ("turning the baby"), delivery by the breech, or by Caesarean section.

"Painless Childbirth." *Painless childbirth* has been a goal of obstetrics since the middle of the nineteenth century, shortly after the discovery of ether as a surgical anesthetic. In 1853 Queen Victoria accepted obstetric anesthesia during the birth of her seventh child—and women everywhere have since demanded painless childbirth. The Queen got intermittent doses of chloroform, just enough at each labor pang to ease the pain but not enough to make her unconscious.

A great variety of anesthetic agents are now available for obstetric anesthesia and analgesia (painkilling without loss of consciousness). Used with discretion they have relatively little effect on the baby. Present-day *"twilight sleep"* is produced by a mixture of an analgesic (painkilling) drug, such as Demerol, with an amnesic drug, like scopolamine, that temporarily wipes out memory. Other methods are nerve-blocking injections of local anesthetics in the pelvic region, for example, caudal anesthesia, in which injections are made at the tail end of the spinal cord.

Education for childbirth is another direction of effort to reduce labor pains. These are the techniques that have been given the name *"natural childbirth."* Their aim is to reduce false fears about childbirth and thus greatly diminish the pains associated with it. In many cases, it may help to reduce pains, but it rarely eliminates them. Hypnotism has also been tried in a few selected cases of childbirth.

Needless fear of childbirth has been bred into many young women by their families and associates—and blithely accepted by their husbands. A classic cartoon shows a young husband and his wife, who is ready for delivery, entering the admitting office of a hospital. The caption reads, "Honey, are you sure you want to go through with this?" Some women (and men) fear childbirth because they heard their mothers and other female relatives complain of it. Others fear childbirth because it is associated with what Gutt-macher calls "the larger, terrifying fear of sex." Childbirth is no picnic, but abnormal, neurotic fear undoubtedly tightens up the muscles employed in childbirth and makes it seem more difficult.

Abortion. A high percentage of pregnancies—perhaps one-third—terminate in abortion, a word of ugly connotation. When applied to induced, criminal abortions ("illegal operations"), this connotation is correct. However, it should be noted that there are also therapeutic abortions and spontaneous abortions. Scientifically, abortion may be defined as the "detachment or expulsion of the previable ovum, embryo, or fetus." A therapeutic abortion is generally defined as one undertaken, on appropriate medical indications, "to save the life and health of the mother." If performed in a licensed hospital, two licensed, competent physicians must sign an affirmation and diagnosis. In the late 1960's a wave of legislative activity concerning therapeutic abortion began to sweep through many states; the issue even reached the U.S. Supreme Court. The movement to take abortion out of the realm of law and put it into the hands of the medical profession gained many supporters, who contend that abortion is *solely* a medical problem and that government has no business regulating it.

The terms "spontaneous abortion" and "miscarriage" are synonyms. They describe the involuntary, undesired expulsion and loss of the embryo or fetus and hence the termination of pregnancy through the first seven months (28 weeks) of pregnancy. If this event occurs after the seventh month, it is called premature birth. When an infant is born dead, it is termed a stillbirth.

Miscarriages, or spontaneous abortions, usually occur during the first three months of pregnancy. The causes are imperfectly known and difficult to attribute to specific cases. More than half are owing to some abnormality in the formation or imbedding of the egg. It can be said, however, that falls, jars, violent blows, and other forms of physical trauma must be classed as secondary or precipitating rather than primary causes of miscarriage. Spontaneous abortion is a medical problem; induced abortion a social problem, and an ancient one.

It is the consensus of opinion in the United States today that a criminal, induced abortion is the worst way out of an "unwanted pregnancy." And yet the latest Kinsey figures show that among American wives 17% of pregnancies end in induced abortion.

Sterility. Approximately 1 in 10 to 15 marriages in the United States appears to be sterile; that is, the married couple desire children, have marriage relationships over a period of a year or more, but the wife does not conceive. Much medical research has been directed at this problem of sterility. For a third to a half of the couples who would formerly have been doomed to involuntary childlessness, proper medical treatment now makes conception, pregnancy, and the birth of a healthy child possible.

The causes of sterility, infertility, or barrenness, as it is called, are various. In almost half the cases the husband is at least partially at fault. In very many instances sterility is *relative* rather than absolute. Either mate might be able to have a child with a different partner, or after suitable treatment, or after a lapse of time. Occasionally, a long-childless couple finally manage to adopt a baby and shortly thereafter have a baby of their own.

SUMMARY REVIEW QUESTIONS

1. What is the difference between Victorian and modern attitudes toward pregnancy and childbirth? How do you account for them?
2. How would you describe in some detail the process of life before birth?
3. What temporary anatomical structures—embryo excluded—develop in the uterus during pregnancy? What is the function of each one and what happens to it at childbirth?
4. How is a diagnosis of pregnancy made? Be explicit.
5. How does the "timetable of pregnancy" correlate with the intrauterine life of the infant-to-be?
6. From the standpoint of either (*a*) a prospective father or (*b*) an expectant mother, what do you consider to be the essentials of "adequate prenatal care?"
7. Beginning with the first suspicion of "labor pains," what are the subsequent stages or steps of normal spontaneous delivery of a newborn child?
8. How do you distinguish between (1) spontaneous, (2) induced, (3) therapeutic, and (4) criminal abortion?
9. Are the following statements sense or nonsense? Why? *The process of childbirth is and forever will be a mystery. . . . Childbirth is exclusively a woman's business. . . . Sterility is incurable. . . . A healthy human embryo weighs at least one pound within one month after conception. . . . The very best man in the world/ Must take his child on faith alone;/ The very worst woman in the world/ Knows her child's her own.*
10. What do the following terms mean to you: zygote, embryo, fetus, premature infant, relative sterility, ossification, "natural childbirth," the "quickening," "rabbit test," miscarriage.

Worth Consulting: *The Story of Human Birth* by Alan Guttmacher, M.D. *Childbirth without Fear* by Grantly Dick Read, M.D. *Biography of the Unborn* by Margaret Shea Gilbert. *Expectant Motherhood* by Nicholas Eastman, M.D.

11

THE BIG KILLERS:

HEART DISEASE AND CANCER

I F YOU ARE NOT KILLED MEANWHILE BY ACCI- dent, the chances are 2 out of 3 that you will die either of heart disease or cancer—the two degenerative diseases that are now far and away the big killers of Americans. The older you grow the more likely you are to die of one or the other.

Principal Causes of Death

In 1900 the five principal causes of death in the United States were, in order: (1) tuberculosis, (2) pneumonia, (3) diarrhea and inflammation of intestines, (4) heart disease, and (5) diseases of infancy and malformations.

Today the list of the big killers runs: (1) heart and circulatory diseases, (2) cancer, (3) stroke, (4) accidents, and (5) certain diseases and conditions of early infancy.

The causes of death differ at different ages in life. Accidents, however, top the list from childhood through age 45.

The leading causes of infant mortality (under 1 year of age) now rank as (1) premature birth, (2) postnatal asphyxia and atelectasis, (3) congenital malformations, (4) other diseases of early infancy, and (5) pneumonia and influenza.

Among preschool children (ages 2 through 4) the five chief killers are, in order: accidents, cancer, congenital malformations, pneumonia, gastritis and enteritis.

Elementary and junior-high-school students (ages 5 through 14) succumb, in order, to: acci- dents, cancer, congenital malformations, and pneumonia.

In the senior-high-school and college-age bracket (ages 15 through 24) the picture changes to: accidents, cancer, suicide, heart disease, and murder.

Young adults and parents (ages 25 to 44) die chiefly, in order, from: accidents, heart disease, cancer, suicide, and stroke.

The middle-aged (ages 45 to 64) are fatally stricken with, in order: heart disease, cancer, stroke, accidents, and suicide.

The aged (65 and over) are killed by, in order: heart disease, cancer, stroke, hardening of the arteries, and accidents.

Heart Disease

In the United States heart disease is now responsible for close to 700,000 deaths a year, approximately 40% of all deaths. Related diseases of the circulatory system kill 250,000 more people. In total these conditions are the primary cause of more than one out of every two deaths in the United States.

We must consider diseases of the heart, blood vessels, and kidneys together since they operate that way. Disease or damage in any one of these three sets of organs is sooner or later reflected in the other two. We speak therefore of the *cardiovascularenal* system: "cardio" for heart, "vascular" for blood vessels, and "renal" for kidneys. When we talk about heart disease, we are really talking about cardiovascular diseases.

Over 90% of all cardiovascularenal deaths are associated with hardening of the arteries—(arteriosclerosis and atherosclerosis) and high blood pressure (hypertension). Blood-vessel damage in the brain—commonly called "stroke"—accounts for about 200,000 deaths a year in the United States.

At any given time somewhere between 10 and 11 million people in the United States are walking around with cardiovascularenal disease. (Only about 5% of the victims are confined to bed.) If you add to the count varicose veins, minor vascular ailments, and unobserved "little strokes," you can calculate that well over 10% of the American population is afflicted with cardiovascularenal ailments.

Discounting the Statistical Picture. Yet, the average person faces no greater risk of dying of heart disease than his grandfather did in 1900. The increase in cardiovascular deaths reflects the success of medicine and public health in preventing earlier deaths from infectious diseases. It also reflects the increased life span of the American population. Approximately two-thirds of cardiovascularenal deaths occur after the age of 65. The death rate from cardiovascular disease has remained constant for the last twenty years.

The hardworking circulatory system is usually the first to wear out as life forces diminish. When we announce that cardiovascularenal diseases account for 55% of the total mortality in the United States, we must also remember that the final total is 100%. Man is mortal. If the Angel of Death were not now using this big cardiovascularenal scythe, he could equally well use others, and more painful ones, as he has in the past. Indeed it has been stated that a high percentage of deaths from stroke is an index of a generally healthy community.

The real problem in cardiovascularenal diseases is the effective treatment and management of patients who come down with these conditions in the prime of life, or earlier. Here great advances have been and still are being made.

It was not so long ago that cardiovascular syphilis accounted for 25% of all heart disease. Today it is considerably less than 1%. Rheumatic heart disease is also on the wane, thanks largely to improved antibiotics, used effectively and widely as a preventive measure. Rheumatic fever control programs, now in operation in many states, afford an excellent example of the wedding of personal and community health.

Research Developments. The dramatic highlights of recent research progress in cardiovascularenal diseases lie in the fields of heart surgery, the discovery and development of new drugs, and in a better practical understanding of the treatment of the *complications* of high blood pressure and hardening of the arteries. The causes of these vascular conditions, however, still remain obscure and unproved.

Entirely new and life-saving types of heart surgery are now being routinely developed. These have been made possible by new pumping machines, "artificial hearts," that keep up the blood circulation of the body during an operation on the heart, and by techniques for actually stopping the heart. The surgeon can now work with a heart that lies still instead of wiggling and jumping out of his hands.

A triumph in heart surgery came in 1968. Surgeons then succeeded in transplanting a "healthy" heart from one person, just deceased, to another person whose heart was so barely competent that early death could be predicted. Many patients did not live too long after the operation, for they were "bad risk" patients to begin with. However, Dr. Christian Barnard of the Union of South Africa succeeded in transplanting a human heart into a 69-year-old dentist, Philip Blaiberg, who lived for many months after the operation.

Just a few years ago there were no drugs that could safely and effectively reduce blood pressure. Now there are scores—including reserpine and other rauwolfia derivatives.

The complications of hardening arteries can also now be better managed with newly developed drugs. Among them are anticoagulants, drugs which help prevent the formation of blood clots; other drugs which forestall or suppress abnormal heart rhythms, the fatal flutter that sometimes follows heart attacks; and drugs which dilate the arteries of the heart, so that new pathways of circulation can be opened.

High Blood Pressure. Blood pressure represents the force of the blood beating back against the walls of the blood vessels. High blood pressure (hypertension) means added pressure on these walls. This makes the heart pump harder, eventually weakening it, and it increases the risk that blood vessels will break. In hypertension the systolic blood pressure may creep over the 200 (millimeters of mercury) mark. This might not be too serious if the blood vessels and the rest of the cardiovascularenal system could take it. Some people's can, but most cannot. Something has to give—commonly an artery in the heart or brain.

If you do have a tendency toward high blood pressure, there is a good chance that you inherited it. This will be especially true if you are short and stocky in build, plump, and "just can't sit still." The average life expectancy of an individual who suffers from high blood pressure is around 20 years from the onset of the disease. However, in any given case, the outcome of the raised blood pressure will depend on three factors: (1) how high the pressure goes, which is the least important of the three factors; (2) how long it stays up—the number of months or years is an important but not the decisive factor; and (3) how well the blood vessels can take it—this is the crux of the matter. Here too heredity counts. You may inherit blood vessels that can take the higher pressure and not break.

Frequent nosebleeds or, in women, excessive menstrual flow (menorrhagia) sometimes indicate that blood vessels cannot take high pressure very well. Other common, but not necessarily definitive, symptoms of high blood pressure include: headaches, fatigue, dizziness, lightheadedness, vertigo (you seem to be spinning around or the world is spinning around you, and a blackout sometimes follows), and a tendency to easy and blotchy blushing, often accompanied by rumbling of the bowels.

Hardening and Fattening of the Arteries. If death from heart or blood-vessel disease has to be pinned on to a specific cause, the right one is usually hardening of the arteries (arteriosclerosis) or fattening of the same (atherosclerosis). It will be remembered that each artery or arteriole has three coats or layers: an inner lining, thin and smooth as mucous membrane and called the intima; a middle layer, the media; and an outer layer, the adventitia. These living tissues get their nourishment from tiny capillaries and from the blood plasma they are carrying. The middle and outer layers of the arteries and arterioles are subject to hardening—getting arteriosclerotic. Sometimes they get as hard as pipe-stems.

Something else happens to the inner lining. It fattens. In more exact terms it suffers from *atherosclerosis*. It loses its smoothness; it becomes thickened, roughened and studded with little projections, which are primarily fat (lipid) particles.

The accumulation of these fat particles on the inner lining of the arteries has several unfortunate consequences. In the first place it narrows the bore or diameter of a vessel, clogging it up like a deposit of lime or rust inside a water pipe. This decreases the amount of blood that the vessel can carry and therefore increases the pressure necessary to force it through. Second, these extraneous fat particles stuck in the arterial walls invite the formation of blood clots.

Blood tends to clot far more easily when in contact with rough or scarred surfaces. If a clot stays where it forms on the inside of a blood vessel, it is called a *thrombus*. If it breaks away, it becomes an *embolus*. Both thrombi and emboli can clog blood vessels.

The fatty material that tends to stick in the inner walls of the arteries is primarily the chemical substance known as cholesterol, although fatty substances, notably triglycerides, are also involved. One important explanation of the mechanism by which atherosclerosis occurs begins with the obvious fact that fats (or lipids) cannot be dissolved in water. These fats can only be brought into water solution, and thus managed by the blood stream (plasma) and other body tissues when they are combined with proteins; thus they become "lipoproteins."

These are relatively large molecules and unstable in the sense that the bond between the fat and the protein is not always a strong one. These larger molecules may tend to get stuck in certain artery walls; furthermore, after they are stuck, the protein tends to get washed away by the blood plasma, while the fat particles of the molecule remain in the artery wall—and make trouble.

With the facts at hand, it is probably fair to consider atherosclerosis itself a metabolic disease, or at least a metabolic defect in the body's handling of certain fats (lipids) and lipoproteins. It should be noted that atherosclerosis is rare in women before the menopause. This may be attributed to the large quantities of female sex hormone in their bodies. Indeed, it has been shown that the administration of female sex hormone to *men* will inhibit atherosclerosis; but this process has a feminizing effect and reduces libido—to which the men object.

The relationship of female sex hormones to the inhibition of atherosclerosis and the importance of the relationship of atherosclerosis to cardiovascular disease and deaths explains why heart disease kills one and a half times as many men as women. Between the ages of 45 and 65 nearly three times as many men as women die of heart disease.

Types of Heart Disease

There are at least 20 kinds of *organic* heart disease that actually affect the heart muscle, the valves of the heart, or its inner or outer linings. There are also a number of functional disorders of the heart in which its function or action is altered. Heart trouble may be primary, or secondary to other diseases. The most common and serious forms of organic heart disease are those affecting the coronary arteries, which supply blood to the heart.

A *heart attack* is usually a case of *coronary thrombosis,* described below. *Heart failure* may be a late consequence of this or other conditions. This group of heart troubles is predominantly, but not exclusively, associated with the middle and later years of life.

Infections present the second large class of causes of organic heart disease. *Rheumatic fever,* or rheumatic heart disease, associated with certain streptococcal ("strep") infections, heads the list. Syphilis, diphtheria, tuberculosis, typhoid fever, and other infections can also injure the heart. Fortunately, these diseases can usually be treated (or prevented) before they cause heart damage.

Congenital heart defects, which develop before birth and are usually discovered shortly thereafter, account for about 2% of all heart defects. "Blue babies" have a congenital defect that permits the bluer venous blood to mix with arterial blood. Surgical operation for the correction of this condition is now commonplace.

Functional murmurs of the heart, sometimes heard through the physician's stethoscope, have little, if any, significance and should not be taken as a focus of worry. Some people also suffer from an irritable heart; they become acutely conscious of premature or extra beats of the heart. Generally speaking, this condition is not serious in the absence of organic lesions.

Other functional disorders of the heart include disturbances of psychic or emotional origin. In these cases the patient fears and believes that he has heart disease when he does not. He nevertheless develops symptoms associated with it, such as palpitation, shortness of breath, extreme fatigue, and dizzy spells. This condition has many names; for example, in World War I it was labeled "soldier's heart."

Because heart disease can be so specifically classified and so much more accurately diagnosed today, more specific and effective treatment is possible for each kind of heart disease. Not so many years ago coronary thrombosis was often diagnosed as acute indigestion.

Heart Attack. Every minute of the year somebody in the United States has a heart attack. Heart attack is the popular term for what physicians call *coronary thrombosis* (also coronary occlusion, coronary closure, and myocardial infarction). Heart attacks can be suddenly fatal, but the great majority—an estimated 85%—are not. The patient recovers under proper treatment and goes on to live many useful years. A heart attack is not a sentence to permanent invalidism.

The *average* life expectancy following a heart attack is better than 10 years. The younger the victim, the greater the future life expectancy. At least one-third of all heart-attack victims will be able to return to their full schedule of previous work and activity. Another third will have to take life easier than they did before. Still another third will have to take it much easier. Only about 1 victim in 20 will remain a bed-ridden invalid.

Although the attack is sudden, the conditions underlying it have been developing for years. For reasons still obscure, the inner linings (intima) of the arteries have gradually become thickened and roughened, the condition known as *atherosclerosis*. The coronary arteries, which supply blood to the heart, are subject to these changes. The narrowed channel slows down the flow of blood, and the roughened surface provides greater opportunity for a blood clot to form on the wall. This stationary clot is called a thrombus. At the moment such a clot cuts off the blood supply to part of the heart the heart attack occurs.

If a large coronary artery is suddenly closed up, the attack may be fatal. However, in most cases, the blood detours around the blocked artery by way of other blood vessels. This is called *collateral circulation*, and it is the road to recovery.

The condition leading to heart attack is atherosclerosis in the lining of the coronary arteries. Since heart attacks are far more common in men than in women, it has been said, "Women deposit their fat under the skin, while men deposit it in the walls of their coronary arteries." Because the body itself is able to manufacture large amounts of cholesterol from foods that contain none, the use of fat-free or other special diets cannot be depended on to prevent atherosclerosis or heart attack.

Most heart attacks occur while a patient is at rest in bed or working quietly. Vigorous exercise by a person unaccustomed to it may perhaps precipitate the final blood clotting in the coronary artery, but even if he had not exercised strenuously, the chances are the clot would soon have appeared. Hence it is foolish to indict any single event as the cause of a heart attack.

If you ever happen to be present when a heart attack occurs, call a doctor at once. Help the patient take the position that is most comfortable for him. This will probably be halfway between lying down and sitting up. He usually cannot breathe comfortable if he lies flat. Loosen tight clothing, such as collar and belt. See that the patient does not become chilled. Do *not* attempt to lift or carry the victim or give him anything to drink unless a doctor tells you to.

Heart Failure. When the heart is unable to pump blood efficiently to all parts of the body, the condition is described as *heart failure*. It may accompany or be the result of coronary-artery disease or other types of heart disease. Though serious, the condition is not necessarily rapidly fatal; many patients live 10 to 20 years or longer after congestive heart failure is first noted.

The cardinal symptom of heart failure is shortness of breath or difficult breathing (dyspnea). Another common and often early sign of congestive heart failure is swelling of the ankles, although this does not always betoken heart disease. When it is related to heart failure, however, it occurs because the heart is not pumping efficiently enough to get fluids out of the spaces between and within the body cells.

The treatment of the failing heart comprises efforts to reduce its work load, improve its action, and get rid of excess body fluids. Digitalis and diuretic drugs are commonly used. Furthermore, the patient must truly learn to live within his physical means, his cardiac reserve.

Rheumatic Heart Disease. Although by no means yet eliminated, rheumatic fever and its sequel, rheumatic heart disease, no longer pose the threat to life and health they recently did. Scarcely 1 in every 40 cardiovascularenal deaths can now be charged against either acute or chronic rheumatic fever.

Rheumatic fever is a serious disease because the valves of the heart can be damaged and scarred during the acute phase. Scarred valves produce heart murmurs, but they are not necessarily significant. The first attack of the disease usually occurs between the ages of 6 and 8, but it may sometimes be delayed to adolescence or early adulthood. The exact cause of the disease remains unknown, but it is now certain that attacks are associated with streptococcal infections—usually "strep throat." This fact gives an effective means both for treating and preventing the disease. With proper treatment at least two-thirds of the children attacked by rheumatic heart disease recover with little, if any, limitation on their future work and play.

The first step in the prevention of rheumatic heart disease is the prompt treatment of all "strep" infections. The second step is the regular use, often over long periods of time, of small, protective doses of sulfa drugs or antibiotics whenever the threat of strep infections is around. Injections of slow-acting, long-lasting penicillin appear to be particularly useful in preventing reinfection.

Blood-Vessel Surgery. One of the promising new lines of attack on the "villains" of the cardiovascular picture, the blood vessels, is to be found in the development of new surgical techniques (micro-surgery in some cases) to correct defects, evident or developing, in these "lifelines" of the human body. It was once thought that surgery for the relief of vascular disease would be practically impossible, owing to the smallness of the operative field and the narrow margin for error in operating on even the larger blood vessels. There are more than 60,000 miles of blood vessels in the average human body. They range in size from the aorta—which has about the diameter of an ordinary garden hose where it issues from the heart—to tiniest capillaries of so small a bore that only a single blood cell can pass through at a time.

Much of the progress in the new blood-vessel surgery has come from the development of seamless, flexible tubing (vascular prostheses) to replace damaged blood vessels. Greater ability to visualize the blood vessels by X-ray has also aided the operating surgeons. Blood-vessel surgery has already been successfully performed in dealing with aneurysms (balloon-like pouches or sacs that puff up at weak points along the walls of the arterial blood-vessel system), in removing plugs from some arteries, in correcting defects of the aorta with which some infants are born, and in removing blood clots that have formed inside veins. Especially promising is surgery on blood vessels outside the brain because this gives new hope for the treatment of *stroke*.

Protecting Your Heart. *The symptoms of heart disease* have a unique characteristic: in general, the more serious the condition, the more remote from the heart are the symptoms. Periodic medical examinations—including electrocardiograms—offer one line of defense against heart troubles. Prompt attention to any abnormal condition that persists is a second approach. Early treatment of infections and other disease conditions that may eventuate in heart disease offers further protection against it.

Several years ago the question of whether fats (especially hard or saturated fats) should be included in the diet of those who wanted to escape heart diseases was a very live issue. The excitement has somewhat simmered down as it has become apparent that you cannot keep cholesterol out of the bloodstream simply by not ingesting it. The body is quite capable of manufacturing its own cholesterol. In September 1962, the Surgeon General of the U.S. Public Health Service observed that it would probably take a generation to prove whether any diet can reduce deaths due to heart or blood-vessel disease. In October 1962, the American Medical Association issued a press release, as follows:

Dieters who believe they can cut down their blood cholesterol without medical supervision are in for a rude awakening. It can't be done. It could even be dangerous to try. . . . Willy-nilly substitution of a few food items without over-all control of the diet accomplishes little if anything in reducing cholesterol.

Success in reducing blood cholesterol by dietary regulation so far has been achieved only in strictly controlled experimental groups, and use of this method remains largely experimental. The carefully calculated diets used in medical research to lower cholesterol are not yet of practical importance to the general public. The current concern about diet . . . should be directed away from hopeless pursuits to a worthwhile goal that can be attained by most individuals—maintaining normal weight. Overweight is the villain.

The simple rules of hygiene also help in avoiding heart disease. Be moderate in food intake and the use of tobacco and alcohol. Keep your weight within normal limits. Get reasonable amounts of rest and exercise in the rhythm of daily living. Avoid nervous tension so far as possible—and don't worry about getting heart disease.

The advice given in the famous "Regimen of Salerno," a twelfth-century Latin poem here rendered in sixteenth-century English, still applies:

Use three physicians still: first, Doctor Diet,
Next Doctor Merryman and then Doctor Quiet.

Stroke

Stroke is the term generally applied to apoplectic stroke, or apoplexy—the sudden breaking or clogging of a blood vessel in the brain. The effect of this vascular accident is either discouraging brain damage or sudden (and usually quite painless) death. People who are found dead in bed are frequently victims of stroke. Stroke generally occurs late in life and, like other cardiovascularenal damage or fatality, is associated with hardening of the arteries and high blood pressure.

Stroke appears as a sudden loss of consciousness (coma) followed by paralysis, generally of the side of the body opposite the side of the brain affected (hemiplegia). Face, arm, or leg may be paralyzed. A few victims of stroke die immediately; others linger on for a few weeks, if the lesions are extensive. But many recover more or less completely and live for years. The great Louis Pasteur did some of his best work after he had suffered a stroke.

Dr. Walter Alvarez has called attention to the frequency of "little strokes," which often go unrecognized for what they really are: brain damage. The victims of little strokes do not fall unconscious, but they lose their former mental sharpness. This is sometimes mistaken for or called senile dementia or "softening of the brain."

It is estimated that there are almost 2 million victims of stroke alive in the United States. The problem with most of these people, partially paralyzed hemiplegics, is to rehabilitate them so that they can still get much out of life.

Cancer

While cancer is a frightening word, the facts about it, as we shall see, are less fearful than the image of the disease.

Cancer begins insidiously and kills slowly—sometimes painfully, often expensively, and over half the time *needlessly*. It is the second great killer of Americans. Yet death from cancer is not inevitable. To a greater degree than with many other diseases it can be said that cancer is curable.

For example, if you had been present in the U.S. Senate Chamber in Washington, D.C., on April 1, 1958, you would have witnessed the first "Cured Cancer Congress" ever assembled. Men, women, and children gathered there were living testimony of many different types of cancer that can now be cured if caught in time. They represented 800,000 other living Americans who had already been saved from untimely death from cancer. (A "cured" cancer case is one in which the patient survives for at least five years without evidence of the recurrence of the disease.)

There is a blacker side to the cancer picture, but the occasion of the first "Cured Cancer Congress," sponsored by the American Cancer Society, dramatically illustrated that among all the major personal and community health problems cancer is susceptible of the earliest and most substantial improvement. Why?

Cancer Is Curable. Cancer untreated, or treated too late, is almost universally fatal. However, cancer treated in time and properly—by surgery and radiation—can be cured in at least one out of every two cases and usually in a much higher percentage. Here is the tragic and yet hopeful cancer story told in percentages:

CANCER STRIKES ONE IN FOUR

OF EVERY 24 PEOPLE

SIX WILL HAVE CANCER

TWO ARE SAVED
by treatment

ONE DIES
who could have been saved
by earlier diagnosis

THREE DIE
of types of cancer that
future research must control

Cancer of the breast and uterus, which account for most cancers in women, can be cured in 80% of the patients afflicted. But only 45% of the breast cancers and of the uterine cancers, are being cured now.

The same sad story in percentages applies equally to the other common sites of cancer in the male and female bodies. Skin cancer—the most obvious and accessible form of cancer—can be cured in 95% of all cases, but the present percentage of cure is only 90%. Rectal cancer can be cured in 70% of the cases, but only 35% are cured. When cancer of the mouth, evident both to dentist and physician, is a small lesion confined to the oral cavity, a 65% cure rate is possible; the present cure rate is only 35%. Lung cancer patients present the sorriest picture of all; 35% could be cured; only 5% are cured. The basic reason for the difference between what is and what could be lies in delay on the part of the patients in seeking early medical diagnosis and treatment.

What Is Cancer? Cancer is usually described as a degenerative disease. Its incidence, like that of heart disease, increases sharply with age. While cancer does occur at earlier ages, and even in children, the vast majority of cases occur after age 45. Most college students, therefore, first become personally aware of the cancer tragedy when it strikes their aging parents, relatives, and family friends. It is sometimes one of the bitterest of tragedies of youth to have to stand by helplessly for months while a beloved parent or relative, cancer-struck, expensively hospitalized, and beyond hope of cure by surgery or radiation, wastes away.

Cancer is not really one disease; it is a whole class of diseases with one characteristic in common: irregular cell growth. Cancer is primarily a disease of cells rather than of body parts or systems.

Microscopically, a great many different varieties of cancer can be identified. Cancer is therefore a *group* of diseases characterized by abnormal, uncontrolled, "lawless" growth of body cells. Plants and animals are also subject to cancerous growths.

Cells are the fundamental units of all living matter. In the normal process of growth and repair, cells grow and take their places in the economy of the body according to what may be called the "rules of nature." Cell growth and development is an extremely complicated process whose central secrets have not yet been fathomed.

Sometimes, for reasons still unknown, a cell or group of cells breaks the ordinary rules of nature. They behave in a disorderly way; they grow wildly. There is no place for them in the normal structure and function of the body. Like weeds in a garden, they crowd out normal, useful cells and steal their food supply. When enough of these wild cells cluster together, they can sometimes be felt as a lump. Unless the growth of these abnormal cancer cells can be checked by some means (usually outside intervention), they oust so many normal cells that eventually the body can no longer function and the victim dies. For example, when cancer cells invade the stomach, they crowd out the specialized stomach cells necessary for digesting food. Hence the patient eventually starves to death.

Cancer cells can start in any part of the body, but some sites are more favored. Unfortunately these cells rarely remain where they originate. Clusters or clumps of cancer cells break off and travel in the blood stream to other parts of the body—from the breast to the armpits, for example. This spread of cancer cells is called *metastasis*.

Cancer cells are definitely different from ordinary cells, and these differences can be observed in tiny sections of tissue removed from the body by surgical techniques (biopsy) and examined under a microscope. Identifying cancer cells is an important part of the job of the pathologist.

Not all new growths are *malignant,* as cancerous growths are described. Many, if not most, new growths are *benign.* They do not spread wildly; they can be safely removed. Since benign tumors are so common, the presence of a lump should not awake wild, unrealistic fear. It should simply send you promptly to a physician. *Tumor* is another word for new growth or swelling.

Where Does Cancer Usually Strike? Nearly one-third of the cases begin in the alimentary canal, most commonly the stomach. The genito-urinary system appears to be the next most vulnerable site (mainly the uterus in women and the prostate gland in men); about one-fifth of the cases begin in these sites. The breast is the third most common area, accounting for about 10% of the cases. Next come the blood-forming organs, where leukemia originates. The rest of the cases occur in the respiratory system, mainly the lung; in the urinary system, most frequently the bladder; in the brain and spinal cord; and on the skin. There are significant differences between men and women in the most important sites of cancer attack. For example, fatal cancer of the breast is 90 times more frequent in women; fatal respiratory (lung) cancer is 6 times more frequent in men, although the rate for women is rising.

What Causes Cancer? Nobody yet knows. However, many contributing and predisposing factors have been sorted out. One of the best known is prolonged irritation by chemical, physical, or thermal (heat) exposures. It has been abundantly demonstrated that coal tars are carcinogenic (cancer-invoking) agents. However, there are many other potential carcinogens in the environment, including solar rays, X-rays, and radioactive substances. For example, prolonged exposure to sun and wind seems to predispose to skin cancer. Certainly skin cancer is more common among outdoor workers, like ranchers and sailors, than among housewives.

Research has wiped out many cancer superstitions, giving assurance that there are many things that *don't* cause cancer. Dismiss the notions that cancer is caused by any specific kind of food or beverage, by blows or violence, by bacteria, or by such far-fetched circumstances as kissing, cooking in aluminum pots, or contact with animals.

Cancer is definitely not a germ (bacterial) disease; it is neither contagious nor communicable. You cannot "catch" cancer from cancer patients.

Many lines of research into possible causes are now under way. In essence they must deal with the factors that cause cells to grow and break down (cell metabolism). Among the factors being investigated are the chemical composition of cells, cell nutrition, the effects of viruses, hormones, and enzymes on the cells, environmental stresses, and the problem of heredity.

Cancer research is now a gigantic, multi-million-dollar annual undertaking. In 1959, for example, the federal government alone appropriated over $75 million for this purpose. But no specific "breakthrough" into discovery of the multiple causes of cancer then seemed imminent. Important progress, however, has been made in the development of cytologic techniques (examination of cells removed from the body) for the earlier diagnosis of cancer.

Is Cancer Inherited? This is an extremely complex question. With inbred strains of mice, elaborate patterns of the hereditary influences in cancer have been worked out. However, it cannot be assumed arbitrarily that what applies to inbred mice necessarily applies to man. There are no such pure, inbred strains of the human species. It is possible that a tendency to develop cancer can be inherited by human beings. However, it does not now appear that heredity is the critical or most important factor in human cancer. Dr. Clarence Cook Little, an outstanding authority in cancer research, has summed up the situation: "The role which heredity plays is so complex, so well concealed, and so difficult of evaluation that it is both unnecessary and unwise for individuals to consider it a personal problem."

Cancer Treatment. Cancer is treated by two basic and approved methods: (1) surgery and (2) radiation, which includes the use of X-ray, radium, and radioactive isotopes. Other methods of treatment are constantly being tested by research teams, and many become the subject of popular reports. However, legitimate scientific experiment should be distinguished from the false claims of cancer quacks, who advertise and promise cures.

Surgery, X-ray, radium, and radioisotopes are used alone or in any combination, depending on the particular case. The aim of surgery is to remove all cancer cells. Modern surgery, including extensive preoperative preparation and postoperative care, has made it possible to invade deeper and deeper recesses of the body to cut out cancerous tissue. Lung surgery affords a remarkable example.

Radiation treatment depends on the fact that many types of cancer cells are more radiosensitive than normal cells; they are destroyed while nearby normal cells are not severely injured. However, great caution is required in administering radiation treatment, and normal cells are shielded so far as possible from the rays. A radio-active isotope, cobalt 60, is now frequently used in place of radium or X-rays for radiation treatment.

Cancer Research

Chemotherapy in Cancer. For many years researchers have followed thousands of leads in the search for a drug that will affect the course of cancer once it attacks the human body. Notable progress was recorded in 1961 in the search for a drug.

The drug methotrexate was found to be effective in arresting some 50% of the cases of a highly malignant tumor, choriocarinoma, which originates in the pregnant uterus. In one series of 63 women with choriocarinoma, 30 of them lost all traces of their disease and on the last check-up had been well for periods up to five years.

This particular form of cancer is itself exceedingly rare, and its cure means little in the overall cancer picture. However, the effectiveness of methotrexate represents a forward step in the search for chemical agents that will block cancer.

Other drugs have helped reduce virulence of breast cancer and have helped prevent further spread of breast cancer after surgery.

New Remedies and Old. An ancient cancer remedy, for example, was found in 1962 to contain a chemical that slows the growth of tumors in mice.

The tumor-inhibiting chemical, called aristolochic acid, was isolated from a plant grown in Madras, India, known as *Aristolochia indica*. Species of this plant in the Mediterranean area were supposedly used as cancer remedies by the ancient Greeks and Romans.

The acid is unrelated to any drug presently used against cancer, and if further tests are successful a whole family of similar compounds will by synthesized and tested, according to Professor S. Morris Kupchan of the University of Wisconsin, who conducted this investigation.

The National Cancer Institute of the U.S. Public Health Service's National Institutes of Health at Bethesda, Maryland has reported progress in the chemotherapy (chemical treatment) of cancer. Its report, "Progress Against Cancer—1961," called special attention to definite (though limited) success in the treatment of advanced breast cancer. The report stated:

One of the standard agents for the treatment of advanced breast cancer (in women) is the male sex hormone called testosterone propionate. About 25 to 30% of patients who receive this drug experience objective responses to it—that is, the spread of their disease is halted temporarily, the size of the tumor itself is reduced, and the need for painkilling drugs is minimized

However, this potent male hormone produces masculinizing effects that are often so distressing to the female patient that the treatment has to be abandoned. A new compound has been developed which has virtually the same anticancer action as the other but is much less masculinizing. This new agent is now available on (physician's) prescription and is coming into progressively wider use.

Virus Research. The possibility that some if not all forms of cancer in man might be caused by viruses, and that these viruses might be rendered and harmless by drugs, became one of the most intriguing prospects before cancer investigators in the mid-1960's. If research in this area proves successful and lives up to its early promise, it opens up the possibility of definite and effective control, through prevention or treatment, of whole categories of malignant disease, such as leukemia, which are now either invariably fatal or poorly responsive to any other treatments so far devised.

"Progress Against Cancer—1961" pointed out: "We are moving into virus-cancer research with the human problem in mind because of the mounting, undisputed scientific evidence that many cancers in animals are caused by viruses. . . . The investigation of viruses in relation to human cancer must be based on what is learned about viruses and cancer in animals. . . . There is a possibility that a vaccine against virus-caused animal cancer may emerge from large-scale laboratory operations. This would be of great importance in the event that even one form of human cancer should prove to be caused by a virus."

Progress in research against cancer continues on an international scale. There is an International Union Against Cancer, a world-wide organization on this vital subject.

In all this research, however, one must not forget the unfortunate cancer patient—still the victim of the disease. Many patients who suffer from the disease become so depressed at the very presence of this potential killer that they lose all heart to live. Their deaths, according to some clinicians, may be attributed as much to loss of morale as to the cancer process. For these people in particular the new research in cancer therapy offers a priceless thread of hope.

"Time Is of the Essence." This standard legal phrase might well be applied to the entire problem of cancer control. Delay on the part of the patient in seeking a medical check-up for "minor" symptoms is the greatest single factor in the causation of early, untimely deaths from cancer. Untimely? Cancer is the leading cause of death in women between the ages of 25 and 55.

Why the delay? Ignorance, fear, superstition, and false modesty are the principal reasons. Too many people are still ignorant of the present high curability of cancer, and fear that a visit to a doctor's office will mean hearing a "death sentence" pronounced in terms of a diagnosis of cancer.

Personal Protection against Cancer. You cannot escape the undesirable growth of cancer cells in your body, but you have many ways of escaping damage or death from them. Make sure that, if cancer strikes, you discover it early and get treatment promptly. Cancer can be diagnosed only by a physician. Your problem is simply to make sure that you get to the doctor in time for him to make an early diagnosis.

Monthly self-examination of the breasts is also to be recommended to women over 35. These are the findings that should send her promptly to the doctor: painless lump in either breast, best felt with fingers held flat and pressed against the breast; change in shape of either breast; one breast higher than the other; nipple retracted or discharging; skin dimpled or pulled in; glands in the armpit enlarged.

An intelligent person should be equipped with a high "index of suspicion" against early cancer. This does not mean, however, a constant fear of cancer (cancerophobia, as it is sometimes called). He should be aware of the common danger signals of disease, which include those that may betoken cancer.

The American Cancer Society has provided a list of seven danger signals of cancer. These are not signs by which a layman can make a diagnosis of cancer. Their purpose is to get the person in whom one or more signals are noted to a physician for investigation and diagnosis.

The danger signals:[1]

1. Unusual bleeding or discharge.

2. A lump or thickening in the breast or elsewhere.

3. A sore that does not heal.

4. Persistent change in bowel or bladder habits.

5. Persistent hoarseness or cough.

6. Persistent indigestion or difficulty in swallowing.

7. Change in a wart or mole.

If any of these danger signals last for two weeks or more, you should be sure to see your doctor for diagnosis—or reassurance.

Some Cancer Comments (by Site). *Breast Cancer.* Leading cause of cancer deaths in women. Danger signal is lump or thickening in the breast which can be detected in annual check-up or as the result of monthly breast self-examination.

Colon and Rectum Cancer. Considered detectable and highly curable when digital and proctoscopic examinations are included in routine check-ups, which should be at least annually. Danger signal is change in bowel habits or rectal bleeding.

Kidney and Bladder Cancer. Almost always preceded by urinary difficulty or bleeding, for which reasons you should see a doctor. Annual check-up with urinalysis is a safeguard against this condition.

Lung Cancer. Now the leading cause of cancer

[1] From *Cancer Facts and Figures,* New York: American Cancer Society, 1962, p. 3.

death among men—cigarette smoking is charged with being the chief cause. Get protection by annual check-up, with chest X-ray, and by giving up or never starting smoking. Danger signal is a persistent cough or lingering respiratory ailment.

Mouth, Larynx, and Pharynx Cancer. Many more lives should be saved because the mouth is easily accessible to visual examination by physicians and dentists. An annual check-up, including examination of the larynx, is a safeguard. Danger signals include a sore that does not heal, difficulty in swallowing, and hoarseness.

Prostate Cancer. Occurs mainly in men over 60. It can be detected by palpation and urinalysis at annual check-up. Danger signal is urinary difficulty.

Skin Cancer. Readily detected by observation and diagnosed by simple biopsy. Annual check-up recommended. Overexposure of skin to sun should be avoided. Danger signals include a sore that does not heal or change in a wart or mole.

Stomach Cancer. There has been a 40% decline in deaths from stomach cancer in the last 20 years—for reasons yet unknown. The condition can be detected in an annual check-up. Indigestion is the prime danger signal.

Uterine Cancer. Mortality of uterine cancer has also declined 40% in the last 20 years. The chances of reducing it to a negligible cause of death are enhanced by widespread use of the "pap" (Papanicolau) smear for its early detection. Safeguard against uterine cancer is annual check-up, including pelvic examination and "pap" smear.

Leukemia. Leukemia is cancer of blood-forming tissues; it is characterized by abnormal production of immature white blood cells. Acute leukemia mainly strikes children, in whom it can be treated by drugs that may extend life from a few months to a few years. Chronic leukemias usually occur after age 25 and progress more slowly.

Lymphomas. These diseases arise in the lymph system and include Hodgkin's disease and lymphosarcoma. Some patients with lymphatic cancers can lead normal lives for many years. If drugs or vaccines to cure or prevent cancer are found, the cancer experts believe that they will first be successful in treating leukemia and lymphomas.

Pain is not a signal of early cancer; when it occurs, the condition may be well along. If the seven danger signals are heeded and a physician promptly consulted, chances of untimely death from cancer are greatly reduced.

The college student who has learned the true facts about cancer and heart disease has a lifelong responsibility as a citizen for spreading this information to others. The educated must be the educators.

As with the figures for heart disease, the doleful statistics on cancer incidence and deaths in the United States can be read two ways. True enough, over half a million new cases of cancer are reported annually in the United States, and over a quarter of a million deaths from cancer occur. But cancer is principally a degenerative disease and a disease of old age. Increase in cancer deaths is a price American society pays for having eliminated many other causes of disease and thus having lengthened average life span from around 47 years in 1900 to around 70 years at the present time.

A National Program for Conquest of Heart Disease, Cancer, and Stroke. The federal government has taken important, recent steps toward the "conquest of heart disease, cancer, and stroke." A President's [Lyndon B. Johnson's] commission on heart disease, cancer, and stroke was appointed in March 1964, and rendered a first report in December 1964. Its primary recommendation was the establishment of a national network of Regional Heart Disease, Cancer, and Stroke Centers for clinical investigation, teaching, and patient care in universities, hospitals, research institutes, and other institutions across the country. Specifically the commission recommended that over a 5 year period there be established 25 centers for heart disease, 20 for cancer, and 15 for stroke. By 1970 a total of 55 Regional Medical Programs for the treatment of these conditions were in operation.

In addition, the commission recommended the establishment of another national network of Diagnostic and Treatment Stations in communities across the nation to bring the highest medical skills in heart disease, cancer, and stroke within the reach of every citizen. Specifically, the commission asked for 150 such stations to be established over a period of five years for heart disease, 200 for cancer, and 100 for stroke.

Altogether the commission made 33 recommendations for steps necessary in its opinion to make a successful, nationwide thrust at heart disease, cancer, and stroke. Among them were the establishment of a national stroke program unit, of a national cervical cancer detection program, of statewide programs for heart disease control and of biomedical research institutes. The commission further recommended expanded education and training of health manpower, such as training of health technicians and specialists in health communication; and additional facilities and resources, such as more medical libraries and a national medical audiovisual center.

To put all these recommendations into effect over a five-year period would cost billions of dollars. But this would be a small outlay in comparison with the annual losses from these three diseases, which now account for more than 70% of the annual death toll in the United States. Dr. Michael E. DeBakey, chairman of the President's Commission, stated that the heavy losses which these three diseases inflict on our economy are close to $40 billion a year in lost productivity and lost taxes due to premature disability and death.[2]

Implementation of all the Commission's recommendations would undoubtedly increase the average length of life of American citizens. It might even change the order of the principal causes of death in the United States. But it would not eliminate the three conditions against which it is directed. Man is mortal. If he doesn't die

[2] *National Program to Conquer Heart Disease, Cancer and Stroke: A Report to the President by the President's Commission on Heart Disease, Cancer and Stroke.* Washington, D.C.: U.S. Government Printing Office (December 1964).

of heart disease, cancer, or stroke, he will have to die of other causes.

Smoking

Tobacco smoking has had its proponents and opponents ever since it was first introduced—from America to Europe. One of its first opponents was King James I of England, who in 1615 issued a "Counterblaste against Tobacco," in which he called it a "filthy habit . . . dangerous to the lungs."

In spite of the terms of criticism, tobacco smoking was until recently something that you could take or leave without undue worry that smoking presented any obvious risk to life or health. The situation is no longer so clear-cut. Physicians and other scientists have already demonstrated the hazards in smoking, especially cigarette smoking, although some controversy over this subject continues. Cigarette packs must now be labeled "hazardous to health." Over 100,000 physicians have given up smoking in recent years.

On the basis of its own and other statistical studies, the American Cancer Society is convinced of the risk of cigarette smoking as a cause of lung cancer. Already in 1962 the Society issued the following statement:

Another cancer risk you can avoid is excessive cigarette smoking. Research findings have convinced most scientists and the American Cancer Society that cigarette smoking is a cause of lung cancer. . . . Facts show that the more cigarettes smoked, the greater the risk of lung cancer. Ingrained personal habits are hard to change and you alone can decide whether to smoke or not to smoke.

Smoking and Health: U.S. Public Health Service Report. Cigarette smoking is a health hazard of sufficient importance in the United States to warrant appropriate remedial action. So concluded and reported an advisory committee to the Surgeon General of the U.S. Public Health Service in January, 1964. The statement was part of a 387-page, detailed report and study, published under the title *Smoking and Health.* To get an official view about tobacco smoking in the United States, it will be worthwhile to quote directly and indirectly from this extensive report,[3] as follows:

Nearly 70 million people in the United States consume tobacco regularly, principally in the form of cigarettes. While per capita consumption of other forms of tobacco has gone down, cigarette consumption has increased and stood at 3986 per person in 1961. It is estimated that roughly two-thirds of the men and one-third of the women over 18 smoke.

In order to judge whether smoking and other uses of tobacco are injurious to health or related to specific diseases, the Surgeon General's committee evaluated three main kinds of scientific evidence: (1) animal experiments, (2) clinical and autopsy studies, and (3) population studies. In the course of the animal experiments seven cancer-producing (carcinogenic) compounds were noted in the tobacco smoke and tars. The clinical and autopsy study on thousands of patients showed that many kinds of damage to body functions and to organs, cells, and tissues occur more frequently and severely in smokers. The population (epidemological) studies were both retrospective, looking back on what had happened to smokers, and prospective, getting smoking histories—or non-smoking histories—and then comparing what happened in the future.

The retrospective studies revealed several things; namely, that proportionately more cigarette smokers are found among lung cancer patients than among control populations without cancer; and that specific symptoms and signs—chronic cough, sputum production, breathlessness, chest illness, and decreased lung function—consistently show more often in cigarette smokers than in non-smokers.

[3] *Smoking and Health;* report of the Advisory Committee to the Surgeon General of the Public Health Service, U.S. Department of Health, Education, and Welfare, Public Health Service, Public Health Service Publication 1103. [For sale by the Superintendent of Documents, U.S. Government Printing Office, Washington, D.C. Price $1.25.]

The seven prospective studies examined by the Surgeon General's Committee included 1,123,000 men who provided usable histories of smoking habits and other data. A total of 37,391 men died during subsequent months or years of the studies. Tabulations in these studies were set up to permit ready comparison of the mortality experience of smokers and non-smokers. By these figures, the mortality rate for male cigarette smokers compared with non-smokers for all causes of death taken together is 1.68, representing a total death rate nearly 70% higher than for non-smokers. An excess mortality (over what would have been expected) was also noted sharply in a number of specific disease conditions among the smokers. For example, the mortality ratio of cigarette smokers to non-smokers was particularly high for such conditions as cancer of the lung (10.8), bronchitis and emphysema (6.1), cancer of the larynx (5.4), other circulatory diseases (2.6), and coronary artery disease (1.7).

The Surgeon General's Committee recognized that no simple cause-and-effect relationship is likely to exist between a complex product like tobacco smoke and a specific disease entity in the variable human organism. It also recognized that often the coexistence of several factors is required for the occurrence of a disease. Nevertheless, the Committee found these things:

¶ Cigarette smoking is associated with a 70% increase in the age-specific death rates of males. The total number of excess deaths cannot be accurately estimated.

¶ Cigarette smoking is causally related to lung cancer in men; the magnitude of the effect of cigarette smoking far outweighs all other factors. The data for women, though less extensive, point in the same direction. The risk of developing lung cancer increases with duration of smoking and the number of cigarettes smoked per day; it diminishes by discontinuing smoking. In comparison with non-smokers, average male smokers of cigarettes have approximately a nine- to tenfold risk of developing lung cancer and heavy smokers at least a twentyfold risk.

¶ Cigarette smoking is the most important of the causes of chronic bronchitis in the United States, and it increases the risk of dying from chronic bronchitis and emphysema.

¶ Cigarette smoking is associated with a reduction in ventilation function. Among males, cigarette smokers have a greater prevalence of breathlessness than non-smokers.

¶ Cough, sputum production, or the two combined are consistently more frequent among cigarette smokers than among non-smokers.

¶ Male cigarette smokers have a higher death rate from coronary artery disease than non-smoking males, but it is not clear that the association has causal significance.

¶ Women who smoke cigarettes during pregnancy tend to have babies of lower birth weight. [But] it is not known whether this decrease in birth weight has any influence on the biological fitness of the newborn.

¶ No clear-cut "smoker's personality" has emerged from the studies.

¶ Overwhelming evidence points to the conclusion that smoking—its beginning, habituation, and occasional discontinuation—is to a large extent psychologically and socially determined. This does not rule out physiological factors especially in respect to habituation, nor the existence of predisposing constitutional or hereditary factors.

Physiological Effects of Smoking. Smoke, a product of combustion, is a mixture of gases, various vaporized chemicals, and millions of minute particles of ash and other solids. These are drawn into the nose, throat, and lungs during smoking. The smoke includes some vaporized nicotine, a toxic substance found in tobacco, although much of it is destroyed by heat. . . . A smoker gets more nicotine and tar if he smokes a short butt.

Pathologists have found that smoking affects both the respiratory system and the circulatory system. For example, it has been found to thicken the lining membranes of air passages and to obstruct them with secretions.

To smoke or not to smoke is a matter of individual choice. Most authorities would agree that never smoking was preferable; and further, that

THE INJURY that cigarette smoking does to the tiny air sacs of the lungs is illustrated here. The top drawing represents normal lungs; in the bottom drawing, continuous smoking has caused the air sacs to balloon outward. Eventually their walls break down, resulting in difficulty in breathing and frequently in emphysema, a serious disabling disease. (Illustration courtesy of American Cancer Society)

moderation was a must. The American Medical Association has stated: "If you haven't started the habit, you should carefully consider all the facts concerning your future health before doing so."

Further Opinions on Smoking. In June 1964, the House of Delegates of the American Medical Association adopted a reference committee report which said that the American Medical Association "is on record and does recognize a significant relationship between cigarette smoking and the incidence of lung cancer and certain other diseases and that cigarette smoking is a serious

health hazard." The report went on to urge that the AMA should develop programs to disseminate educational material on the hazards of smoking "to all age groups through all available means of communication."

The American Heart Association has also given some pertinent answers to questions about the relationship between cigarette smoking and the circulatory system.

Are there more heart attacks among smokers than non-smokers? The heart attack rate [is] three times as high as in nonsmokers, pipe and cigar smokers, and former cigarette smokers.

Are there more deaths from heart attacks among smokers? The average increase is 70%. It can be estimated that about 60,000 men (40 to 69 years of age) die prematurely in the United States each year from heart attacks associated with smoking.

Does cigarette smoking cause heart disease? It has not been proved that cigarette smoking is a direct *cause* of heart disease. However, studies strongly suggest that it contributes to or speeds up the development of coronary artery disease which leads to heart attacks.

How does smoking affect the circulatory system? In most people who have been tested, smoking makes the heart beat faster, raises the blood pressure, and narrows the blood vessels of the skin, especially in the fingers and toes.

Social and Psychological Effects. Many social and psychological factors related to tobacco smoking have been noted. For example, many young people begin smoking in imitation of older people, sometimes those just a few years older. Smoking may offer many psychological satisfactions. For example, it may satisfy the infantile desire to have something in the mouth; the infant sucks his thumb if nothing better is available. In some cases lighting up a cigarette may be a means of relaxation; in others, it may represent an act of self-expression. To still others the cigarette represents a kind of "reward" that the smoker can offer himself whenever he wishes.

Tobacco smoking begins early in American youth. By the time they reach their senior year in high school, 40 to 55% of all children are found to have done some smoking. By the time they leave high school one in every four boys (25%) and one in every 8 girls (12.5%) are smokers. The boys are the heavier smokers. An equal if not greater number of young people take up smoking in their college years. It may be recalled that about 65% of American men and 35% of American women do smoke.

Present Status. Tobacco manufacturers are trying to reduce the hazards of smoking by modifying tobacco, cutting down its nicotine content, and filtering out the tars. They have also initiated research to isolate harmful substances so that those who smoke may continue to smoke safely. The results to date have not been too encouraging.

. So long as millions of Americans continue to smoke, it cannot be assumed that the last word on the tobacco controversy has been said. Millions of dollars are being granted annually by the U.S. Public Health Service, the American Medical Association, and others for further study of tobacco and smoking. One hope is that this research will come up with a truly "safe cigarette." The filtertips currently used on cigarettes are not considered to be an adequate safeguard.

The United States government has put itself in an awkward position in the tobacco controversy. One branch of the government (U.S. Public Health Service) condemns cigarettes while another branch (Department of Agriculture) supports the price of tobacco, and still a third (Bureau of Internal Revenue) collects large amounts in taxes from the sale of tobacco.

A National Clearinghouse for Smoking and Health has been established in the U.S. Public Health Service. It serves an important educational and coordinating function. It was one among many organizations concerned with a World Conference on Smoking & Health, sponsored by the National Interagency Council on Smoking and Health, and held in New York in September, 1967. The Summary of the Proceedings of this conference is a mine of useful information on the proved relationship of smoking and diseases of the heart and lungs.

On the basis of statistical evidence now available, it can be categorically stated, "Don't smoke." Tempered by current practice and professional experience, this categorical statement might be modified thus: "Don't start smoking. Don't smoke excessively. Don't inhale."

SUMMARY REVIEW QUESTIONS

1. What are the principal causes of death in the United States today? What were they in 1900? Why the difference? What are the principal causes of death in the college age bracket?
2. What reasons, if any, are there for believing that the present statistical picture of heart disease and associated conditions is not so frightening as it might appear if taken at face value?
3. Why is heart disease more properly described as cardiovascularenal disease? What relationship does it have to high blood pressure, hardening of the arteries, and kidney disease?
4. What is a heart attack? What is its *immediate* cause? What are the possible outcomes of a heart attack? What is heart failure? What is rheumatic heart disease? How, if at all, can it be prevented?
5. What is the difference between arteriosclerosis and atherosclerosis? In what way may these conditions be responsible for various forms of cardiovascular disease? To what extent is a fat-free diet a protection against such diseases?
6. What is a stroke? What are the usual outcomes of this event? In what areas does new hope for stroke victims lie? What grounds are there for saying that a high death rate from stroke is an index of a generally healthy community?

7. What is cancer? How does it actually kill and cripple? How does it spread? Is it inherited? How is it treated? What are the new hopes for cancer treatment?

8. What is your attitude toward cancer? Have the facts you now have about it changed your attitude from what it used to be? If so, in what way? If not, why not? Do you think your attitude is different from your parents' attitude? If so, why; if not, why not?

9. What are the seven danger signals of cancer? What should you do when any of these warning signals flash?

10. What are some (name at least six) of the most common sites of cancer in the human body? What specific protective measures, if any, can be taken to minimize the risk of cancer occurring or progressing at each of these sites?

11. What are the arguments for and against tobacco smoking? What arguments against smoking impress you most strongly? How would you defend your personal decision to smoke?

12. In light of the fact that nearly 70 million people in the United States smoke—principally cigarettes—what practical and workable measures would you suggest for decreasing, if not elliminating, the smoking habit?

13. Do you think the present statistical picture of "big killers" of Americans is likely to change during your lifetime? Why or why not?

14. Are the following statements sense or nonsense? Why? *Cancer is curable. . . . Women deposit their fat under the skin while men deposit it in their coronary arteries. . . . A heart attack is a sentence of death or permanent invalidism. . . . Eating food cooked in aluminum pots and pans is the cause of cancer. . . . A man is as old as his arteries. . . . The satisfactions of smoking are worth the risks.*

15. What do the following terms mean to you: cholesterol, lipoproteins, hypertension, vascular accident, aneurysm, malignant, benign tumor, metastasis, chemotherapy, "Counterblaste against Tobacco"?

Worth Studying Further: *You and Your Heart* by H. M. Marvin, M.D., and others. *Common Sense Coronary Care and Prevention* by Peter Steincrohn, M.D. *The Truth About Cancer* by Charles S. Cameron, M.D. *Cancer* by R. J. C. Harris. *Smoking and Health:* Report of the Advisory Committee to the Surgeon General of the U.S. Public Health Service. *Tobacco and Health* by G. James and T. Rosenthal.

12

ACCIDENT PREVENTION—SAFETY

I N THE THREE SECONDS IT WILL TAKE YOU TO read this sentence, somewhere in the United States somebody has been seriously hurt in an accident. In the five minutes that it will take you to read this page and part of the next, someone has been killed in an accident. More Americans have been killed in traffic accidents than in all the nation's wars.

The accident picture in this country is so grim that we tend to repress knowledge of it. We often react by saying that the topic of accidents is boring—until we ourselves are somehow caught. Then, often too late, we want to know what caused the accident and how it could have been prevented. Not wanting to talk about accidents is quite a common reaction.

We should not want to live constantly with the threat of death by violence hanging over our heads. Reasonable safety-mindedness is fine; rational steps to avoid accidents can then be taken. But overanxiety or constant fear about being involved in an accident is a symptom of mental disturbance and sometimes mental illness.

In this chapter we shall deal with the highlights of the broad subject of accident prevention and safety education. The emphasis will be on the prevention of motor-vehicle accidents, since they are the greatest single hazard to young men and women. There are, of course, many points of view from which the subject of accident prevention can be considered; the traffic policeman has one point of view, the safety engineer another, the accident statistician a third, and so on.

However, since all statistical records reveal that the "human element" is the great unpredictable factor in accidents, or, in more obvious terms, that the cause of accidents is people, we shall direct our discussion largely to the kind of people who are most liable to have accidents and to the psychological, *unconscious* drives and circumstances most likely to bring them on. Far too many accidents, we shall see, only *appear* as accidents. They were *purposeful* attempts at self-injury or self-destruction. These accidents can be prevented only by attention to the mental health of the individual *before* he would otherwise be involved in them.

Even today there is still a good bit of superstition about the causes and prevention of accidents. Many people still carry charms, such as a rabbit's foot, or wear amulets to ward off accidents. Even more carry in their minds a vague belief in some magic formula that will save them from harm, from accident, from violence.

When an accident happens to them, they may attribute it to "gremlins"—invisible imps of disaster first "noticed" by British aviators during World War II. This explanation is not so foolish as it looks at first glance; it is an externalization of the fact that the fundamental causes of accidents are *people,* often ourselves. Since we are unwilling to admit this horrible, guilt-producing thought to ourselves or others, we conveniently project the blame for accidents on the gremlins.

We speak glibly of the "causes" of accidents. Our safety engineers have gone a long way in identifying the *scenes* of accidents, the places and the situations in which they are most likely to occur. Much can be done with this information to prevent future accidents; for example, the accident record on a particular street intersection may make it imperative to install stop lights. But neither the engineers nor the accident statisticians can tell us why a particular accident has happened or is going to happen.

The reason is this. Accidents have causes; but the causes are often so personal, so obscure, so complex, so unrelated to the scene of the accident that we cannot see or find an explanation until after the tragedy has occurred

Accident Proneness

Accidents can happen to anybody, but the fact is that some people are more liable to accidents than others. They can sometimes be identified by their accident records and, with greater difficulty, by their personality patterns. It is easier to label a person "accident prone" than to prove it. Nevertheless, where careful records are kept, as in some industries, it soon becomes evident that the greatest number of accidents cluster around a comparatively few people who are called—rightly or wrongly—accident prone.

It appears that the person who has already had an accident is most likely to have another; further, the person who has lots of little accidents appears to be going to meet a big one. Uncorrected defects of sense organs, poor vision, and partial deafness, for instance, account for some cases of accident proneness. But modern psychiatry offers a deeper explanation.

Some psychiatrists believe that most truly accident-prone persons unconsciously wish to have accidents happen to them, for the accident victim at least gets sympathy. Having an accident resolves intolerable conflicts in his unconsious mind, just as drinking does for the alcoholic. A repeated pattern of accidents, not just an occasional accident, can be considered a poor and damaging pattern of life adjustment that accident-prone people are internally driven to find and accept. This escape into accidents is possible because having an accident is still socially acceptable.

Every accident-prone individual has his own specific personality structure and unconscious motivations, but psychoanalytic study has revealed some of the broad emotional characteristics of the type, thus:

He was often brought up in a strict home. He deeply resented parental authority and often flouted it. He carries this resentment of authority into early adult life; he hates bosses, policemen, and all other symbols of authority. Seeking his own pleasure, he is a law unto himself. Many people admire him for daring, bravado, and the air of excitement he creates. But he himself rarely feels strong emotional attachments to other people. His school and work records are likely to be spotty; he tries to escape responsibility and the association with authority that it entails.

As an adult, he usually responds to stimuli with action rather than thought. But he is more likely to respond quickly and impulsively to his own inner needs and feelings than to the realistic facts and situations that confront him. He looks to accidents as solutions of his emotional torments because the accidents may bring him love and sympathy—and sometimes money—without requiring the assumption of responsibility or exertion on his part.

The broad-stroke picture of this personality type fits the description of social misfits other than the accident-prone individual. Dr. H. Flanders Dunbar, an authority on psychosomatic medicine, says: "When this personality pattern is set beside those of other groups in the population, it turns out to match very precisely that of the juvenile delinquent and the adult criminal. The behavior characteristics of the persistent breaker of laws is virtually identical with that of the persistent breaker of bones—right up to the point where the one commits a crime and the other has an accident."[1]

What Accident Statistics Tell Us

Every year in the United States somewhere between 9 million and 10 million people are accidentally injured and somewhere between

[1] H. Flanders Dunbar, *Mind and Body: Psychosomatic Medicine,* (New York: Random House, 1947).

90,000 and 100,000 are killed by accident. Around 350,000 people are permanently disabled to some extent by accidents every year. For many years the accident death rate in the United States remained almost constant (at about 72 deaths per 100,000 population). It is an amazing fact that, when organized safety efforts or other conditions push the death rate from accidents down at one point of the compass, it appears to rise up at other points. For example, during World War II, when auto driving was restricted, the motor-vehicle accident death rate declined. At the same time, since war production and military training were being pushed, the industrial accident death rate increased, the military training accident death rate (especially airplane accidents) increased, and the over-all accident death rates during the war years were just about the same as before. The postwar trend was substantially downward. The accidental death rate fell to a low of 50 (per 100,000 population) in 1961.

Yet it is fair to assume that, without organized safety efforts and continuing safety education, America's accident record would be even more shocking than it is. After diseases of the heart, blood vessels, and kidneys (the cardiovascular-enal diseases), and cancer, accidents are the fourth principal cause of death in the United States. *In school and college years, from five to twenty-five, they are the first cause of death.*

We often think of accidents in terms of catas-trophes, because these are the events that make newspaper headlines. A catastrophe, statistically speaking, is an accident in which five or more lives are lost. However, a careful record of national catastrophes reveals that less than 2% of all accidental deaths occur in them.

Another key fact is that only about 10% of the catastrophes are due to the uncontrollable forces of nature—floods, hurricanes, tornadoes, and the like. Your chances of being struck fatally by lightning during any year, for example, are only about two in a million—even less if you are a city-dwelling woman. Ninety percent of the head-line catastrophes are the result of some kind of human failure or neglect, engendering confla-grations, explosions, railroad wrecks, airplane crashes, mine accidents, building cave-ins, ma-rine accidents, and the like.

But, wherever you turn in the accident picture, the failure in the human factor stares you in the face. For example, in traffic accidents, defects in the vehicle are reported in less than 10% of the cases. That is why it has been often stated, with-out serious challenge, that 90% of all accidents are preventable. Yet fatal and crippling accidents continue to occur daily. Over the years, un-heralded, unspectacular, foolish accidents out-strip catastrophes fiftyfold; and as a cause of death they outrun the sum of war deaths, mur-der, suicide, and legal executions combined by a ratio of at least 4 to 1.

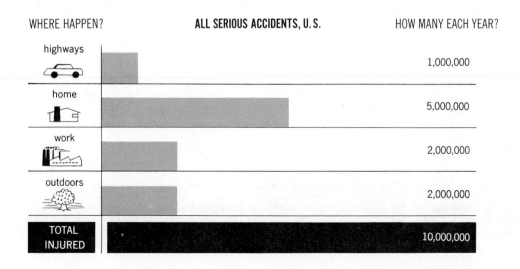

WHERE HAPPEN?	ALL SERIOUS ACCIDENTS, U.S.	HOW MANY EACH YEAR?
highways		1,000,000
home		5,000,000
work		2,000,000
outdoors		2,000,000
TOTAL INJURED		10,000,000

A Philosophy of Accidents. We often speak of the accident problem in purely numerical terms, forgetting both the human and philosophical concept behind the word "accident." Material on the psychology of accidents has been included in this chapter, but a Frenchman, Professor Jean L' Hirondel, of Caen, speaking at the 1962 International Conference on Health and Health Education put the accident problem in its proper philosophical perspective in the following terms: (Translation from the French original by this author.)

Accidents are only one aspect of the human drama and the constant struggle of man against the universe [about him].

Three kinds of perils menace us:

1. Those arising from ourselves and especially from the imperfections of our bodies;

2. Perils presented by other human beings;

3. Finally, the attack [or agression] of the elements of nature outside man [on man], where such elements can be schematically identified, namely:

—the attacks of microbes and viruses; these are the infectious diseases; and

—the aggression [or violence] of physical agents; these precisely are accidents.

Even with such "classifications," so to speak, it is often difficult to give a precise definition or description of an "accident." [For example:]

A hunting "accident" may be accident, suicide, or murder depending upon the motivation of the protagonist [the man who fired the gun].

Snakebite [with the injection of venom] is termed an accident. The toxins [spread through the body] by microbes are said to cause a disease.

Frostbite [or freezing to death] is called an accident, but injury to the lungs [pneumopathology] due to cold is classified as an illness.

FATAL ACCIDENTS IN U.S.

HOW KILLED? | | HOW MANY EACH YEAR?

motor vehicles — 35,000 / 40,000

falls — 28,000 / 30,000

burns — 8,000 / 10,000

drowning — 6,000 / 8,000

railroad — 3,000 / 4,000

firearms — 2,000 / 3,000

gas poisoning — 2,000 / 2,500

poisoning (except gas) — 2,000 / 2,500

all others — 10,000 / 12,000

TOTAL ACCIDENTS — 96,000 / 112,000

FATAL ACCIDENTS IN U.S.

WHERE KILLED?   HOW MANY EACH YEAR?

highways	35,000 / 40,000
home	30,000 / 35,000
work	15,000 / 18,000
outdoors	16,000 / 19,000
TOTAL KILLED	96,000 / 112,000

With this philosophy, Professor Hirondel concludes that accidents are a check on the development of mankind by the forces that both surround (threaten) and motivate him. He quotes the Biblical injunction of the Lord to Adam: "People the earth and subdue it."

The International Conference dealt in practical as well as philosophical concepts of accident prevention. "The National Child Cycling Proficiency Scheme in the United Kingdom," submitted on behalf of the Royal Society for the Prevention of Accidents, advised that if you teach 10-, 11-, and 12-year-olds how to ride bicycles safely, you will save them from millions of motor vehicle accidents when they are allowed to drive cars eight to ten years later.

Prevention of Motor Vehicle Accidents

There are enough automobiles in the United States so that every man, woman, and child could be riding simultaneously. Yet in 1895 there were just four gasoline motorcars in the country—a Ford, a Haynes, a Duryea, and an imported Benz. People were shocked that these cars could travel at a speed of 11 miles an hour; automobiles have since been clocked at a speed of over 600 miles per hour.

With more than 83 million powerful cars on the streets and roads, and probably 100 to 125

million drivers, it is a traffic problem of first magnitude to keep them out of each other's fenders. The modern automobile is a powerful instrument; but the driver is its brain. Without a driver, a motorcar is useless. But with a careless, thoughtless, inexperienced driver, it can become an instrument of death and a tool of destruction.

Practically all college men and a high percentage of college women know how to drive, or think they do. Actually there are great differences in skills and attitudes. Many are excellent drivers all the time and enjoy respect for their ability. Still more are fair to good drivers, with occasional lapses into trouble. A few are poor and dangerous drivers, partly responsible for the high fatal accident involvement rates recorded in drivers under 25 years of age. Sample studies indicate that the safest drivers are the 35 to 50 age group. Younger drivers, between 16 and 25, are involved in fatal accidents much more often.

What does it take to be a good driver—one whose invitations to ride with him are more welcomed than feared? First and foremost, a proper *attitude* toward driving, its risks, responsibilities, and opportunities. After that, mental and physical fitness, knowledge, judgment, skills, and habits based on good instruction and intelligent experience.

What Makes a Good Driver? *Knowledge.* An important part of the knowledge that makes a good driver is that of the physical and physio-

TRAFFIC ACCIDENTS are caused by people, who are frequently driven into them by unconscious motivations—such as regression, an infantile disregard for personal safety or the rights of others. Motor vehicle accidents are the principal cause of death in the college-age population.

logical laws or principles that govern the motion of the car and the driver behind the wheel. The most fundamental traffic laws are the laws of nature: gravity, friction, force of impact, and centrifugal force.

The entire control of a moving automobile depends on the grip which four small areas of tire surface have on the roadway at any given moment. These four points of contact are no bigger than the palm of the hand which grips the steering wheel. The coefficient of friction between tires and roadway is itself dependent on many factors, including the condition of the tires, the condition of the brakes and brake pressure, and the kind and condition of the road surface, which is often further dependent on weather conditions. A good driver knows and respects all these conditions. He is also aware of the centrifugal force that operates on curves; this force inexorably tends to push the moving car off the road, just as a rock whirled on a string tends to break the string.

Most important, the good driver is aware of the tremendous amount of kinetic energy developed by a moving automobile and the real difficulty of changing its motion—specifically, stopping the car. Modern engineering genius has made it seem deceptively simple to stop an automobile. Only when the car collides with something or someone else before stopping is the poor driver jolted into a realization of what a powerful force he was directing.

The kinetic energy packed into the moving automobile is a function of the weight of the car and the speed at which it is being driven. Speed too high for driving conditions is usually the killing factor in motor-vehicle accidents; it is associated with fatal accidents more than twice as often as any other observed factors. The relationship of speed to death in auto accidents has been worked out by A. N. Kerr, a California mechanical engineer, in terms of *danger units*. At a speed of 25 miles per hour an automobile has developed 1 danger unit of kinetic energy. This amount of energy also represents just about the "shock limit" of a human being, the equivalent of a fall from a second-story window.

At 25 miles per hour an automobile can be stopped within an average street's width, and if it turned over upon hitting an obstacle, it would roll over only once. As speed is increased, danger units increase, but the danger increases faster than the speed. In fact, the danger units are proportional to the square of the speed. Thus, at 35 miles the car packs 2 danger units; at 50 miles, 4 danger units; at 75 miles, 9 danger units. The human body was never engineered to take such shocks.

Just as there are danger units packed in the momentum of a moving automobile, we can likewise speak of a danger zone always projected in front of it. This danger zone can be easily pictured by imagining the hood of the car stretched out ahead of it for literally hundreds of feet. The good driver is always aware of this danger zone and knows the various factors that determine its length. Both physical and physiological factors are involved. The danger zone is the distance ahead within which the car can be brought to a complete stop.

The actual stopping distance is the sum of the braking distance *plus* the reaction-time distance. The braking distance depends upon pure physical laws already mentioned, the factors affecting the coefficient of friction. The braking distance is the distance the car will travel after the brakes are applied. At 10 miles per hour, on a hard-surfaced road with brakes in "good" condition, it is 7.5 feet; at 25 miles, 46.9 feet; at 60 miles, 270 feet.

But, before you even begin to push your foot down on the brake pedal, the foot must respond

DANGER ZONE AHEAD OF A MOVING AUTOMOBILE *

Stopping distance calculated at the following speeds:

Miles per hour	Distance in feet before car stops
10	18.5
20	52.0
25	74.4
30	100.5
35	130.4
40	164.0
50	242.5
60	336.0

Stopping distance is sum of (1) braking distance, calculated for brakes that just meet the requirements of the Uniform Vehicle Code (44.5 percent efficient); and (2) braking-reaction-time distance, calculated at an average of three-fourths of a second.

*This table is an abridgement from Table I, "Stopping Distances," in *The Driver*, first volume in the Sportsmanlike Driving Series published by the American Automobile Association, Washington, D.C., 1946, p. 30.

to a signal from your brain. This takes time; the nerve impulse must travel from the original stimulus on eye or ear to the brain and from the brain to the leg and foot muscles. The length of time required for this action is called the braking reaction time. It varies in different individuals, and in the same individual at different times. It can be measured with a fair degree of accuracy by various testing devices. Under ordinary driving conditions the average braking reaction time is about $\frac{3}{4}$ second. A car traveling 25 miles per hour will have moved ahead about 27 feet in that split second.

However, even young people with comparatively fast reaction times on ordinary tests slow down under many conditions, notably fatigue; drinking of alcoholic beverages; inattention owing to daydreaming, conversation, or listening to an auto radio; eye strain; low visibility; and indecision possibly reflecting emotional strains. The good driver knows all this and guards against most of these hazards.

If he is drowsy or tired while driving, he pulls off the road and takes a nap. If he drinks, he doesn't drive. If he finds himself distracted by "back-seat driving" or other conversation, he refuses to go on until it stops. If he is required to wear glasses while driving, he always wears them. He constantly takes visibility conditions into account; he slows down at intersections; he does not pass cars on hills; he doesn't overdrive his lights, that is, he doesn't drive at night or in a fog at a speed which makes the inescapable danger zone ahead of him greater than the distance he can see ahead.

Daydreaming and indecision are more difficult factors to control. About the only possible advice that can be given here is not to drive on days that you find yourself acting absent-minded or feeling "jittery." Physical condition is a factor in safe driving; sometimes a toothache may be at the root of an auto accident.

Sound Driving Practices and Habits. The good driver is habitually aware of adverse driving conditions and their effect on shortening the danger zone ahead of his car. He compensates for these adversities by driving more slowly. For example, he knows that, when he is wide awake and alert and his car and tires in tiptop shape, he can safely drive at 50 miles per hour on a hard, smooth, dry, level, straight road in clear daylight. He further recognizes that changes in any combination of these conditions will require proportionate reduction in speed. Thus, when feeling fatigued and driving at night with fogged-up headlights on a wet pavement with a 5% down grade and then suddenly subjected to the glare of oncoming headlights which cut his visibility to only 100 feet, the good driver habitually reduces his speed to about 15 miles an hour.

Three "C's" can be used to describe the habits of the good driver: *C*ourtesy, *C*ommonsense, and *C*aution. Courtesy on the highway undoubtedly prevents many accidents; some authorities believe that, if it were commonly practiced, highway accidents could be cut in half.

Rude, discourteous, unsportsmanlike violation of driving rules is associated with a high percentage of accidents. In one reported series of accidents, for example, the drivers involved were guilty of the following violations of sportsmanlike driving rules: demanding the right of way (11%), exceeding speed limit or safe speed (8%), driving on the wrong side of the roadway (6%), disregarding warning signs and signals (4%), passing improperly (3%), turning improperly (3%), driving while under the influence of alcohol (3%), following too closely (2%), failing to signal or giving improper signal (2%), parking or starting improperly (2%). To sum up, in 56% of these traffic accidents, the offending drivers did not observe courtesy, caution, or common sense. Afoot, where it is more annoying than dangerous, no one is permitted to use the sidewalks as rudely and bumptiously as many drivers use the highway.

The character of the good, safe driver can be summed up in his observance of these six habits:

¶ Through experience under instruction, he has developed mechanical and technical skill in controlling his car.

¶ He knows what to expect of his car under both favorable and adverse driving conditions.

¶ He avoids taking foolish chances; he *never* overdrives the danger zone projecting ahead of his car.

¶ He has a courteous and sportsmanlike regard for the rights of all other users of the public highway, including pedestrians, bicyclists and motorcyclists, and other motorists.

¶ He signals his intentions to all persons who may be affected by the course of the car of which he is the brain; he does not expect other people to be mind readers.

¶ He is alert for the mistakes of other people, and he does what he can to compensate for them; he does not demand the right of way to his own or anyone else's hurt.

The Unconscious Causes of Auto Accidents

Attitudes. The good driver, as we have described him, always knows what he is doing when he is at the wheel of his car. His safe driving habits are "automatic" reactions or responses to stimuli without interference or misdirection by unconscious motivations of which he himself is not aware. Under conditions of emotional stress, an ordinarily good driver may become temporarily a poor and dangerous driver. The big pool of poor drivers, however, and the still-wider stream of "accident-prone" persons, is made up of individuals who do not really know what they are doing because they are unaware of or will not accept the deep unconscious motivations, the dangerously overworked mental mechanisms, that control their attitudes and their conduct.

To understand the attitudes which make some people exceptionally bad risks as auto drivers, it must be frankly recognized that in modern American society the automobile is regarded as more than a cheap and convenient means of transportation and its value is measured in terms other than either the weight of metal in it or even its cost in dollars.

The automobile is used as a symbol of many factors in the life of the American individual. The kind of car a man drives is often taken as a measure of his status or prestige in the community, although this is by no means universally so. Equally true, the right of a young man to drive the family car is a token of the independence he has achieved and a measure of the degree of maturity and responsibility which his family thinks he has attained.

The more basic fact is that almost every single mental mechanism of which the human mind is capable can be expressed in feeling and action related to driving or owning an automobile. The car becomes not only an extension of the ego; it also symbolizes other family relationships, and it substitutes for both love and hate objects. Many people become poor, dangerous, accident-prone drivers because they use the role of driving as an outlet for subconscious reactions whose origins have nothing to do with the realistic act of transporting themselves from one place to another.

We will not repeat the list of the mental mechanisms here (see pages 17–21). We shall simply give a few examples of how they relate to bad driving and auto accidents:

Repression. A poor driver may really hate driving because, for example, he may be trying to repress memory of an auto accident of which he was once a cause, a victim, or a witness.

Identification. A poor driver may identify the act of driving a car with a family member, usually a father, toward whom he still has unresolved aggressions. He may subconsciously want to hurt his father by getting into an accident and hurting his car.

Extroversion. Some people "drive like mad" in a hopeless attempt to escape inner conflicts. Reckless driving is an excellent example of unreflective action.

Fantasy. Daydreams of attaining an unassailable height of power often incorporate fantasies of driving or riding in a long, sleek automobile with limitless speed and power. The car rides easily over all obstacles and opposition, and there is no one powerful enough to bid the driver to stop. Confusing fantasy with fact, the driver steps on the accelerator and sometimes speeds to his death.

Rationalization. The poor driver invariably rationalizes the factors that led him into an accident. He was driving too fast, he asserts, not because he started for an appointment too late but because "he absolutely promised to be on time."

Regression. Almost every type of regressive, childish behavior can occur in that driver whose infantile ego reasserts itself in hogging the road, insisting on the right of way, double parking, speeding—all with an infant's complete disregard for the rights and presence of other people. This can be a fatal form of emotional infantilism.

Projection. The poor driver projects the blame for his accidents onto everything and everyone except himself. His accidents are *always* "the other fellow's fault," or they were caused by bad roads, poor visibility, faulty brakes, or any other driving condition for which the driver himself failed to make proper allowance.

Isolation. The driver who segregates and isolates his thinking and feeling into logic-tight compartments is often the most dangerous and hopeless of the lot of poor drivers. He honestly cannot see that his demoniac conduct behind the wheel is completely at odds with his polite and often mild-mannered conduct in other situations. So he continues to charge pedestrians, speed up when another car tries to pass him, and take chances in passing other cars.

Symbolization. The false "sense of power" that this poor driver gets when he steps on the gas symbolizes the feeling of importance he would like to have but has failed to achieve in other areas of living. For him especially the car symbolizes the ego, and he shows off by reckless driving.

Substitution (or Displacement). In this class of poor drivers we sometimes find the introverted, over-obedient child who was afraid to talk back to his parents, the henpecked husband, and the Mr. Milquetoast who doesn't dare speak up to his boss. He displaces his hidden feelings of resentment against them by madcap driving and a cavalier disregard for the rights of others. He weaves carelessly in and out of traffic lanes; he shows other cars his dust. After all, they can't talk back.

Inferiority Feelings. Many a poor driver handles his car with an attitude of superiority that represents overcompensation of the wrong kind for feelings of inferiority and inadequacy. Driving makes him feel like the proverbial "Mister Big," and he shows it in many ways. He won't move over when other cars want to pass him; if they finally do succeed in passing, he immediately speeds up to overtake them and "get even."

Highway Safety A Mental Health Problem. Accident records incontrovertibly show that it is the drivers with poor attitudes who have the most accidents. Highway safety thus becomes in great part a problem of mental health. The poor and dangerous driver, unfortunately, does not usually recognize himself as such. His unconscious reactions and motivations toward the automobile are part of his total personality pattern.

From a personal standpoint, you can make yourself a better driver by understanding your personality pattern in all respects and thus becoming a more mature individual. From the standpoint of the public safety, however, since the poor driver is a menace to others as well as himself, the problem must be approached differently. Only a few, bad-risk drivers are weeded out by checking their repeated accident records and refusing them further driving privileges or a driver's license.

Theoretically, it might be possible to test all drivers for mental and emotional difficulties before they were allowed to get on the road and cause accidents; but this task of plumbing the unconscious minds of probably 115 million automobile drivers is far beyond the practical resources of public safety officials. Only the crudest beginnings have been made, and then only in a few states, by refusing licenses to people with frank mental illnesses and mental deficiencies.

An Engineering Problem. It is clearly recognized that highway safety is also an engineering problem. This takes into consideration the design and construction of motor vehicles themselves and the design and upkeep of the streets and highways on which they ride. Important, relatively recent engineering contributions to automobile safety are the seat belt and harness. Prop-

erly installed and used regularly, they can cut death and accident injury tolls. The National Safety Council estimates that if everyone used seat belts and/or harnesses regularly, at least 5000 lives a year could be saved and the number of serious injuries could be reduced by one third.

Are automobiles today designed with the maximum concern for the safety of their drivers and passengers? It is often claimed that they are not. Such an attack was made in 1966 in the book, *Unsafe at Any Speed,* by Ralph Nader, a young Washington attorney. Some of the safety factors that he recommended have since been incorporated in the design of new automobiles.

Cost of Accidents. The immediate and accumulating costs (e.g., loss of earnings) of motor vehicle and other accidents run into billions of dollars a year. The National Safety Council regularly calculates the money costs of all types of accidents involving deaths and injuries in the United States. The estimated cost for the year 1963 was $16.5 billion. This figure includes wage losses, medical fees, and hospital expenses, insurance costs, property damage and destruction (e.g., fire), and production losses. About half the total costs were charged against motor vehicle accidents; about a third against work accidents. In 1963 the total number of disabling accidental injuries reported was over 10 million; the number of deaths 101,000.

Young men between the ages of 16 and 25 are most likely to be involved in auto accidents. They, or their parents, pay for this hazard in the form of much higher insurance rates. An insurance company[2] has averaged out the projected accident record, and costs of these accidents, 50 years ahead, for a young man who starts driving at age 16. By the time he is 23 he will probably have had 4 accidents, 1 involving injury; by 40 he will have had 9 accidents, 3 with injuries; at 66, a total of 13 accidents, with 4 injuries, costing altogether about $6500. Assuming that the young man at 23 takes a 23-year-old bride, who also

[2] Kemper Insurance Company, quoted in editorial in *Safety Education,* A National Safety Council Publication (January 1964), p. 22.

has been driving since she was 16, and that they have three children, plus grandchildren, the lifetime grand total at age 66 for this *one* man and his family will be 38 accidents, 12 involving injuries, at a cost of about $19,000.

Motorcycle Accidents. An increasing number of motor vehicle accidents can be assigned to motorcycles and their smaller versions, the motorscooter and motorized bicycle. In 1967 it was estimated that unless the upward trend of motorcycle registrations and fatal motorcycle accidents abated, somewhere between 4000 and 5000 motorcycle deaths could be expected annually in the 1970's. (About 1 in 7 of these would be with the lighter vehicles, which are rapidly increasing in number.)

The U.S. Bureau of Public Roads estimates that there will be a total of at least 5 million motorcycles registered and on the roads in 1970. This would bring about a ratio of one motorcycle to every 40 people. In Europe, where motorcycles have long been more popular, the ratios in seven countries run from 1 in 9 persons to 1 in 29.

The hazards of motorcycling are made evident by observing the statistics on motorcycle accident fatalities. The number of passengers and drivers killed per 100,000 motorcycles registered was $2\frac{1}{2}$ times the corresponding rate for all other types of motor vehicles. The National Safety Council estimates that the accidental death rate for motorcyclists ranges between 20 and 40 per 100 million vehicle miles, compared with 5.6 for drivers, passengers, and pedestrians in all motor vehicles.

Experience is of prime importance for safe handling of motorcycles, motorscooters, and motorized bicycles. In one British study it was shown that drivers under age 21 with less than 6 months experience had higher accident rates than those with more than 6 months experience. A Minnesota hospital study of motorcycle accident injuries found that 1 in 5 of the injured persons had been riding a motorcycle for only the first or second time! About $\frac{3}{4}$ of them were on borrowed or rented vehicles.

In a typical motorcycle accident the driver is usually thrown forward so that his head sustains the impact with another vehicle, object, or pavement. Injury to the head occurs in 50% or more motorcycle accidents. Accordingly, motorcycle riders are now wearing more protective headgear (crash helmets), and efforts are now being made to require special drivers' tests and licenses for the motorcycle operators. The highest rates for motorcycle accident deaths occur in the college ages between 15 and 24. About 10% of these are females.

A Word About Pedestrians. Though the poor driver is the central figure in all auto accident records, it should be noted that pedestrians are also sometimes at fault. From 9000 to 12,000 pedestrians of all ages are killed in traffic accidents every year. Some jaywalk to death. There is alcohol on the breath of about 1 in every 5 adult pedestrians killed in traffic accidents. Two out of every three pedestrians killed are either violating traffic laws or acting in a patently unsafe manner. The following simple rules for pedestrians, if obeyed, will save lives:

Cross streets only at crosswalks. Three out of five urban pedestrian deaths occur between intersections.

Watch those first few steps into the street.

Obey stop signs.

Make sure you're clear *before* you attempt to cross a street or road. Learn to judge the speed of approaching automobiles, and don't try to beat them on foot.

Walk on the *left* side of country roads where there are no sidewalks. You will be in a better position to see cars approaching on your own side of the road.

At night on country roads wear or carry some light-colored object so that your visibility in an oncoming driver's eyes will be increased.

Other Kinds of Accidents

Not all fatal accidents occur on the highway. They also take place at work, at play, and, most frequently, at home.

Home Accidents. Over half of the fatal accidents that take place at home strike people over 65, and one-fifth of them happen to children under 5. The highest accident rates are recorded for two-year-old boys. Among the causes of home accidents we must therefore put physical frailty or handicap and poor judgment high on the list, although psychological mechanisms are also at work. Falls are the principal type of fatal home accident. Every home should be repeatedly checked for accident hazards; for example, poor lighting, unsafe electrical fixtures, stairways without railings, slippery floors, scatter rugs that slip underfoot, untidy housekeeping that leaves bundles and objects lying around on floors and staircases.

The kitchen is the most dangerous room in the house, according to accidental-injury records. All types of home accidents occur there: falls, burns, scalds, explosions, internal poisoning, gas poisoning, and suffocation. After the kitchen the chief danger spots around the house, roughly in order of accident frequency, are: outside stairs, inside stairs, living room, porch, bedroom, basement, dining room, bathroom, and hallways. Comparatively few fatal accidents, except for carbon monoxide poisoning, occur in the garage. But the outside yard, statistically speaking, is just as dangerous as the kitchen. The essence of accident prevention in the home is good housekeeping coupled with common sense.

Industrial and Occupational Accidents. More thought is probably given to the prevention of accidents in industry and at work than in any other area. Safety engineering has done a tremendous job in cutting down the risks of injury even in hazardous employments, such as mining and quarrying. The human factor, however, remains the uncontrollable element. Poor housekeeping in the shop and horseplay around machinery are important causes of industrial accidents. So also are improper use of machinery or other equipment and failure to use protective devices. It is significant that proportionately more people are killed working on farms, where they are more or less their own bosses, than working in factories. Because accidents cost money, organized safety work in industry has gone to great pains to identify accident-prone individuals before they hurt themselves or others.

When industrial safety measures were first introduced, it was feared that safety measures, such as wearing goggles, would slow production and cut efficiency. It has turned out, however, that the safe way of doing a job is also the most efficient way.

College Accidents. Lest college students think that problems of environmental health, safety, and occupational health are far removed from their immediate sphere of interest, they may be surprised to learn that only a small percentage of the nation's colleges and universities operate environmental health and safety programs— whose purpose is the conservation of the human and physical resources of the college population. Few colleges even believe such a problem exists. As an example of tragic failure to face up to such problems it is worthwhile to describe a scene from the campus of a midwestern university [*Student Medicine,* **10**:4, 504 (April 1962)]:

Two students who were enrolled in a chemistry course took some chemicals from the laboratory which could be used to make smoke in their dormitory. The chemicals, mixed in the lab and placed in a small sealed jar, exploded when the jar was bumped. The student who bumped the jar was permanently blinded in both eyes. . . .

Outdoor Accidents. Sports accidents kill hundreds of men and boys over fifteen every year. Most of the deaths are accounted for by the so-called "milder sports": swimming, fishing, and hunting. Very few deaths, numerically speaking, result from rough or vigorous sports like football, boxing, wrestling, baseball, and auto racing. This is partly the good result of more adequate supervision of vigorous sports. Responsible coaches and athletic directors take it as their primary jobs to instruct team candidates in skills that will keep them from getting hurt. The first thing a football player must learn, for example, is how to fall properly. Unsupervised recreation is more likely to invite accidents.

Drownings make up the largest category of fatal outdoor accidents. These could be substantially reduced in number if poor swimmers and non-swimmers obeyed water safety rules and stayed out of deep water. Good swimmers most frequently drown when they attempt feats beyond their powers. The same psychology, applies here as in motorcycle accidents, where the expert riders are more likely than the novice riders to try stunts leading to fatal accidents. Experience sometimes induces overconfidence and carelessness.

Organizing for Safety

Consistent and organized safety efforts have over the years reduced the toll of accidents that might otherwise have been rung up. The water safety programs of the American Red Cross is an example. Reduction in Fourth of July fireworks accidents as a result of legal restrictions on the sale of fireworks is another example. Public safety departments, including traffic policemen and fire inspectors, are constantly at work to reduce accident and fire hazards.

Many national organizations cooperate in safety promotion and accident prevention efforts; among them may be listed the National Safety Council, the American Automobile Association, the American Red Cross, the National Board of Fire Underwriters, the National Committee for Traffic Safety, and the International Association of Chiefs of Police—Safety Division. They emphasize in varying degrees what safety workers call the "three E's" essential to the public safety: Engineering, Enforcement, and Education. But in the final analysis it is up to the individual who wants to beat the law of averages concerning the occurrence of accidents to educate himself to be above average in alertness, safety-mindedness, and self-possessed maturity.

Emergency Medical Identification

One positive step that the safety-minded individual can now take, if he requires it, is to provide himself with adequate emergency medical identification. Probably 40 million people in the United States have physical conditions or disabilities serious enough to warrant wearing or carrying emergency medical identification.

Emergency medical identification is provided

STANDARD (American Medical Association) symbol for emergency medical identification devices.

by medallions, bracelets, lockets, purse and wallet cards, and other signal devices warning of physical conditions, such as diabetes or penicillin sensitivity, afflicting the particular individual. Then, if he is ever found unconscious, the police officer or attending physician will immediately know what to do—or often, very importantly, what *not* to do—for him. Epileptics and diabetics are sometimes mistaken for drunks; the emergency identification device immediately sets the record straight.

Following pioneering efforts by such organizations as the Medic-Alert Foundation, the American Medical Association in 1963 adopted a standard symbol for emergency medical identification. It is a hexagon enclosing a six-pointed "star of life" on which is emblazoned the staff of Aesculapius, symbol of medicine (see illustration). The American Medical Association (Emergency Identification, 535 N. Dearborn St., Chicago, Ill.) will upon request supply a list of manufacturers and vendors of emergency signal devices.

Who needs emergency medical identification? Essentially people with "hidden" medical problems who might fail, without it, to receive proper first-aid and emergency treatment. Your physician is the one to determine finally whether you should wear or carry emergency medical identification. The records of the Medic-Alert Foundation, compiled since 1956, show that there are over 200 specific conditions in which emergency identification is extremely important, if not imperative. These conditions include: *diseases,* such as diabetes, epilepsy, hemophilia, myasthenia gravis, multiple sclerosis, glaucoma, and amnesia; *allergies* to penicillin, horse serum (in tetanus antitoxin), insect bites, and a long list of common drugs; *medications* being currently taken, such as antabuse, cortisone, and digitalis; *previous surgery,* such as the laryngectomy which creates the "neck breather"; and various *miscellaneous conditions,* for instance, contact lenses, deafmutism, practices like skin and scuba diving which may cause "the bends." For individuals in all these major categories, emergency medical identification may be life-saving.

SUMMARY REVIEW QUESTIONS

1. What are the primary causes of accidents? How and where, therefore, should efforts to promote safety begin?
2. What are the characteristics of the "accident-prone" individual? With what other types of characters can this individual be compared? Why?
3. What accident statistics quoted in this chapter registered most vividly on your mind? Quote them.
4. What are the characteristics of a good automobile driver? What makes a poor driver?
5. What are some of the unconscious causes of automobile accidents? In what ways, if any, are these unconscious causes related to the symbolic roles which the automobile plays in American life?
6. What are some simple safety rules for pedestrians? (Give at least five.)
7. Why is "poor housekeeping" such an important cause of accidents at home and at work? How does "good housekeeping" serve to prevent accidents?
8. What are the "most dangerous" rooms in a house or home? What is the relative order of frequency of accidents in all the different rooms of a house (most frequent site of accident first)? Why should the list run in approximately the order you have given?
9. What can be done to prevent various types of sports and outdoor accidents? Whose responsibility is it?
10. With reference to safety and accident prevention, what are the "three E's"? The "three C's"?
11. Are the following statements sense or nonsense? Why? *Safety first. . . . Accidents are necessary. . . . The safest place is home. . . . If you drink, don't drive; if you drive, don't drink. . . . Accidents are an insignificant cause of death and injury among college students. . . . A good driver can afford to take chances on the road.*
12. What do the following terms mean to you: gremlins, safety engineering, catastrophe, stopping distance, danger unit, shock limit (of a human being), RoSPA, jaywalk, scatter rugs, reaction time?

Worth Looking Into: *Accident Facts,* published annually by the National Safety Council. *Sports Illustrated Book of Safe Driving* by the Editors of *Sports Illustrated. First Aid Textbook* by the American National Red Cross. *Life Saving and Water Safety* by the American National Red Cross.

13

HEALTH FRAUDS

WE HAVE DELIBERATELY RESERVED MATE-rial on medical misinformation and health rackets to such a late point in this text because it should serve as a kind of summary and review of everything that has gone before. To be an intelligent health-fraud-and-nonsense detective, you must first have a solid background of legitimate, scientific health and medical information. It is difficult today to escape exposure to unreliable, misleading, and even dangerous health and medical misinformation. But you should now be able to begin to detect the difference, and join the fight against quacks and nonsense.

Identifying Medical Misinformation

The rest of this chapter is devoted to the exposition of certain perennial health rackets, frauds, fads, and hoaxes. They can be described as expensive and often dangerous nonsense which needlessly increase medical costs. There are some guidelines for detecting these health rackets.

Incredible amounts of health and medical information—and misinformation—find their way into print in newspapers, magazines, brochures, pamphlets, leaflets, and books, are broadcast in television and radio programs, or pass by word of mouth. People are hungry for this kind of information. A survey on science news, conducted in 1958 for the National Association of Science Writers and New York University, revealed that 42% of the men and women interviewed wanted more medical news. Women, whose medical bills are higher, wanted even more than men. The

survey also indicated that people get most of their medical news from newspapers (64%) and television (41%).

For the most part this is reliable news. Yet on many occasions an experiment is reported as a cure, a hope stretched into a promise, a research lead twisted into a clinical result, or a sensational headline made out of a routine finding. The fallacies in this type of medical misinformation are difficult to detect.

The best, but not an infallible, test for the accuracy of medical news is to look to its *source* rather than the medium in which it is published. If the news emanates from a convention of a recognized medical or voluntary health organization, or scientific society, from the official publication of such an organization, from a university, or from a well-known hospital, and if it is written or bylined by an established science writer or reporter, the story is probably reliable and worth credence. If the information is released by an insurance company or a well-recognized pharmaceutical company, its credibility is also high. However, the statements of self-styled "doctors"—not M.D.'s—fly-by-night companies with pills, powders, or other remedies, systems, or devices to sell directly to the public should be viewed with judicious suspicion.

The most reliable single source of information on medical subjects is still your own physician. He better than anyone else can tell you whether some newly reported remedy is really appropriate for you. Many of them are not. Often they are dressed up with meaningless statistics—the better to fool you.

Fighting Health Frauds and Rackets

Although no area of human suffering is exempt, the areas in which the health racketeers most blithely ply their trade are food and nutrition fads, weight-reducing schemes, cosmetic quackery, dental nonsense, mental-health cults, cancer hoaxes, and drug panaceas for the "relief" of minor, annoying, or non-existent chronic illnesses. They don't dare legally to say "cure." But, ah, to "be regular"! To escape the "misery" of colds, piles, and rheumatism!

Among the types of products often dangerously and ridiculously "puffed" are stomach tablets, "tonics" with and without alcohol, liver pills, breath sweeteners, eyewashes, cough medicines, cold "preventives," and laxatives. As for so-called "testimonial advertising," the kind that reads, "I took a bottle of your medicine and now feel like a million dollars," the Bureau of Investigation of the American Medical Association has collected numerous examples of such testimonials that appeared in the same issue, and sometimes

on the same page of a newspaper, as the obituary notice of the testimonial giver. It should be made clear, however, that advertising abuses of public confidence are limited to a small minority of the drug industry and that the majority has made strong efforts to tone down the offenders.

Probably the most tragic of health frauds and hoaxes are alleged cancer cures. These seem to attract devoted followers who defend them to the death. Yet in 1956 the Federal Food and Drug Administration was forced to issue an official public warning against one cancer hoax as worthless and "dangerous to those who rely on it instead of obtaining competent medical treatment." Many so-called "cured" cancer patients treated by quacks never had cancer in the first place.

One of the most amusing of the modern hoaxes, expensive but not dangerous, is the "royal-jelly" cosmetic nonsense. "Royal jelly" is the substance that queen bees feed on; it is a well-investigated mixture of common proteins and vitamin B complex. Some astute merchandisers have discovered that if you put 20 cents' worth of royal jelly in an ounce (10 cents' worth) of cold cream, you can sell the combination for $10 an ounce as a skin beautifier. The secretary of the American Medical Association's Committee on Cosmetics has stated several times that the committee has *no* evidence that royal jelly "in any way affects the cosmetic appearance of the skin."

Lines of Protection against Fraud. The situation today is not so blatant or scandalous as it was a few decades ago. In 1938, partly as a result of a series of deaths from an inadequately tested "elixir of sulfanilamide," Congress passed long-overdue laws strengthening the original pure food and drug laws of 1906 and giving the Federal Trade Commission (FTC) increased jurisdiction over advertising claims of foods, drugs, and cosmetics. Since then the drug and pharmaceutical industries have for the most part cleaned house.

As more powerful and effective drugs are introduced into medical practice, increased precautions in testing them for both direct effects and side effects are called for. Realistically this is a joint responsibility of the pharmaceutical manufacturers, the medical profession, and the governmental agencies that license the use of new drugs. More stringent criteria for testing drugs are constantly being developed, but there have been some tragic examples in the use of drugs whose possible side-effects were not sufficiently explored in advance. One relatively recent example was the tranquilizer, thalidomide, the use of which by pregnant women in the early stages of pregnancy resulted in deformed babies. It should be emphasized that drugs prescribed by physicians are (with the rarest exceptions, as noted above) safe under the conditions of prescribed use. The patient who far more frequently gets into trouble is the one who prescribes drugs for himself.

No unsafe drug can now be legally marketed in the United States, though many foreign countries do not enjoy such protection. The enforcement of the pure food and drug laws is in the hands of the Federal Food and Drug Administration, which cooperates with the American Medical Association and leading universities in establishing standards for drug safety.

The flagrant type of drug and cosmetic scandals which were sensationally exposed in the United States in the 1930's, in such books as *100 Million Guinea Pigs,* have for the most part disappeared. Still, subtle abuses of public confidence continue to arise. In 1951 the *Journal of the American Medical Association* still felt called upon to castigate some advertising of home remedies in the following words—which have not lost their cogency when applied to some of the publication and television advertising still with us today.

Undoubtedly the untruths are not as blatant as a few decades ago [in the heyday of proprietary medicine advertising], but clever writing and careful display more than compensate for the limitations on deliberate fabrication. . . . The advertising copywriters probably are well aware that comparatively few people read fine print when large bold-face words are near by to distract their attention.

Superlatives appear to be the order of the day. . . . By clever wording, promises are suggested which leave the reader believing that his health and other problems can now be solved without risk of failure. . . . It is time to clean up advertising.[1]

As far back as 1957, the chief inspector of the U.S. Post Office Department was moved to declare: "Medical frauds are today more lucrative than any other criminal activity." He cited weight-reducing schemes as the most profitable racket. A subcommittee of the U.S. House of Representatives found that in the city of Washington, D.C., alone the public was "wasting about a million dollars annually on useless and sometimes dangerous reducing drugs, pills, candies, and gums." The door-to-door vitamin subscription racket is also a juicy plum for its promoters.

A spokesman for the American Dental Association's Council on Dental Therapeutics addressed another House subcommittee in 1958. He described false toothpaste advertising as "reckless" and "vicious" and gave a host of specific examples. He named one dentifrice advertising campaign as "outright deception," called another "not only misleading and deceptive but also harmful to the public," and said of a third, "If [this toothpaste] is claimed to have twice the decay-germ-killing power [of others], then [its] advertisements may be considered twice as misleading."

The FDA is Getting Tougher. Its hand strengthened considerably by extensive (and admittedly sometimes controversial) U.S. Congressional subcommittee hearings (the Kefauver committee) in 1960 and 1961, and by new enforcement laws passed in 1962, the Federal Food and Drug Administration (FDA) moved forward more sternly than ever before in the mid-sixties to enforce laws against quackery and stamp out fraudulent and racketeering practices. It began to name names and take successful court action against notorious quacks and charlatans, their

---

[1] *JAMA* (editorial), March 31, 1951.

publications, "drugs," "health foods," and fake devices.

In 1962, for example, the FDA undertook a nationwide seizure campaign against a fake diagnostic machine, of which some 5000 had reputedly been sold at a price of $875 each in preceding years. This machine was supposed to diagnose a long list of serious medical conditions; all it actually did was to measure the amount of perspiration on the skin of the unlucky patient hitched up to its electrodes.

In 1962, also, the deputy director of Bureau of Enforcement of the FDA could say with confidence:

The quacks are being challenged on many fronts by a growing number of individuals and organizations. Public health officials no longer fear the quacks and are speaking out against them at the risk of time-consuming and costly damage suits. . . . We in the Food and Drug Administration are not only talking about the quacks but we are being specific and naming names. . . . The time is gone:
 . . . when a self-styled nutritionist can use the air to spread his false teachings and promote nutritional products, without being challenged;
 . . . when a health food propagandist can use the printing press to flood the country with nutritional nonsense, without being challenged;
 . . . when a health writer can use the daily press to spread false medical theories that are used to promote the sale of sea water for the treatment of serious diseases, without being challenged;
 . . . when doorstep diagnosticians like the thousands of salesmen of health foods can use the privacy of the home to sell their wares for the treatment of every known and unknown disease condition, without being challenged;
 . . . when the publications of physicians containing unorthodox and unproven theories can be used in commercial promotions of foods or drugs, without being challenged;
 . . . when charlatans can sell worthless articles for the treatment of cancer and arthritis, without being challenged;
 . . . when promoters can launch nationwide promotions of unproven articles for the treatment of any disease condition, without being challenged;
 . . . when our food manufacturers and drug manufacturers can promote their products by meaningless,

confusing, and false nutritional and therapeutic claims, without being challenged.

Yes, we have challenged all these and many more to prove their theories in the Federal courts where they move from the sunny land of the copy writer to the cold, objective atmosphere of scientific fact.

The FDA's Role. The Federal Food and Drug Administration (FDA, an agency of the Department of Health, Education, and Welfare) has a large and varied task. Its main job is to enforce the Federal Food, Drug, and Cosmetic Act. To this end it makes sure that foods are safe, pure, wholesome, and made under sanitary conditions. It checks all drugs and therapeutic devices to be sure that they are safe for their intended purposes. It checks cosmetics to be sure that they are safe and prepared from appropriate ingredients. Finally, it scans the labels of all these products to be certain that they are honestly and informatively labeled and packaged.

To give a good hint on how the FDA carries out its manifold responsibilities for purity, quality, and labeling of foods, drugs and cosmetics, we have listed a few of the many specific things the FDA does:

1. Makes periodic inspections of food, drug, device, and cosmetics establishments and tests samples from interstate shipments of these products.

2. Assists industry in voluntary compliance with the law and in setting up controls to prevent violations.

3. Requires manufacturers to prove the safety and effectiveness of "new" drugs before they are put on sale to the public.

4. Tests every batch (except for exemptions) of antibiotic drugs and insulin for safety and effectiveness before they are sold. The manufacturers pay for such tests.

5. Enforces the law against illegal sales of prescription drugs.

6. Sets up standards of identity, quality, and fill of a container for food products in line with the congressional mandate "to promote honesty and fair dealing in the interest of consumers."

7. Passes on the safety of food additives, and checks to see that safety rules are followed.

8. Sets safe limits on the amount of pesticide residues that may remain on food crops, and checks shipments to see that these limits are observed.

9. Passes on the safety of colors for use in foods, drugs, or cosmetics, and tests and certifies each batch manufactured.

10. Checks imports of foods, drugs, devices, and cosmetics to make sure they comply with the laws of the United States.

In addition to its Washington, D.C., headquarters, the FDA has 18 district offices, where it can perform scientific analyses and investigations of the multifold products it is required to check. The FDA has about 800 scientifically trained inspectors in the field. Its cost to taxpayers (for 1962–1963) was estimated at 15 cents a person, representing a total appropriation from Congress of $28,280,000. Products covered by laws enforced by the FDA have a sales value of more than $117 billion! They are disbursed in probably 100,000 factories and warehouses and about 700,000 retail establishments.

During the sixties, in an average year, 60,000 establishment inspections were made, and 75,000 samples of products made in the United States were collected for analysis. An additional 15,000 samples were collected from shipments offered for importation into the country. It can be seen that this adds up to coverage of only a fraction of the foods and drugs bought by the American public. Enforcement of the food and drug laws must therefore be intelligently selective.

Though they have been notably rewritten and modernized on several occasions since—notably in 1938—the first federal "pure food and drug laws" actually date back to 1906. Dr. Harvey W. Wiley led the crusade for the new law and later undertook its enforcement. It is hard for us to realize the shocking conditions under which food was being commercially manufactured at the turn of the century and the bland, useless "cure-all" promises of that day's patent medicines.

State law enforcement officials are also getting tougher on the health racketeers. The New York State Attorney General, for instance, has taken legal steps to bar many shady fund-raising schemes in the name of health from plying their profitable promotional charlatanry. In at least one case the Attorney General demonstrated to the satisfaction of the courts that shady promoters were pocketing 90% of the funds raised for an apparently worthy, but secretly racketeered, health cause.

"Patent Medicines." Half of the drugs sold over the counter in the nation's nearly 60,000 drugstores can be purchased without a doctor's prescription. Sales of these drugs reach a volume of over $1 billion a year. Some of these drugs are heavily advertised; others are not. None of these products is likely to be directly harmful, except insofar as they delay treatment of the causes rather than the symptoms of a specific disease.

It is still common to speak of these non-prescription drugs as "patent medicines." Few of them are actually patented, because that requires a public registration of the exact content, proportion, and mode of manufacture of the drug. So-called secret-formula drugs are properly described as *proprietary drugs*. Their chief value is in their advertised brand name. Any competent pharmacological chemist can break their "secret" formulas.

There are no secret, undiscovered remedies for disease available for sale in drugstores or by mail. No matter how heavily and fancily advertised, they contain some old-fashioned drug long known to medicine or some new drug in such tiny doses as to be impotent. You can find this out by reading the fine print on the label. The real "miracle drugs" are not for sale without a prescription. Nor are they heavily advertised to the public.

The most widely sold "over-the-counter" medication remains aspirin, cheap in ordinary tablet form but often inflated in price when combined with other questionably useful ingredients and sold under a trade name. Aspirin production in the United States reached an all-time high in 1963, when nearly 30 million pounds were manufactured. The public paid a record $350 million for straight aspirin tablets and mixed ingredient products that year. Something like 16 *billion* aspirin tablets were consumed!

Practically all non-prescription analgesics ("painkillers") contain aspirin as their only, or chief, active ingredient. The London *Lancet* counted and published a list of 322 of these mixed-ingredient pain relievers, each sold under its own brand name!

The sums paid for aspirin *alone* in its various guises equalled 10% of the total sum ($3.5 billion) paid by the American public in 1963 for *all* prescription drugs, including the so-called wonder drugs.

The source of effect in some non-prescription remedies is alcohol. Many of the so-called "women's tonics," at one time very popular in "dry" states, had a comparatively high proportion of alcohol and represented a socially acceptable way for a professed teetotaler to take a drink.

An occasional dispenser of unreliable medical information is the "counter-prescribing druggist." Ethical pharmacists, it must be remembered, eschew and condemn this practice, but there remain a few clerks who are flattered to answer the question, "Hey, doc, what can you give me for a cold?" The person who expects to get reliable medical information for the price of a bottle of medicine is gambling dangerously with his health.

"Kind" friends and relatives, because they enjoy our personal trust, are often as dangerous health advisers as the few unscrupulous advertisers. Avoid them like poison, for that is what their suggestions frequently amount to.

The purchasers of quack products are not always aware that they are being victimized. Just one company had 75,000 agents using pseudo-scientific vitamin literature to sell its products! After proving that it contained false claims, the FDA destroyed 50 tons of this literature in the Chicago area alone. The quacks have no hesitation about claiming that their products are good for diseases and conditions that no legitimate remedies can cure—for example, cancer, multiple sclerosis, muscular dystrophy, Parkinson's disease, cataracts, cirrhosis, baldness, and sterility. To cure one of these conditions, the luckless victim is often given nothing more than a bottle of seawater—at a price of $3.75 or higher. The peddler argues that taking a little seawater a day is providing the body with a "chemical smorgasbord" and that its "rich" supply of minerals has a "vaccinative" effect against so-called deficiency diseases!

The American public apparently has a high degree of gullibility when it comes to reaching for useless, valueless health products. At the National Congress on Medical Quackery, jointly sponsored by the FDA and the AMA in Washington, D.C., in December 1963, it was conservatively estimated that the public wastes at least $1 billion a year on falsely promoted, worthless or dangerous products or methods of treating disease. Over half this was considered to be wasted on falsely promoted vitamin products and health foods. The FDA has records of protein products that contain little or no protein; cholesterol capsules that do not prevent cardiovascular disease; high potency vitamins which are *im*potent. On the regulatory front the FDA brings scores of legal actions. But an active educational and informational program is more rewarding.

Folly of Self-Medication. *He who has himself for a physician has a fool for a patient.* Except by physicians, who never treat themselves and rarely minister even to their own families, this ancient and appropriate warning is still lavishly disregarded.

Why do so many people continue to fall chronic victims to false or at least exaggerated hopes and claims that some particular remedy is "good for whatever ails them"? The remedy may be a heavily advertised specialty sold in drugstores, a "natural" food not commonly found in the American dietary, or even a nauseous herb concoction cooked on the kitchen stove according to a recipe that "grandmother brought from the old country."

The answer lies in the mental mechanisms. The victims first project all their troubles on "poor health," and secondly identify and idealize their salvation with their faith in a particular remedy.

They feel better, they say, if they take the medicine—or the exercises, or the mechanical treatment, or whatever other nonsense is offered them. The astonishing part is that they often feel better! But only for a short while.

This fact has long been recognized in the practice of medicine by the occasional prescription of *placebos,* sugar pills or bitter medicines that have no real effect on body functions. Vitamins sometimes serve as self-prescribed placebos.

Quacks, Cults, and Fads. Many of the same psychological factors which drive individuals to the danger and folly of self-medication also push them into the arms of irregular healing cults and outright quacks. And the same unhappy results often obtain. The strength and persistence of healing cults and quacks throughout the centuries lie in several facts:

At least eight out of ten cases of illness are self-limited. The patient will recover regardless of what is done or not done for him. Recovery follows treatment; therefore treatment caused recovery. That is what the quacks and cults persuade their patients, who gratefully swallow their utterly fallacious reasoning.

There is still an element of mystery—facts beyond present knowledge—in how recovery from disease is brought about by the healing force of nature (*vis mediatrix naturae*). The quack and cult exploit this mystery. They practice magic in modern dress and make irrational appeal to superstition and fear of demonic powers, sometimes recounted in a pseudoscientific vocabulary.

In the United States, at least, the general standard of living is high enough so that many people can afford to patronize irregular healers at good fees. These charlatans prey upon human ignorance. Often they "cure" diseases that never existed in the first place, such as "lost manhood." One stigma of the healing cult is its belief in a single "cause" or a single "treatment" for all varieties of disease.

It is, of course, illegal to practice medicine in the United States without a state license to do so. To this extent, certainly, the public is protected from irregular, untrained, self-styled doctors. But weird healing cults tend to spring up from time to time without claiming to practice medicine. They sometimes put forth extremely fancy names and set up elaborate establishments and machinery to draw business to themselves. They advertise. Perhaps the most protective single piece of advice that can be given to the person who wants to stay out of the hands of quacks and charlatans is to avoid any practitioner who publicly advertises his ability to heal or cure.

The truth is that there is nothing that a charlatan (or group of them) can do for a patient that a doctor of medicine—M.D.—cannot do better and more safely. Certainly the M.D. is far better trained in the rational diagnosis of disease, and there is less chance of a serious underlying source of pathology being missed while idle manipulations go on to relieve surface symptoms.

Some distinction, perhaps, should be made between fads and cults. A fad becomes a cult when its founder sets up a school to teach others how to practice a system of healing which the founder is already purveying directly to the public. Food faddists are legion, each with his own special brand of diet. Bulgarian buttermilk or yogurt is an old standby. The food faddists rarely, however, set up schools but instead make their money through books, lectures, and direct sale or endorsement of foods. Safflower seed, its oil, and other derivatives, are among the newer nutritional "gimmicks."

Very few licensed physicians have ever fallen into out-and-out quackery; the very unusualness of this situation has made such rare falls from grace both newsworthy and historical. When controversy over a medical treatment gets into the newspapers, there is usually some politician or editor trying to make a case or a story out of a dangerous fallacy.

Don't waste too much sympathy on the "persecuted" innovator who uses newspaper publicity and the courts to advertise products and methods whose worth he has been unable to prove to his professional colleagues through professional channels always open. Fakes and quacks thrive on the publicity arising out of lawsuits.

We cannot predict under what fancy names

or titles or claims the fads and cults of the future will be established. We can only predict that they will occur. Quackery is a classical example of history repeating itself.

We also venture to predict that the ads of the fads of the future, like those of the present, will be heavily interlarded with false phrases like "Science says" and "Doctors prove" and that they will wave meaningless statistics under their readers' noses.

How to Lie with Statistics

In his highly entertaining but thoroughly sound little book, *How to Lie with Statistics,* Darrell Huff has pointed out a number of statistical tricks which, he says, the crooks already know and honest men must learn in self-defense. He calls attention to biased samples, meaningless averages, purposeful omissions ("the little figures that are not there"), apples-and-peaches comparisons, illogical correlations ("semi-attached figures"), the *post hoc, propter hoc* fallacy (this happened after that; therefore this caused that), the cut-off ("gee whiz") graph, the deceptive map, and the two-dimensional picture to express three-dimensional facts.

If you want to analyze a statistical statement, says Huff, ask questions: Who says so? How does he know? What's missing? Did somebody change the subject? Does it all make sense? He cites, among scores of amusing examples an "amazing new dentrifice" headline ("23% FEWER CAVITIES") based on just *six* experimental cases, a "proof" that railroad travel is "dangerous" (the "proof" omitted to say that 95% of the fatalities were among hobos riding the rods), and a nonsense demonstration that milk causes cancer (more people drink milk, more people get cancer; therefore, milk causes cancer).

Huff points out that many a statistic is "false on its face." "It gets by," he says, "only because the magic numbers bring about a suspension of common sense." A *New Yorker* cartoon amusingly makes the same point. A tough tycoon is shown saying to his yesman, "All right, then, get another *independent* laboratory report." The moral is plain: buyer, voter, patient, BEWARE!

Sources of Reliable Information. Your own knowledge, intelligence, and common sense must be your first and best line of protection against health frauds and rackets. If you are unsure of your ground, however, and skeptical about some of the things you hear and see, you can obtain reliable, accurate, unbiased information from the following sources:

1. Your own physician.
2. Officers of your local county medical society, or your public health officer.
3. Your local Better Business Bureau.
4. The American Medical Association, 535 North Dearborn Street, Chicago, Illinois.
5. The Federal Food and Drug Administration, Washington 25, D.C.
6. The Federal Trade Commission, Washington 25, D.C.
7. Local chapters or national headquarters of voluntary health agencies or professional societies (e.g., National Foundation, American Dental Association) on questions which fall within their particular sphere.

Health frauds and rackets, quacks and charlatans provide an alarmingly interesting chapter in the long history of human gullibility. You may expect to meet again in modern dress the fakery associated with such ancient princes of quackery as Valentine Greatrakes, Elisha Perkins (and his magnetic tractors), Mesmer (parlor hypnotist), Cagliostro, and Sylvester Graham (who gave his name to graham crackers).

SUMMARY REVIEW QUESTIONS

1. What are the best tests for the accuracy and reliability of medical news? Where does this news usually appear? Why is medical news so popular?

2. What are some of the perennial health rackets to which the American public is exposed? (Give at least six examples.) Why do these rackets persist?

3. What legal protection against health frauds and rackets does the American public now have? How did this come about? What other protection is possible? What is the role of the FDA?

4. How would you distinguish between health rackets and (*a*) health cults, (*b*) health fads, and (*c*) health quacks? How, if at all, would you defend any one of these as being "more innocent" than the others?

5. How can you lie with statistics? (Give at least six examples.)

6. Are the following statements sense or nonsense? Why? . . . *He who has himself for a physician has a fool for a patient. . . . Seawater is a good remedy for many minor illnesses. . . . Vitamins every day keep the doctor away. . . . You can prove anything with statistics.*

7. What do the following terms mean to you: consumer health, socialized medicine, shaman, Federal Trade Commission (FTC), quackery, patent medicine, yogurt, *post hoc, propter hoc*?

Worth Looking Into: *How To Lie With Statistics* by Darrell Huff. *Devils, Drugs, and Doctors* by Howard W. Haggard, M.D. *The Medicine Show* by the Editors of Consumer Reports. *Folk and Modern Medicine* by Don James.

PART FIVE ENVIRONMENTAL HEALTH

14

ENVIRONMENTAL HEALTH
AND MEDICINE

MAN, THE THINKING ANIMAL, WHO HAS obtained—almost—complete dominion over the beasts of the field, birds, insects, fish, and other creatures of the deep, nevertheless remains subject to the biological, physical, and social environment that he has created for himself. As human beings have increasingly triumphed over their "natural" enemies of climate, pestilence, and famine, they have created a man-made environment which introduces new hazards to human health.[1]

The accident rate of the human race has probably remained constant since the first caveman fell out of a tree when he tried to climb it and reach for a succulent fruit. But the present day-by-day instrument of violence and death in the most "civilized" countries of the world has in the 20th century become the motor vehicle (see Chapter 12).

We have largely conquered, or are on the way to conquering, epidemic and communicable disease, but in the process of liquidating insect pests, predators, and vectors of disease we now run a risk of upsetting the cycles of nature (the ecology of parts of the globe) to the extent that we may be endangering our eventual food supply.

We wittingly, or unwittingly, pollute the waters we must live by and the air we must breathe. We take into our lungs, air saturated with hydrocarbons from the exhaust of motor vehicles, from the smoke of industrial plants, and from tobacco.

We have developed marvelous new life-saving drugs—the antibiotics, for example—but we often use them unwisely, giving our enemies—microbes like the staphylococcus—a chance to adjust to their antibiotic enemies. The phrase "iatrogenic disease" (disease caused by medical treatment) has come into prominence in recent years. The classic example is blindness owing to retrolental fibroplasia, caused by giving too much oxygen to premature infants whose lives would not be saved without some added oxygen in their early days of life. This, however, is only to repeat in more sophisticated language an ancient saying which probably has a counterpart in all languages and cultures: "The remedy is worse than the disease."

[1] This chapter derives some of its most important concepts from the International Conference on Health and Health Education, held from June 30 to July 7, 1962 in Philadelphia, under the sponsorship of the International Union for Health Education (IUHE) in collaboration with the World Health Organization (WHO) and at the invitation of the American National Council for Health Education of the Public (ANCHEP). The writer attended this conference and had the privilege of serving as a member of the leadership team among the technical study groups devoted to "Health Education of College and University Students." The conference—the largest of its kind ever held—was conducted in three languages, English, French, and Spanish, with simultaneous translations provided. Approximately 1200 delegates from 60 countries arond the world attended the conference. It was obvious that people from the so-called "over-developed" nations had much to learn from delegates from the so-called "underdeveloped," or better, "developing," countries.

We have a new science of aerospace medicine and a new concept of molecular disease, which promise breakthroughs within a decade or two for conquest over the degenerative and chronic diseases which afflct millions of inhabitants of the globe. But we have not yet licked such down-to-earth problems, whose methods of control are well known, as malaria, tuberculosis, the venereal diseases, and juvenile delinquency.

Further study of man in his biologic, physical, and social environment is certainly indicated—and this is a problem (or set of problems) to which every student of this text may eventually hope to make his own contribution. In presenting this material on environmental health, on which volumes can be and have been written, we must limit ourselves to just a few of the most significant and sometimes man-made hazards to human health, notably accidents; water, food and air pollution; pesticides; radiological health; and world health.

Man's Physical Environment

As Dr. Abel Wolman, speaking at the International Conference on Health and Health Education in Philadelphia in 1962 said: "Within the last ten years, the 'environment' has been rediscovered. [But] man, as an ecological animal, has shown throughout his history a remarkable capacity for adaptation to his external and internal environment. He is, in fact, a result of these persistent and continuing adjustments. The physical environment [however] is only a part of his total constellation. Other impacts are simultaneously at work."

Dr. Wolman has listed as the four main categories which encompass our concept of the physical environment: water, air, earth, and food. He has also pointed out that these categories have been elaborated historically into other subdivisions which at different times in human history have primarily engaged scientific and even political concern. Among these subdivided categories, some of which are current and brand new, others of which represent ancient but still unsolved problems, he lists: water supply and

wastes, food and milk, insect vectors, air, radiation, housing and occupied space, accidents, industry, noise, recreational areas, urbanization, and outer space.

Dr. Wolman has properly cautioned that in reaching for the stars we do not neglect and forget the problems that are underfoot. This too may be considered ancient, though still valid advice, for we have the legend of the ancient Greek philosopher who was so entranced at gazing at the stars that he fell into a well.

Changes in Man's Social Environment

Whatever else historians of the future may say about the twentieth century, they cannot overlook the fact that it is the period of most rapid social change that has been recorded (to date) in human history. The revolutions in communication, transportation, and public health that science and technology have wrought have forever changed the social environment of the globe. And they have affected the juvenile on the streets of New York, London, Moscow, and Paris just as much as they have changed the lives of the native of an emergent Africa.

Dr. Margaret Read, formerly professor of education at the University of London, made the valid suggestion that we keep in mind the three following principles when we look at twentieth-century peoples in their social environment, especially where the emphasis of the century is on areas of rapid social change:

1. The first principle is that the nature of social groups in a society determine the relationships and responsibilities arising from kinship patterns, from patterns of authority depending on knowledge, status, and age, from patterns of making a livelihood based on the environment. [There is an] overriding mutual dependence of individuals upon each other within an accepted pattern of relationships and behavior.

2. The second principle is that [today's] winds of change blow without regard for existing patterns of livelihood and social grouping. Some changes may be directed from above as part of a government program. Others arise from a considered or sponta-

neous desire in a community to alter its way of living. In either case the total social environment is affected in some way or other, and nutrition, child care, homemaking, and personal security are inextricably bound together in the process of change.

3. The third principle is that in all changing cultures, adult human beings can choose between acceptance and rejection, between conformity and nonconformity. This fundamental trait in human behavior appears whether an individual is conforming to traditional practices or to new ones. When a health educator is impatient because, as he says, "people do not readily learn from him," he has to see his program as the community sees it, offering perhaps certain improvements, but demanding a break with traditional custom. Choice in these circumstances involves individuals and communities in a careful and considered weighing up of many related aspects of social living.

Environmental Health: The Range

Environmental health, which possibly derives from the term, "environmental sanitation," represents man's effort to control all those factors in his physical environment which "exercise, or may exercise, a deleterious effect on his physical, mental or social well-being." Taken literally, and as a whole, this is a large order. However, when it is broken down by specific projects, it is well within the realm of official and government agencies. It must also be recognized that much greater progress has been made in some parts of the world than in others.

Environmental sanitation, as we understand the term today, began in England in the mid-nineteenth century when Sir Edwin Chadwick established the first sanitary commission and Dr. Southwood Smith organized a "Health of Towns Association." In the United States the great motivators toward better environmental sanitation were Lemuel Shattuck, Stephen Smith, and, somewhat later, William Thompson Sedgwick. Shattuck was a Boston publisher. His famous "Shattuck Report," as the "Report of the Sanitary Commission of Massachusetts: 1850" has become known, set the stage for a new era of public-health work in the United States. Stephen

Smith was a New Yorker; he called strong attention to the health abominations, such as pigsties next to schools, in the metropolis.

Sedgwick, long a professor at the Massachusetts Institute of Technology, was one of the great apostles of the "sanitary awakening" which swept America in the 1890's. He taught that "the common drinking cup is anathema," which it is, and that "dirt is dangerous," which is not necessarily so true as he believed. The causes of disease, as we have seen, are multiple.

Environmental health today is a matter of broad and complex scope. In one way or another it relates to practically all of man's activities. Major efforts, both by governmental and non-governmental agencies, must be made to attack the environmental health problems resulting from the rapid growth of our highly technological civilization. New problems must continually be studied and more thoroughly understood if measures for their control and ultimate prevention are to be developed. Environmental health is still an open-end topic and in some respects raises more questions than it answers. It is related to many public health and community health services already in operation (e.g., water supply), but it gives a new focus for many of these activities.

A wide range of scientific and operating personnel is necessary to put working programs of environmental health into effect. Biologists, physicians, physical scientists, social scientists, engineers, mathematicians, and members of other scientific disciplines are required for the effort. Among the things they must do is undertake joint research on problems of common interest from many points of view (e.g., air-pollution control); yet they must provide unified mathematical, statistical, data-processing service (together with techniques for information storage and retrieval) and develop new instruments and analytical laboratory procedures for getting a fresh handhold on both old and new problems. This may seem a somewhat abstract approach but it is an essential process for applying the vitalized new concept of environmental health to concrete problems of great diversity.

It would be impossible within the brief scope of these chapters, or of this book as a whole, to cover all the facets of environmental health. We shall therefore present some of the most important and representative areas. Among the topics of environmental health we shall discuss are air pollution, water supply and pollution control, radiological health (protection from radiation), and occupational health. We shall have to pay less attention to problems of milk and food protection and distribution, environmental engineering, and pest control. We can only mention that the field also cultivates analytical methods and instrumentation, mathematical and statistical approaches to environment, and the underlying sciences of pharmacology, toxicology (study of poisons), physiology, and biochemistry.

The field of environmental health already employs the interest and services of many people, although more will be needed. It was estimated that in the United States in the 1960's between 30,000 and 35,000 scientists, engineers, and other professionals were engaged in environmental health activities. These included individuals in the water and sewage fields, in state and local health departments, teaching, research, public works, and in private and consulting practice.

The Historical Pathway.[2] In its narrow sense environmental health is the offspring of public health, which represented, historically, man's effort to protect himself and his community against disease—for centuries primarily against communicable disease. Environmental health broadens the field enormously. It seeks to identify and provide positive protection for healthy individuals against adverse influences that crop up in an expanding society, which is becoming ever more technical and complex.

There have been unprecedented improvements in public health, community health, and environmental health practices and accomplishments in the twentieth century. On a worldwide basis, however, the progress has been spotty. The United States, Great Britain, and Western Europe took giant strides toward health protec-

[2]George Rosen, *A History of Public Health*, (New York: MD Publications, 1958).

tion in the twentieth century. It is fair to say, however, that the so-called underdeveloped nations, at least in an economic and technological sense, are often back in the nineteenth century. They still face problems of preventable diseases which the more fortunate countries learned to cope with 50 to 75 years ago.

The technological advances in the more fortunate countries, however, have brought new problems; for example, automobile accidents. It is another interesting fact that whereas these countries formerly had to deal with water, air, and food contaminated chiefly by *bacteria*, they now have to deal with these elements actually or potentially polluted by *chemicals*. Expanding industrialism brings technical, social, economic, and eventually health problems that must be faced; for example, housing, atmospheric pollution, and use of radioactive materials.

Some Key Questions for the Future

It would be hard to pinpoint exactly the environmental health problems now emerging in the United States and elsewhere. The types of problems can perhaps best be hinted at by asking ourselves some pointed questions. In these questions we give substance to the nature and future of environmental health problems.

How fast will the American and other populations grow during the remainder of the twentieth century?

What special plans must we make for the increasing percentages of older people in our own and other populations?

How can we accommodate ourselves to the ever-expanding complexity of our technology? (How, for example, do we handle the problems and displacements created by automation?)

What will the development of new industries do to our society and environment?

How risky is increasing reliance on nuclear power?

How large and what kind of agricultural efforts must we put forth to feed our populations?

What hazards may arise from the introduction of new chemicals into our food, water, air, clothing, tools, and even toys?

What will be the results of urban sprawl, forming huge metropolitan areas?

What will changes in communication and transportation do to us? (Are we going to have to learn to live with the sonic booms of faster and faster aircraft?)

What will we do with our increased leisure time? What sort of recreation facilities must we plan for?

The health risks, or opportunities, implicit in these questions are obviously greater in some instances than others, but taken altogether the questions suggest the eruption of many diverse problems in environmental health. They will have to be identified and solved—hopefully before they become too acute.

Environmental Health and Medicine. We cannot deny that we live in an era of change— progress if we want to make it so. The twentieth century is not the nineteenth century; nor is the second half of the twentieth century exactly commensurate with the first; to name but one crucial difference—the population explosion. Our outlook on health, its preservation and restoration, and our attitude about the practice of medicine, with as much emphasis on preventive medicine as curative medicine, are being revised as we breast the multiple currents of the present decade.

It has been very wisely said that man's health today depends on his aptitude to meet unexpected challenges in an environment being constantly transformed. From birth, and even before, the human being begins a life struggle to adapt himself to a shifting environment and to an equilibrium which is constantly being threatened. The mass and speed of development of new scientific knowledge, in medical as well as other sciences, have had a strong impact on the present social evolution of man. This advancement has given medicine itself added roles and responsibilities; it must play both an educative and social mission along with and indeed as part of its

preventive and healing tasks. This is the essence of environmental medicine. It is practiced not only by physicians but also by public health officers, nurses, educators, technicians, sanitarians, and others. Physicians must treat patients and communities as a whole; and they need the help of everyone else with technical knowledge toward this end.

The twentieth century has boldly set the welfare of the human race as its goal. There are, unfortunately, some stumbling blocks on the path. Today's medical weapons create some new dangers. We cannot expect to wipe out all change and struggle. Education must play an increasing role in helping man to adapt to changing conditions.

In this broad pattern of environmental health and medicine it becomes difficult to formulate a definition of "health." Perhaps as good a definition as we can essay in words is this: Health is a fullness of life, the balanced output, the total harmony in as close accord as possible with the evolving demands of the environment. More briefly, we can say that health is a product of harmony, more or less perfect, between man and his environment: biological, physical, social, and ideological. These are separated here for the sake of analysis; he faces them as a unified whole with many facets. And he must master them—or at least keep them from mastering him.

Physical environment was the first of the environments that man had to master for his survival. This he has managed on an ever-increasing scale. Consider the topography that man has had to conquer: earth, oceans, rivers, mountains, deserts, lakes, swamps. With this geography have come mighty forces of weather to be mastered. Hidden in these physical surroundings were also useful sources of energy, water power, steam, electricity, and nuclear energy, which man finally captured for himself. Now the human race has extended its physical conquests beyond Earth and set out on a conquest of space.

Two historical facts should be noted. Whatever tools, instruments, or artifacts man has created, these technological creations have become an integral part of his environment and pointed to his future. Whatever has increased man's communication and mobility has influenced his appreciation of and loyalty to enlarged areas of physical environment. Thus, sociologically, man has advanced from the tribe, the horde, the village to the modern state, to the international alliance (United Nations), and to outer space.

The *biological environment* of man consists of the animals he has tamed or not, the plants and trees he has cultivated or not, fish, insects (who were recognized as a bother but not as a danger until the nineteenth century), and microbes (including viruses). The ability to master his biological environment, on the one hand to produce food and on the other to minimize disease, has been one of man's new and big steps forward. Of utmost importance was the germ theory of the nineteenth century, which, attached to the twentieth-century recognition that most diseases are the result not of a single cause but of many conditions, has led the way to annihilating a number of disease-producing biological agents. Biologists tell us further that a nuclear catastrophe would upset the biological environment and leave the globe in command of enormously radio-resistant insects, like the cockroach and various bacteria.

The *social environment* of mankind is other people. Mankind now has the largest social environment of its history, and the outcome of this fact is uncertain. The social environment of man has been organized, split up, and sub-divided to provide the political, economic, social, and educational institutions that man manipulates in the conduct of his activities. Since the mental health of living individuals in society must evolve out of and take form from the social institutions of mankind, the social environment of man must remain one of the great banks in which the treasure of human personalities is stored up. The phrase, "a sick society," would describe an unhealthy social environment.

The *ideological environment* is nothing but the set of ideas with which individuals and groups of individuals of varying sizes surround and encase themselves and sometimes worship. A man's ideological world reflects what he believes he represents and stands for in the universe. He may be willing to fight and indeed die for this ideal. It may be the most powerful motivating force to get him to change factors in his physical, biological, and social environment. You can win a man by appealing to his ideals. The advancement of environmental health for the mass of mankind can probably be achieved most effectively by this technique.

The Rediscovery of the Environment

From his earliest history man has been compelled to conform to various environments. However, he also has a record of efforts to tamper with and change elements in his environment, i.e., the men who "captured" fire and invented the earliest tools that made hunting, fishing and killing more efficient. Around 7000 B.C., some primitive men discovered how to sow seeds and domesticate animals and—with this knowledge spread to groups of men all over the world—gradually established the agricultural revolution. Hunters and food-gatherers became farmers and herdsmen, a social revolution occurring with the technical one. We can read in detail about the "industrial revolution," which began in the late eighteenth century and is not over yet. Industry, however, has succeeded agriculture as the chief productive factor in our society; and the relative number of farmers is constantly shrinking. Many—but it cannot be said all—of the problems which mankind faces today stem from the industrial revolution.

We have only to glance about us, at least in the technically advanced countries of the world, to see how grossly and how eagerly man has sought to alter different phases of his present environment. There is no hint that he is going to stop trying to tamper with his environment. We may distinguish, perhaps, between minimal, subsistence economies, where a relatively stable adaptation to the environment is the desiderata, and technologically advanced, industrial economies, where in general whatever is "new" is gauged as "good" and where time for adjustment and adaptation to change is not always sufficiently allowed. On this point there is wisdom in a *Summary Report to the President* of the Committee on Natural Resources of the National Academy of Science, which said:

It is apparent that man must concern himself with a variety of changes in the environment, both those caused by human beings and those reflecting man's responses. Some are good; some may be very harmful. That we often do not have any clear-cut idea of their impact on man, or of man's response, is cause for concern. It would seem unwise to continue to tamper without concurrently striving to determine the real and lasting effects of our actions.

With its new tools (for example, nuclear energy, pesticides) and new ideologies (for instance, communism, "suburban living") the human race in recent decades has begun to bump up against its various environments as it has not done in several centuries. Indeed looking at the immediate past, with its developments in communication, transportation, medicine, and public health (the germ theory of disease), it looked hopefully—but falsely—for a few years as if mankind might become free of dependence on its various environments. This was not to be. The interaction between man and his environments has reached a new and critical stage, which has led to a rediscovery and new awareness of the environment.

We are now facing up to questions and problems that we had left more or less slumbering for many years. This is not to say that there were not always some forward-looking men and groups who recognized and investigated what we now again call environmental health problems; but it is to say that the crucial and rising importance of these problems was not fairly evaluated. Why bother about a few puffs of lingering smoke on the horizon? But how do you relieve a city bathed in "smog"? The fundamental questions about environmental health and medicine are quite simple to ask: What do we know about our environment? What, if anything, are we doing to alter it? How can we adapt to it? If not, how can we adjust it to our own benefit? What laws must we make and live by to manage

our environment most successfully? These are simple questions; but the answers are complex, extensive, and usually variant from locality to locality.

The trend toward rediscovery of the importance of the environment in human health and medicine has been emphasized by the number of special conferences and seminars that have been held on this topic and its subtopics, and also by the fact that the U.S. Public Health Service has established an Environmental Control Administration in its Consumer Protection and Environmental Health Service. Legislative proposals, budget increases, and political emphasis have been laid upon environmental health and medicine in recent years. This has been most markedly true in the most heavily industrialized countries but it has also been impressive in less developed regions where an inevitable advance in urbanization has been creating an environmental impact upon health. In whatever country it is located, the large and enlarging city evolves new environmental health problems. Against some of these problems education is the only, and it it is frequently the best, weapon.

Choices in Environmental Health Programs. The choices of environmental health programs to be undertaken in different localities throughout the world vary greatly and depend upon many criteria of need, awareness, and readiness. The dilemma now confronting the environmental health worker or committee is a surfeit of challenges along with a deficit of scientific understanding and underpinning in some highly significant areas of physical environment. In the days when infectious diseases were the principal challenge to the health officer, courses of action could be more clearcut because the nature of the diseases, their modes of transmission, and the techniques for their control were for the most part reasonably well understood.

Today we face a situation, at least in industrialized and urbanized nations, where contamination of land, air, water, and food is frequently easily demonstrable. However, it is much more difficult to show the positively deleterious health results which stem from these more subtle, long-term, and often symbiotic circumstances. It is not enough to know that a possibly hostile physical environment exists. It is more important to be able to evaluate this potentially harmful physical impact so that the wisest measures for its control can be undertaken.

In many areas of the world, with multimillions of inhabitants, infectious diseases that are controllable are still the prime hazards. For these areas environmental sanitation is the easy and obvious choice of environmental health activity. It makes little sense to go pursuing the carcinogenic (cancer-producing) risks of drinking water in a country where half the people do not have bacteriologically safe water in their homes and three-quarters lack anything but the most primitive means of excreta disposal. Sanitation is the first step here. Its techniques are simple, well known, and proved. They are somewhat expensive, but no-where near so costly as the loss of life their absence engenders.

On the easily proved premise that it is often difficult to get people to do what is good for them, Dr. Abel Wolman in 1958 evolved a well-defined set of criteria which might be used for initiating and making choices between suggested environmental health programs in a given community. The program chosen for action in the attack on the environment, he said, should have as many as possible of the following characteristics: (1) It should be a program that can be dramatically "sold" to the community. (2) It gives more than reasonable expectation of easy and prompt execution. (3) It requires minimum expenditure of time and energy for promotion. (4) It brings potentially the greatest public health, comfort, and economic returns. (5) It affects the greatest number of people. (6) It rests to a major extent upon the resources of the people. (7) It requires the minimum education of all the people. (8) It has a strong scientific and technological basis. (9) It requires little or no additional research. (10) It is most timely.

As we review Dr. Wolman's criteria we are reawakened to the vital influence of the social and ideological environment on the physical and biological. In the *practice* of environmental medicine we must make wise choices of programs that work. And yet, because it intersects so many of the advancing frontiers of human life in so many areas of the globe, we cannot expect the same certainties from the practice of environmental medicine that we enjoy from curative medicine (which has its own kinds of uncertainties). We do not have final answers in the broad fields of environmental health and medicine; but we are under obligation to look for these answers and give the ones that have so far been evolved in the various subdivisions of this broad and vital subject.

Pollutions and Contaminations. In one sense we can say that environmental medicine is partly the never-ending struggle against pollutions and contaminations that threaten human health. It is the battle both to prevent them and to eliminate, or at least minimize, them. In this broad and realistic definition environmental medicine touches on and intersects many other established areas of medical practice and scientific research—for example, public health, preventive medicine, industrial medicine, bacteriology, climatology, engineering, and radiant energy (radiology).

The *major* pollutions with which environmental health and medicine now deal are *water* pollution, *air* pollution, *land* pollutuon (bacteriological and chemical), *noise,* and *food* contamination. Some of these pollutions, in some areas of the globe, including the United States, have relatively recently risen or rerisen to new levels of hazard and significance. We shall deal with the impact of these major—and often new—pollutions in our last two chapters. Here we shall consider other problems that fall into the field of environmental health and medicine: occupational health, environmental engineering, international quarantine.

Occupational Health and Industrial Medicine

The civilian labor force in the United States numbers between 75 and 80 million people, of whom about 4 million are unemployed at any given time. To protect and improve the health of this working population is the role of occupational health and industrial medicine in the United States. Other countries have commensurate responsibilities. It is a task which falls in the province of environmental health and medicine, since the workers spend such a large part of their lives in their working environments. The cooperation of labor, management, and government, and the intercession of both departments of health and departments of labor are necessary to prevent and control occupational diseases, and other health hazards at work, and to promote preventive health services for employees.

Occupation has a significant influence on health, and health has a considerable influence on production. But the value and importance of the everyday practice of occupational health has not yet reached a high state of appreciation. Of the 53 million wage and salary workers in U.S. industry, for example, fewer than 15 million work in establishments with in-plant health services; that is, where a physician and/or nurse is on hand to supply health services. And this is a good record in comparison to most other countries!

The major occupations at which people in the United States now work, as estimated in millions by the U.S. Bureau of Labor Statistics, is about as follows:

Operatives and kindred workers	12,668,000
Clerical and kindred workers	10,564,000
Craftsmen, foremen, and kindred workers	9,283,000
Professional, technical, and kindred workers	7,695,000
Managers, officials, and proprietors (except farm)	7,206,000
Service workers (except private household)	6,978,000
Sales workers	4,344,000
Laborers (except farm and mine)	4,128,000
Farm laborers and foremen	3,082,000
Farmers and farm managers	2,541,000
Private household workers	2,364,000
Total	70,851,000

It is significant to note what a relatively small part of the United States working population is engaged in agriculture—scarcely 5.6 million men and women, or barely 8% of the working population. Again this is in sharp contrast with most of the rest of the world.

The cost in days and dollars of time lost from work as the result of illness and/or accident is appalling. In the United States in 1962, for example, it was calculated that "currently employed" people lost a total of 394 million days from work as the result of illness or accident; and the cost in wages was more than $7 billion! These figures can be put in other ways: On any average working day in 1962 in the United States, 1.3 million working people, or about 2% of all civilian employees, were too sick or disabled to go to work. The number of days lost from work for health reasons in 1962 was more than 20 times as great as the days lost from industrial disputes.

Not all of this time lost can be charged against the industrial environment. Growing problems in health as related to occupation and employment also stem from the changes in the age-composition of the working force. Nevertheless a tremendous amount of investigation of working-environment is still requisite to minimize its hazards. It is not always easy to identify an occupationally related disease; and the mechanisms for reporting and analyzing the incidence and prevalence of such diseases are not yet adequate. Furthermore, rapid technological changes in modern industry are constantly giving rise to new risks and new environmental health problems.

Industry has not shirked its responsibilities. In addition to individual corporate investments in the search for, study of, and elimination of plant hazards, the 4000 + member Industrial Medical Association and the American Industrial Hygiene Association work toward healthier working conditions. Government agencies and departments also play an important role. The Occupational Health and Safety Unit of the U.S. Public Health Service, for example, has established an Occupational Health Information Exchange, a facility that provides for exchange of information on the hazards of industrial products and processes and the methods for their control. This bureau also conducts clinical, environmental, and toxicological studies of factors that might affect the health of workers. It provides technical and consultative services at many levels and generally encourages the development of safe, healthy working conditions.

Occupational Disease—The Historical Conspectus. Medical history, dating back at least to Agricola in the mid-sixteenth century, affords numerous examples of specific, dramatic, and killing occupational diseases that turned out to be caused by one or a small group of environmental factors. In this list we can put such disabling and fatal diseases as lead, mercury, phosphorus, and radium poisoning, tar cancers (e.g. "chimney-sweep's cancer" of the scrotum observed by Sir Percival Pott in the eighteenth century), and silico-tuberculosis. New industrial materials, however, produce new hazards that have to be ferreted out by careful medical and scientific detective work. Except in rare, and really accidental, circumstances, the day of occupational diseases that dramatically kill and maim their victims is probably over. Instead, the working environment may evoke residual diseases and disablements that operate slowly and subtly and may be confused with "normal" processes of aging. The involvement of a given individual may be less, but a great many more people will be involved. Multiple factors, difficult to isolate and demonstrate, will probably each add some burden to the physiology of the exposed worker. Half of today's workers already have some physiological impairment.

With the introduction of labor-saving machinery and automation, heavy physical labor to get the world's work done will decline in importance. This is true even in underdeveloped, largely agricultural areas, where the introduction of even simple farm machinery, long used in technologically advanced countries, saves a tremendous amount of back-breaking physical labor.

On the other hand the psychological stresses on many jobs are increasing and can be expected to continue doing so. As one example, the operators in airport control rooms, plant control rooms, communication centers, and emergency installations are under increasing pressure to handle and interpret masses of incoming information in split-second fashion. Their mental health, which reflects their social environment, is as crucial to their jobs as their physical health. Management will have to become increasingly alert to the evolution of jobs, arising from advancing modern technologies, that would put some men to work under conditions of stress which are beyond the extreme limits of their capacity for adjustment. Jobs must be broken down; men fitted to jobs.

Challenges Ahead in Occupational Health. As with all other fields of environmental health, it is obvious that occupational health is a relatively new endeavor with many challenges ahead. The assignment, difficult to work out in detail, may be simply stated as follows: The future development of occupational health demands (1) a recognition of the environmental factors and potential risks associated with each of the wide variety of human occupations; (2) an appraisal of the favorable and unfavorable factors, and the specific risks, on human health; (3) the working out of means to minimize and eliminate the risks, real or potential, and the unfavorable factors; and (4) the assurance that the available knowledge for promoting and protecting the human factor in industry and agriculture is in fact applied.

Some of the specific challenges that must be met in the future development of occupational health and industrial medicine may be briefly pointed up here:

Evaluation of Trends. Because of the complexity of industrial processes and the changing character of jobs and workers it will be necessary to keep comprehensive and useful records of all trends or developments in industry which might have a health aspect.

Clinical and Epidemiological Studies. A great many "industrial" diseases already recognized still have much to be learned about them. Workers exposed to cotton and other vegetable fibers, to coal dust, to asbestos, to other industrial dusts, to irritant gases, mists, or fumes should be studied—especially to obtain quantitative data of long-term effects of such exposures on the lungs.

Toxicology Studies. There is no *systematic* survey of new materials released to the public—especially by smaller companies. On the other hand many of the larger chemical firms do a considerable amount of study, which should be encouraged. Recent commendable examples are the studies on the toxicology of vanadium, ozone, nitrogen peroxide, fluoride, oil mists, and intermetallic compounds.

Stress Evaluation Studies. More exact measurements, by new methods, must be made of the physiological effort and psychological stress used in work. These processes constitute the basic mechanisms on which the abnormal stresses of the environment operate to produce disease, sometimes by slow but inevitable steps. Effects of heat, climate ("thermal stress"), noise, vibration, and tolerance to chemicals must be investigated.

Monitoring Instruments. There is need for the development of more sensitive monitoring instruments to keep track of various aspects of the physical environment, such as radiant heat, vibration, noise, pressure, and dust counts.

Development of Standards for Working Environment. Determination of the optimal environmental conditions to be recommended for the health, efficient productivity, and possibly "happiness" of the workers is an essential concomitant to the continuing advancement of occupational health programs. Standards mean goals and progress.

Environmental Engineering

Environmental engineering, a relatively new term, may be described as sophisticated sanitary engineering. In a way environmental engineering is the wedding of urban (or metropolitan) planning and "human engineering" to old-fashioned sanitary engineering, whose original responsibilities do not disappear but rather become enlarged. Environmental engineering deals with problems encountered at each of the four successive levels of public health concern with the environment, enumerated by the American Public Health Association as follows:

1. Insuring the elements of simple survival.
2. Prevention of disease and poisoning.
3. Maintaining an environment suited to man's efficient performance.
4. Preservation of comfort and the enjoyment of living.

Among the challenges which environmental engineering faces are these: more basic knowledge of the effects of *waste* on man, both physical and social effects; more efficient and economic means of water supply, collection, treatment, and distribution; more effective methods of sewage treatment, including onsite disposal; better drainage; more useful and acceptable means for the collection and disposal of garbage and refuse; more healthful housing within the means of those who need it; establishment of health criteria and guidelines for urban renewal, zoning, open space usage, and accident prevention.

The metropolitan factor is the key element in modern environmental engineering. The problems of safeguarding man's life and livelihood, especially in the United States but increasingly so all over the world, stem largely from the fact that modern man wants to live in cities or right next to them, in suburbs. Over 70% of the United States population now lives in urban areas. There are more than 200 Standard Metropolitan Statistical Areas in the United States and the number is increasing annually. Twenty-seven of these metropolitan areas are interstate, including in terms of population the largest such area in the world—the New York City—Northern New Jersey metropolitan area, with an estimated population of 15 million people. Many problems in environmental engineering would be much easier to solve if they were not magnified and complicated by the urban dimensions in which they must be faced.

There are, however, persistent problems in smaller magnitudes. For example: The installation of approximately 300,000 individual sewage disposal systems every year in suburban and rural areas creates both personal and community health problems. In 90% of the 9000 communities of the United States with populations over 1000, the facilities for refuse disposal are inadequate. To safeguard the health of 1.5 million travelers daily on interstate carriers requires the environmental engineering supervision of the construction, maintenance, and operation of 5000 conveyances and the approval and certification of 4500 sources of water, milk, and food. To be sure that shellfish (produced in 22 states), milk (produced in 40), and certain other foods are free of disease-producing microorganisms and other contaminants when they move in interstate commerce requires an elaborate system of governmental inspection and certification.

The environmental engineer today must be able to handle the problems of environmental health posed by the urbanization and suburbanization of American society. The nature and trend of the population concentration in a given area, the economic and social patterns of these people, their cultural and ethnic traditions, the public and private social institutions with which they live—all these factors enter into the environmental health problems they pose. Consideration of these factors becomes especially important when changes have to be made.

As one example of air pollution, consider Los Angeles. Studies there showed that 69% of the hydrocarbons deposited in the air each day came from automobiles, trucks, and buses. Thus it was obvious that the environmental engineering problem of air pollution is related to commuting habits and patterns, and also to industrial and recreational locations.

New Challenges to Environmental Engineering. Every day brings new challenges to environmental engineering in the area of housing and occupied space, urban and recreational land use, public water supplies from the water-works' intake to the consumer's tap, the accumulation and disposal of solid wastes, the design of safer roads and traffic systems, and many other areas of concern to human safety and welfare. New hazards appear. For example:

Until not so many years ago the principal cleansing agent used in the United States was *soap*. Discharged in waste water, the "used" soap was acted upon by biological agents which changed it into harmless substances that eventually disappeared. Then came detergents. By 1958 people in the United States were using nearly 4 billion pounds of detergents a year. Detergents are discharged to the environment generally by way of drainage to surface or ground waters. The chemicals in them, chiefly the foaming agent which was originally alkyl benzene sulfonate, resist bacteriological and biological decomposition. They passed readily through the usual water and sewage treatment processes. Hence environmental engineers found themselves challenged by the presence of detergents, which had come from great distances, in individual and municipal water supplies.

One approach to this problem has been at the level of "human engineering," persuading and requiring manufacturers of detergents to switch to chemical formulas which decompose more readily under biological action. The members of the Soap and Detergents Association agreed that by January 1, 1966, all alkyl benzene sulfonate would be eliminated from their formulas and products. New "soft" detergents will still not be as decomposable as old-fashioned soap, but they are a great improvement over the hard detergents from a public-health and water-supply point of view.

Other chemical contaminants besides detergents have been occasionally found in public water supplies in recent years. These include such insecticides and pesticides as DDT, aldrin, lindane, dieldrin, diphenyl ether, tetralin, and acetophenone. The new question for environmental engineering that has appeared is whether any of these chemical contaminants are present in water supplies in quantities sufficient to make them potential cancer-producing agents.

The environmental engineer must face these obvious facts: Regardless of political boundaries, air, water, and land resources are fixed. As populations increase, there is less of each for every individual. In some places, especially metropolitan areas, this may create pressures and problems. Increasing populations also mean increasing amounts of waste products (human, agricultural, industrial). Concentrated in and around limited—metropolitan—areas these waste products could eventually choke growth and lead to urban stagnation. The environmental engineer must immediately make plans for the disposal of increasing amounts of waste products.

One of the great practical problems that the environmental engineer faces is to increase the world's supply of potable water. In the final analysis the oceans are the source of virtually all the world's water. They are also a potential source of a great deal larger percentage of the world's food supply than has yet been drawn from them. Chemical processes have been developed for converting fish into odorless, tasteless, nutritious flour; and better methods are being devised for harvesting and converting into human food the billions of microscopic plants and animals—plankton—floating in the seas.

The engineers have gone *directly* to the oceans for increased supplies of fresh water. They have developed large installations to purify seawater. The methods include distillation, freezing and membrane solar distillation. To improve the processes and reduce the costs engineers and chemists are seeking new membrane materials and installing metals, such as titanium and alloys of nickel, which have greater resistance to corrosion. With brackish water the methods used for purification are electrodialysis and solvent extraction. For powering the new desalinization plants, it looks as if nuclear energy will be a practical and economical source of power. The world's (then) largest freeze-desalination plan for the production of "fresh water" was completed at Wrightsville Beach, N.C., in the spring of 1964.

International Quarantine. Quarantine—40-day detention of a vessel suspected of carrying plague—was introduced at Italian seaports in the fourteenth century. This was probably one of the most important concepts and techniques of public and environmental health ever invented. Note that the restriction was put upon a *premise*—the

suspected vessel—and not directly upon people. The practice of international (and local) quarantine, with changes based on improved medical knowledge, advances in communication and modes of transportation, and greatly increased numbers of travelers remains part of the environmental health program of every nation. The object of the programs is to prevent the introduction into and the spread throughout the country of quarantinable diseases or any other illnesses that present a significant threat to the public health. The International Sanitary Regulations and the operations of the World Health Organization simplify the everyday practice of international quarantine. It is practiced more diligently and faithfully in some countries than in others. We shall use the figures and practices of the United States as representative of international quarantine.

The increase in international travel, especially in the volume and speed of air transport, has intensified quarantine problems. Medical inspections of arriving aliens continue to increase as a result of more travel for business and pleasure, exchange programs, and immigration, as permitted. There are medical aspects of immigration legislation. The examination *abroad* of alien applicants for visas, who number nearly 200,000 a year, requires the direct services of the U.S. Public Health Service or the supervision of local physicians.

Medical examinations are also required of all the other aliens, something over 3 million a year, who enter the United States. Over 300,000 migratory farm laborers in addition are examined at U.S. Reception Centers near the Mexican border. Where necessary, a smallpox vaccination is given.

The U.S. Foreign Quarantine Service carries out authorized inspection and vaccination programs covering people and certain imports at various points of entry into the country. The object is to prevent the introduction of quarantinable or certain other communicable diseases. Insect and rodent control programs are conducted on ships and airplanes in port areas. A ship sanitation program is also carried out. The headquarters office of the foreign quarantine service collects, analyzes, and disseminates data on worldwide communicable disease prevalence and immunity requirements.

The magnitude of the foreign quarantine service can be seen from these figures for a recent year. Over 400 ports of entry ("points of coverage") were covered. More than 65,000 aircraft inspections were performed and in about one-third of the cases (nearly 20,000) the aircraft were treated for insects. About 33,000 ship inspections were performed. The number of individuals inspected on aircraft was about 2.7 million, on vessels about 2 million, on land via the Mexican border about 1.4 million.

International quarantine as practiced by the United States and other countries is the direct, and largely successful, attempt to keep the diseases prevalent in one environment out of another.

SUMMARY REVIEW QUESTIONS

1. In what three environments does modern civilized man exist? In which of these three have the greatest changes occured in the twentieth century? What are some of these changes and their underlying causes?

2. What is the range of environmental health as we understand it today? What are some of the most important problems (name at least six) with which environmental health and medicine must presently grapple? What are some of the environmental health problems now emerging with which we shall have to deal more vigorously in the future?

3. How do you interpret the phrase, "the rediscovery of the environment"? What events of the eighteenth and nineteenth century are partially, if not largely, responsible for the twentieth century's environmental health problems?

4. On what basis must public health authorities and many other professionals concerned with environmental health make wise and rational choices of programs to improve environmental health conditions? What factors of location will strongly influence priorities in choices of programs?

5. In what ways may work or occupation injure or endanger health? Can you give some specific examples (at least three) of occupational diseases and tell how they were brought on?

6. What are some of the specific challenges that must be met by safety engineers, industrial physicians, business management, government experts, and others in the future development of the fields of occupational health and industrial medicine? Where is the most attention paid to providing adequate protective measures for workers? The least attention?

7. What are some (name at least four) of the major problems and challenges in the field of environmental engineering? For what purposes have the environmental engineers gone to the oceans?

8. What present-day factors have magnified the problems of international quarantine? What is the purpose of international quarantine? How, briefly, does the United States operate its foreign quarantine service?

Worth Looking Into: *Man In His Environment,* proceedings of the Fifth International Conference on Health and Health Education, Philadelphia, 1962. *Environmental Health Problems,* report of a committee to the Surgeon General of the United States Public Health Service. *A History of Public Health* by George Rosen, M.D. *The "Shattuck Report,"* report of the Sanitary Commission of Massachusetts, 1850, by Lemuel Shattuck.

15

IMPACT OF THE NEW POLLUTIONS

ONE MEASURE OF THE PROGRESS OF CIVIL-ization might be the progressive removal of hazards from the environment of mankind—physical, biological, psychological, social, and even ideational hazards. We might say, for example, that the ideational hazard of "the divine right of kings" was removed in the eighteenth century, the biological hazard of infectious diseases minimized in the twentieth century.

Historically we can observe an almost fantastic progress in environmental health and medicine from the middle of the nineteenth century to the middle of the twentieth century. It is reflected, among other ways, in the tremendous increases in longevity and life expectancy in the technically and scientifically advanced countries of the globe.

Then, in the middle of the twentieth century, we see a new cloud rising on the horizon. It is a cloud of pollutions; and it is beginning to shadow over some of the bright progress of environmental health and medicine. In many respects it comes as a surprise, an unwelcome surprise. We suddenly find that parts of our environment which we long judged safe and clean and pure are not so. They are polluted, contaminated, distorted. As responsible, intelligent twentieth-century students we cannot run away from the impact of these new pollutions. Indeed we must help to dispel them.

There are three old elements in our environment which now, suddenly, in the mid-twentieth century we discover to be newly polluted and contaminated: air, water, and food. We also come face to face with two major new contaminants: man-made radioactivity and pesticides. The individual who wants to promote and protect his own personal health and contribute to the improvement of community health must realistically know what hazards he faces in the presence of these five new major risks in his environment: (1) air pollution, (2) water pollution, (3) food contamination, (4) pesticides, and (5) radioactivity. We shall provide a full, up-to-date discussion of these five major topics (and a few more related ones) in this and the next chapter.

The impact of the new pollutions is strong. But it is not necessarily fatal. An intelligent attitude toward these new hazards is to listen and learn where the danger really lies; then to take steps as an individual and a citizen to avoid and help reduce it.

Air Pollution

To sustain his life man needs on the average $4\frac{1}{2}$ pounds of water, 2 to 3 pounds of food, and 30 pounds of air, day in day out. He has some choice of food and drink, but he must breathe whatever air is available to him; and in cities, this may well be partially polluted or unclean. The occurrence over the years of several clear-cut air pollution disasters, with out-breaks of sickness and death associated with air pollution, has indicated that this problem, growing in importance, must be faced.

Possibly the first recorded air pollution disaster occurred in the Meuse Valley of Belgium, in 1930, where many people died. In the United

AIR POLLUTION. Smoke from industrial plants and processes is one of the major factors causing smog. (Photograph courtesy of National Air Pollution Administration)

States an air pollution tragedy occurred at Donora, Pennsylvania, in October 1948. Industrial waste so befouled the atmosphere that day was like night; 5000 people fell ill; 17 died. London, England, has reported at least two occasions—December 1952 and December 1962—when it was so blanketed by grime and soot that thousands of "extra deaths" occurred and had to be charged to the occasion.

Far more common than the disasters are the annoyances brought to many cities by their air pollution and smog problems. Los Angeles has suffered from an annoying smog problem for a number of years. One factor in the problem arises from its location, because the mountains east of the coastal plains keep banks of air piled up over the city and county. Under these, man-made pollutants collect from a populous and industrialized city. The Air Pollution Control District of Los Angeles estimates that gasoline-driven vehicles in the county pollute the air daily with 1180 tons of hydrocarbons, 300 tons of nitrogen oxides, and 8950 tons of carbon monoxide. Factories, refineries, and even backyard incinerators contribute to the smoky air pollution.

Speaking at the American Medical Association Congress on Environmental Health in May 1964, S. Smith Griswold, Los Angeles County air pollution control officer, said of the situation

there: "We have a basic understanding of what is polluting our atmosphere. . . . Potentially we have the ability to assure an acceptable standard of air quality. . . . Ignorance and apathy are the real limitations upon the control of air pollution. A community endures air pollution because it lacks leadership and the will to act."

Some of the contaminants in fresh air, which is approximately 78% nitrogen and 21% oxygen, can be visualized as soot, dust, and smoke. There are, however, other contaminants that do not make themselves visible or even smellable. Some of these are the combustion products of gasoline; they intermingle in the atmosphere, and in the presence of sunlight they may form unknown aerosols. This complex chemical mixture, sometimes called synthetic or photochemical smog, seems to pose some menace to health.

Meteorological factors sometimes play a role in bringing about air contamination. Generally speaking, the movement of the great masses of air above us is sufficient to replace stagnant air with fresh air. On occasions, however, these currents fail. Masses of air hover motionless for hours and days and accumulate high concentrations of pollutants. Most serious, usually, is a thermal inversion, in which a layer of warm air forms and acts as a lid over the colder air, which is prevented from dissipating its waste products in the usual manner.

Health and Polluted Air. The studies that were made in London and Donora left evidence that acute air pollution is a serious threat to health, particularly to the health of elderly people who have recently suffered from heart or lung ailments. While direct cause-and-effect relationship between contaminated air and disease has not been shown, nevertheless, there is strong evidence that air pollution is associated with a number of respiratory ailments. Among these are non-specific infectious upper respiratory diseases ("the common cold"), chronic bronchitis, chronic constrictive ventilatory disease, pulmonary emphysema, bronchial asthma, and lung cancer.

Much of the cleansing of the larger airway passages of the lungs is done by ciliary action; little hair-like projections (cilia) with a whip-like motion sweep the larger irritants out of the lung. It has been shown experimentally that this important, protective ciliary action can be slowed down by such air contaminants as sulfur dioxide and synthetic smog. Hence when concentrations of irritants build up in the lungs they must be removed by coughing; other symptoms of respiratory difficulty may soon follow.

Another problem in the air pollution field is that of long-term breathing of only "slightly" polluted air. What will happen if this goes on for 10 to 20 years? The general conviction is that long-term, low-level air pollution can contribute to and aggravate certain diseases. The report of the Panel on Health Considerations at the 1962 National Conference on Air Pollution stated:

It would be a mistake to leave this conference with the impression that there is insufficient evidence for action—now. The evidence that air pollution contributes to the pathogenesis of chronic respiratory disease is overwhelming. The classical concept of one agent being responsible for one disease . . . is an investigational convenience.

An Official U.S. Government Study: Summary. In September 1963 a study of air pollution in the United States was published as a staff report to the Committee on Public Works of the United States Senate. The following summary of this report[1] gives a clear picture of why our problem of air pollution is becoming more serious:

The rapid deterioration of the quality of our air has reached the point at which more effective control measures can no longer be postponed. To underline this point, research continues to provide new evidence that air pollution is objectionable, not only for its esthetic and nuisance effects, which we can see and smell, and its economic damages, which are more varied and costly than we had supposed, but also because of its hazards to health and safety.

Pollution is increasing faster than our population increases, because our rising standard of living results

[1] *A Study of Pollution—Air,* a staff report to the Committee on Public Works, United States Senate (88th Congress, 1st Session). (Washington, D.C.: U.S. Government Printing Office, September 1963).

in greater consumption of energy and goods per person, and our production and transportation activities increase on both accounts.

Technical procedures are available which can prevent the discharge of most contaminants to the air. The application of some of these procedures involves considerable cost. However, failure to use them is now costing the public far more in economic damages, even aside from the nuisances and hazards to health associated with air pollution.

Despite the lack of satisfactory answers to certain specific problems, such as motor vehicle pollution and sulfur oxides from fossil fuels, a significant reduction of pollution from most of our problem sources is now possible through widespread application of proven control principles.

In this country, we have only begun to attack air pollution realistically. The Federal program of research and technical assistance has defined important facets of the problem and provided guidance to States and communities in assessing the nature of their local problem and demonstrating remedial measures.

One-third of the States have established programs to deal with air pollution, but most of these are, so far, quite limited in scope. Local government programs, where they exist, are generally understaffed and without sufficient financial and trained manpower resources to meet their needs properly. Only 34 local programs have annual budgets exceeding $25,000 and 7 of these are in California. . . . In the past decade, despite a 30% increase in urban population, there has been, outside of California, no overall increase in manpower to combat air pollution at the local level.

It has been estimated that in 1961 major air pollution problems existed in 308 urban places. This represents an increase of 84 in a decade. About 7300 places, housing 60% of the population, are confronted with air pollution problems of one kind or another.

The American public looks forward to a growing population, an expanding economy, and an improving state of well-being. Essential to this is clean air. To compensate for past neglect of air quality conservation, a greater effort is required now, by the public, by industry, and by governmental agencies at all levels. The nationwide character of the air pollution problem requires an adequate Federal program to lend assistance, support, and stimulus to State and community programs.

There is a need for the establishment of air quality standards in terms of known and suspected effects on what is necessary for the protection of human health and welfare, agriculture and property.

A number of States do not have air pollution control laws; others have laws which have control authority only, or no control authority, but local option legislation and research and technical assistance authority.

It is quite evident that an aggressive program of research needs to be directed toward providing assistance in developing appropriate State and local air pollution control laws and standards. There is also a need for nationwide enforcement and standards and in addition consideration needs to be given to the international aspect of air pollution.

An International Union of Air Pollution Associations was formed with United States leadership in June, 1964.

The question of air pollution is of greatest concern to residents of large metropolitan and highly industrialized areas, such as the cities of New York, Los Angeles, Philadelphia, and London. With the increasing urbanization of the globe this is becoming a more widespread problem, and its very existence often dictates individual choices of places of residence.

Air pollution occurs wherever industries, cities, and masses of people, moving around in automobiles and otherwise, come together. There are some special cases, such as pollution by volcanic smokes and dusts, as seen in Costa Rica in 1963 and 1964. Air pollution in cities, as we have noted, is usually the result of the emission of a *number* of different gases and particles, notably factory or household smoke and automobile exhausts. It is probable that all metropolitan areas have some limit on their air resources. When and where weather conditions are favorable to dispersal of contaminants, air resources are greater. But even in favored metropolitan areas, acceptable concentration limits of pollutants are sometimes exceeded.

Air pollution affects human life and health and a great many other human interests and activities. We have noted tragic examples in Donora, Pennsylvania, and in London, England. We have also cited increasing evidence that prolonged exposure to even low-level air pollution may aggravate chronic diseases (e.g. bronchitis) which affect large numbers of people. Polluted air also causes enormously costly damage to crops, animals, and buildings.

Some Unresolved Questions About Air Pollution. Hosts of unresolved questions about air pollution remain. To gain perspective on the problem it will be worthwhile to examine a sampling of the observations that have been made and the further lines of research they suggest.

Statistical studies have indicated a higher incidence of lung cancer in urban than in rural areas. The air in cities has been found to contain certain known cancer-producing (carcinogenic) substances, notably benzpyrene. It has therefore been suspected that benzpyrene and related hydrocarbons (aromatic, polycylic hydrocarbons) in the atmosphere may contribute to the causation of lung cancer. It has been shown that experimental animals exposed both to the virus of influenza and inhalation of ozonized gasoline develop epidermoid cancers in the lung. All this information suggests further investigation; it does not provide definite answers.

Since the respiratory tract is the portal of entry for inhaled substances, diseases of this tract are suspected of being made worse by air pollutants. For example, it has been observed that asthmatic attacks occur more frequently on days when there is smog damage to plants; that patients with emphysema (enlarged air sacs) improve when they breathe filtered air after exposure to several days of smog; and that the condition of patients with chronic, obstructive respiratory disease fluctuates with certain air pollutant levels.

The famous song, "Smoke Gets in Your Eyes," may be taken as common evidence of the effects of atmospheric pollutants on the eyes. Smog is another well-known irritant of the eyes; but exactly which constituents of smog have this effect remain to be discovered. Smog is sometimes described as *photochemical* air pollution; that is, the gases and other particulate matter in the atmosphere are altered by the presence of sunlight. This also is a subject for more research.

As cities increase in size, new industries develop and new products are created, the chances are that the problem of air pollution will get worse instead of better in the next generations unless it is vigorously attacked now. Since air pollution, despite its predilection for cities, follows no political boundaries, the over-all attack on it must be organized cooperatively and on a comparatively broad basis. Certainly in the United States there is a role for the federal government.

Practical Attacks on Air Pollution

Some complex research problems must precede the application of new techniques to the control of air pollution. We must, for example, have more knowledge of the interreactions of pollutants in the atmosphere; we must know more about their synergistic (heightened) effect on physical and biological systems; we need better instruments—automatic instrumentation —to find out these other things.

In addition to research efforts, though including them, the present attack on air pollution should embrace the following steps:

¶We must more accurately and completely *appraise* present and potential air-pollution levels in specific localities. This would be mapping the problem and showing the danger points.

¶Local communities must be encouraged and stimulated to participate in *air-pollution abatement.* This may require administrative or legal action, such as industrial zoning, enforcement of nuisance ordinances, or even planning to limit the number of people in some geographic areas.

¶We must *improve methods* and instruments for continuous recording of air pollutants in the more heavily affected geographic localities.

¶We must make more complete and accurate *analyses of weather* conditions on a large scale and correlate them with data on air pollution in specific areas.

¶We must find ways to promote *interjurisdictional agreements* on the control of air pollution, so that touching or distant communities can get together in the solution of the problems that affect all, but that none can solve alone.

In the United States the federal government entered the field of air pollution relatively recently. The first legislation empowering the U.S. Public Health Service to deal with the field as a single entity, in focus, dates back only to 1955. Since then it has been more readily recognized, and translated into laws and appropriations, that air is a national resource we cannot squander.

"Let's Clear the Air": A National Conference. A national conference on air pollution under the title, "Let's Clear The Air," was held in Washington, D.C., in December 1962, under the auspices of the U.S. Public Health Service. On this occasion, Luther L. Terry, Surgeon General of the Public Health Service, said:

The filters in air-sampling devices throughout the country are still coming out black or gray. I am not discouraged, however, for we have reached agreement on a fundamental principle: that it is every man's right to breathe air which is not a hazard to his health or property and that this right must take precedence over a great number of lesser rights, real or imagined. . . .

While everyone cannot be expected to possess detailed knowledge of every aspect of air pollution, it is essential that virtually everyone have a basic understanding of the problem. This understanding is needed by the business man when he plans the design and location of a new factory, by the city council member when he is faced with the task of zoning a city or determining the flow of traffic, by the physician when he treats a patient with respiratory disease and by countless others.

An interesting observation on the variety and complexity of the problem was offered by S. Smith Griswold, control officer of the Air Pollution Control District of the County of Los Angeles, California (whom we have quoted before), as follows:

We have found that few communities have the same total air pollution problem. In Los Angeles 80% of our problem is motor vehicle emission; 20% comes from industry and other sources. In neighboring San Francisco, the problem is approximately 60% vehicular and 40% industrial. In Los Angeles we burn no coal and relatively little fuel oil; in Pittsburgh coal burning was once the major source of air pollution. In Los Angeles our air is very stable; we have light winds and low inversions. In Chicago and Cleveland the winds are brisk and inversions rarely a problem.

Despite the overall dissimilarity, the individual components of the problem are similar and the same correctives may be applied wherever those components are important. A steel furnace in Pittsburgh can be controlled in the same manner as a similar one in Los Angeles. A catalytic [petroleum] cracker in New Jersey can be controlled in the same degree as one in San Francisco.

Crankcase and Exhaust Devices for Automobiles. A statement by letter, from Edmund G. Brown, then governor of the state of California, called attention to the positive and pioneering efforts being made in this state, thus:

In 1959 the State department of public health adopted standards for the amounts of hydrocarbons and carbon monoxide which could be put into the air by the State's present car population. Our goal is to return air in California to 1940 quality. Following this the State legislature, through a special call in 1960, created the Motor Vehicle Pollution Control Board, a 13-man agency, serving without compensation, to test and certify emission control devices.

The board has, to date, certified 15 crankcase emission devices for factory installation. It has approved the principle of these devices for used cars. . . . More than a million cars in our State now have crankcase devices and when another 6 million car owners install them, we shall see a significant reduction in that source of pollution.

The governor's letter also indicated that progress was being made with exhaust control devices, a more complex engineering problem. These tailpipe or afterburner devices are aimed at eliminating 65% of all hydrocarbons and most of the carbon monoxide.

Wolfgang E. Meyer, chairman of a conference panel on "The Automobile, the Truck, and the Bus," confirmed the fact that the automotive engineers and industry had successfully resolved the crankcase emission problem. He pointed, however, to several other problems, among them, the diesel engine. He said:

The diesel engine differs from the gasoline engine in that it uses less volatile fuels, that it operates at higher air-fuel ratios, and that it employs different fuel supply and ignition means. These as well as other factors account for important differences in the combustion process and consequently in exhaust emissions. Diesel exhaust is lower in hydrocarbons and carbon monoxide than that of gasoline engines, but slightly higher in oxides of nitrogen. . . .

Diesel engines, however, present a more serious problem with regard to smoke and odor as compared to gasoline engines. Properly maintained and adjusted diesel engines emit, at their worst, only very faint smoke. The black diesel exhaust smoke that justly causes complaints and concern can be controlled by scrupulous maintenance and retention of the factory adjustment of the fuel system. The causes of diesel odor have not yet been identified conclusively and therefore control methods are still lacking.

Political Aspect to Air Pollution. Despite the generally favorable reception at the national conference to the idea of "clean air," it is fair to note that caution was expressed and even some objection to putting all the recommended practices into effect. A "go-slow" attitude may be expected from those to whom air pollution control will be costly or from those on whose political toes it will step. There is a political aspect to the application of air-pollution control measures.

In a layman's viewpoint on the national conference, Howard K. Smith, well-known radio and television news commentator, touched on the political aspects. He quoted a telegram from the American Medical Association which said in part: "Believing that air pollution can and should be controlled, the American Medical Association endorses the concept of local, State, and Federal joint enterprise." Mr. Smith said he found "great stress on the idea that local government has the primary responsibility for air pollution control." But he asked:

When it comes to air pollution, what is local? An airplane pilot, on the first day of your sessions, talked of seeing the smudge from many cities blending together in a cloud which covered parts of several states. "The wind bloweth where it listeth" and our jurisdictional lines traced on the surface of the earth have little relevance. . . .

Man has within his grasp the control of his environment. Sometimes haltingly, sometimes grudgingly he controls it for the benefit of the greatest number. You who are dealing with the most basic commodity of all are riding the crest of an irresistible wave. We are going to clear the air. Let's clear it now.[2]

Water

Water is essential to human existence; hence most civilizations have been founded where there was an adequate water supply. With increasing world population, increasing water supplies are necessary. The usual water sources are rivers, lakes, wells, dams, and the like. With modern sanitary engineering these have generally been kept as safe sources of water for human consumption. Another phase of environmental engineering has been given over to the sanitary disposal of human and other wastes, so that they do not contaminate the sources of drinking water. Great progress has been made in providing pure water supplies for most urban communities in the United States.

At the 1964 American Medical Association Congress on Environmental Health, Dr. Charles L. Wilbar, Jr., of Harrisburg, Pa., said:

In the minds of some people, including some legislators, it seems that public health aspects of water pollution are being overshadowed by the need to keep the water pure for recreational, industrial, and agricultural purposes. . . . It would seem to me that physicians need also be interested in these aspects of water pollution control while remembering the primary importance of keeping water clean for health purposes.

Since 1900 fresh-water use in the United States has jumped eightfold—from around 40 billion to 325 billion gallons a day. By 1980 it

[2]*National Conference on Air Pollution Proceedings,* (December 10–12, 1962), Public Health Service Publication 1022; Washington, D.C.: U.S. Department of Health, Education, and Welfare, 1963. (For sale by the Superintendent of Documents, U.S. Government Printing Office, Washington 25, D.C., $2.75, 436 pages.)

is estimated that water needs will increase to 600 billion gallons a day—almost equal to the total fresh-water supply in sight. Under these circumstances water will have to be treated for re-use and re-used liberally. Conversion of sea water to fresh, potable water may become a necessity.

The United States has been generally fortunate in its water resources. However, with the rapidly increasing American population and the increased need for water in normal industrial production practices, a new look at America's water reserves, and how she will handle them, is justified. In the 1960's the United States had about 325 billion gallons of water available a day. Through conservation measures it is anticipated that this can be built to 600 billion gallons a day by 1980. If water use doubles from 1980 to the year 2000, it is difficult to see where the extra gallonage is coming from.

As water re-use becomes increasingly necessary, the key factor is *water quality.* This means that pollution wastes will have to be treated at their sources so they do not pollute waters that must be re-used. Improved treatment methods are being tried, because the fact is that there is already a considerable amount of water that could be used over and over again if a means could be found to remove the small but important amount of dissolved materials remaining after subjection to currently available treatment.

An unprecedented population and economic growth in the United States is demanding more water. Industry, the largest user of water, will need twice as much as is presently used by 1980. Those who use it for irrigation, municipal water supplies, and recreation will also be demanding more water. The increasing discharge of pollutants diminishes suitable water supply and hence contributes to the increasing water demands.

The Water Pollution Problem. In the 1880's water pollution made headlines when typhoid and cholera epidemics struck some cities. These diseases were discovered to be carried by waterborne bacteria. It was further discovered, then, that the city's water supply could be rendered safe by purification techniques, such as filtration and chlorination.

For four generations, now, city-dwellers and their suburban friends have been taking pure, safe drinking water for granted. "Just turn on the tap." But the situation is changing. Polluted, dirty water is causing a new and still not completely defined peril to human health. Every glass of water from the faucet is not necessarily clean and potable. New and unusual contaminants are getting into the American water supply. Some are wastes; others are chemicals found in the new pesticides, herbicides, and detergents. These inevitably return to surface or underground waters after they have been washed off croplands, out of barns, or out of kitchens and laundries. Cumulatively they may be hazardous. Drinking water in many communities is beginning to have a definite, unpleasant taste. In the southwestern part of the United States there is the special case of public water supplies, as well as waterholes used by cattle and wildlife, becoming contaminated by salt brine.

These present problems in environmental health and medicine should not come as a complete surprise. After all, in the last 50 years, we have doubled the United States population, tucked two-thirds of it into cities, and raised our industrial production about 900%. In these same years hundreds of thousands of new chemicals have been manufactured and found their way into streams. In some crowded localities water intake has been located dangerously close to sewer outlets. A combination of forces, none of which are rapidly abating, are polluting the waters and bid fair to continue doing so unless remedial measures are adopted.

The three basic uses for water in the United States are (1) municipal, the smallest; (2) agricultural, for irrigation; and (3) industrial, by far the largest. In 1960, industry consumed about *half* the available water, about 160 billion gallons a day; irrigation, about 43%—141 billion gallons; and municipalities, a mere 7%, about 22 billion gallons. By 1980, according to some estimates, industry will be consuming about *two-thirds* of the 600 billion gallons a day then hopefully available, with 166 billion gallons going for irrigation (27%) and a mere 37 billion gallons for municipalities (6%).

The water challenge now before the nation is to complete, as rapidly as possible, engineering works which are necessary to capture 600 to 650 billon gallons of water a day, and furthermore to treat water in such a way that each gallon is usable at least twice. Water re-use is nothing new. The water of the Ohio River, for example, is used 3.7 times before it reaches the Mississippi. But water to be re-used must be of suitable quality. Unfortunately, water-pollution control programs have not developed as rapidly as the need for them. As a result, at least in the United States, pollution has become the Number 1 water resource problem.

What is Pollution? Since water pollution is a far-reaching and increasing problem in environmental health in the United States, it will be worthwhile to go into some detail concerning what is meant by pollution and what is specifically causing it, as well as recommendations in some cases of what can be done about it. "Pollution" may be defined as anything that degrades the quality of water. Water becomes polluted, unsuitable for re-use, when *over*burdened with any of the following things:

1. *Organic wastes,* which are contributed by domestic sewage and industrial wastes of plant and animal origin.

2. *Infectious, disease-producing agents,* also originating in domestic sewage and some kinds of industrial wastes.

3. *Plant nutrients,* which promote nusiance growths such as algae and water weeds.

4. *Synthetic-organic chemicals,* such as detergents and pesticides, potentially toxic, the result of new chemical technology.

5. *Inorganic chemicals* and mineral substances. These result from mining, manufacturing, and oil plant operations. They interfere with natural stream purification, destroy fish, cause "hard water," complicate water treatment processes.

6. *Sediments,* which damage hydroelectric operations, choke streams, destroy fish and spawn.

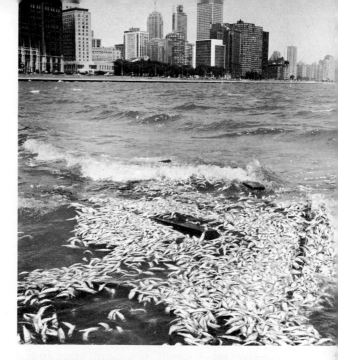

7. *Radioactive* pollution, from mining of radioactive ores and processing them; also from "fall-out,"

8. *Temperature increases,* from power plants and water impounding. Increased temperature may have harmful effects on aquatic life, may reduce water's capacity to assimilate wastes.

Water pollution in the United States is no longer a local affair. Long stretches of streams are degraded. Conventional waste treatments are hard pressed to hold the line against the sheer mass of biological and chemical pollutants entering their intakes. Sewage construction has not matched our population growth and movement. Coastal waters in 23 states are increasingly subject to pollution from waste discharges of coastal cities, a situation adversely affecting shellfishery, finfishery, recreational and waterfront property values, and creating health hazards.

Groundwater pollution, also increasing, is still essentially a local affair, with different causes in different localities. Seawater is intruding to pollute groundwater in a number of coastal states, such as Maryland, New Jersey, Texas, and California. In the oilfields of the Midwest and Southwest brine disposal practices are causing salt pollution of groundwaters, particularly seepage from evaporation pits. In an increasing number of metropolitan suburban areas, where a large part of the population must rely on individual septic tanks for its waste disposal, this has resulted in serious pollution of groundwaters which must basically provide this same population with its water supply. Industrial waste-storage lagoons, improperly located in permeable soils, are also often responsible for local ground water pollution. One of the most hopeful steps on the part of industry, a move encouraged by experience with oil brine, is to look to deep *underground* strata for disposal of highly poisonous, untreatable, or radioactive wastes.

We have been discussing the specialized problems in the United States; but we should point out that most of the world's population uses water supplies that are unsafe and insufficient in quantity, disposes of excreta and waste dangerously, and commits many other sanitary errors. The water pollution hazard is illustrated in a number of South American countries, where diarrheal diseases remain the leading cause of death for children from ages 1 to 4. We have an interesting example of the efforts made in one water-poor South American city of 350,000 (Arequipa, Peru) to improve the quantity and quality of the water supply—and thus reduce gastro-intestinal disease rates. An intelligent plan to pipe pure water to houses was set up, but it met resistance expressed in such phrases as: "Water is a gift from God. Why do we have to pay?" "We prefer river water; it is sweeter." "How can we wash if water is more expensive?"

How Much Water Pollution? Returning to the American scene, it will be worthwhile to investigate how much of what kind of water pollution we suffer and what the prospects are for reducing it. We can state the situation in terms of what we *have* accomplished and what remains to be done.

Municipal Wastes. In 1900 there were only 950

IN THE UNITED STATES pollution has become the major problem in water resources, a situation affecting fishing, recreational, and waterfront property values, and creating health hazards. These dead fish (alewives) are within full view of the magnificent skyline of Chicago. (Photograph by Hays-MONKMEYER) communities in the United States that had provided their citizens, numbering about 24.5 million people, with sewers. Since then the number of communities with sewers has increased to nearly 12,000 and the number of citizens served to about 125 million (60%). About two-thirds of these sewered municipalities have constructed sewage treatment works, serving perhaps 110 million people. At the same time the amount of municipal pollution has increased and is increasing because of more population, obsolescence of older sewage treatment plants, failure to construct needed new sewers, increased interception of industrial wastes by municipal sewers, and greater numbers of water-using devices in the home (automatic laundries, garbage grinders, etc.). Even if we build more sewers and sewage treatment plants at a greatly accelerated rate between now and 1980, we will still have as much municipal waste and pollution reaching the nation's streams as we do now!

Combined Sewer Systems. The discharge of mixed raw sewage and storm water into our streams from combined sewer systems overflows is one of the most harrassing water pollution problems a number of our cities face. Combined sewer systems are a product of mistaken, nineteenth-century engineering concepts. What happens in these old-fashioned combined systems is that a high percentage of raw sewage, sludge, and rainwater runs off directly into the receiving stream without going through the sewage treatment plant. Even occasional, "rainy season" overflows of raw sewage on receiving waters often create serious pollution problems, as exhibited in posting and closing beaches in New York City, Milwaukee, and other areas. There are still about 2000 American communities that depend wholly or partly on combined sewer systems.

Industrial Wastes. There are at least three classes of industrial wastes that rank as water pollutants: (1) organic industrial wastes, (2) inorganic industrial wastes, and (3) new chemical wastes. Some radioactive wastes and "heat pollution" will be considered under this heading.

Industry places a staggering demand on the nation's water resources. It uses water in scores of ways—as a solvent, a coolant, a washing agent, an ingredient, a means of transportation, etc. The amounts of water used sound fantastic. For example, it takes 200 gallons of water to produce a dollar's worth of paper; 1400 gallons to make a dollar's worth of steel. Talking in tons, it takes 320,000 gallons of water to produce a ton of aluminum; 600,000 gallons for a ton of synthetic rubber.

Organic industrial wastes are discarded substances of direct animal or vegetable origin which are originally taken into such industrial processes as fiber or food processing, textile manufacture, papermaking, or kindred industries. The U.S. Public Health Service estimated that in the 1960's the amount of organic industrial wastes, treated and untreated, going into the nation's watercourses was about *double* the total municipal waste load being discharged! If production estimates are valid, the amount of industrial organic waste could double by 1980. It is not suprising under these circumstances that the U.S. Public Health Service also estimates that if industry is to do its fair share in keeping America's water clean, it will have to construct about 6000 first-class sewage treatment plants.

Inorganic industrial wastes originate from such processes as metal pickling, metal finishing, chrome tanning, mining, processing, and manufacturing a wide variety of metal and chemical products; and from mine-acid drainage. Something over 20,000 openings from abandoned or inactive mines account for more than half the total mine-acid discharge in the United States annually. This is estimated at 3.5 million tons of acid every year, disgorged into about 4000 miles of waterways. The acid kills fish, corrodes underwater structures, destroys the recreational value of streams, and makes necessary more extensive and expensive water purification processes for industry and municipalities. In the spring of 1964 the U.S. Public Health Service undertook two extensive projects in West Virginia to locate all mine openings and find effective ways of keeping drainage from entering streams.

Inorganic industrial wastes contain metals

such as iron, chromium, nickel, and copper; salts such as sodium, calcium, and magnesium; acids such as hydrochloric and sulfuric; and a host of other waste compounds. They degrade water quality by causing tastes, odors, and colors; excess saltiness and hardness; and corrosion. Some are toxic or potentially so.

New chemical wastes appear increasingly in our streams and water supplies. They are not removed by and are indeed resistant—and sometimes antagonistic—to present-day water and sewage treatment processes. The new synthetic wastes are present in low concentrations in most waters; but we have no idea what their long-range toxic effects on man and other living organisms may be. Some are known to be highly poisonous to fish and some forms of aquatic life. Others are known to cause persistent tastes and odors. It should be realized that at least half the thousands of new products now manufactured by the synthetic chemical industry were not in production, nor dreamed of, in 1940. With the rapid growth of the synthetic chemical industry a major new water pollution problem has emerged. Not only do the finished products become new chemical pollutants, the by-products in the manufacturing processes also contaminate streams.

Radioactive wastes are a relatively recent factor in the water-pollution problem. They are the result of the growth of our new nuclear technology. The sources of radioactive substances which may be responsible for water pollution are varied. They include mining and refining of radioactive minerals, such as uranium and thorium; escape of refined radioactive substances used in power reactors or for other industrial, medical, or research purposes; and nuclear weapons testing. In the mid-sixties the U.S. Public Health Service national water quality analytical network showed that the radioactivity in the country's lakes and streams was "well below the safe allowable concentration." However, there is always a potential hazard.

Heat pollution, so-called, is caused by the return to water courses from power plants and other industrial sources of relatively large quantities of water heated as the result of being used as a coolant in industrial processes. As water temperature goes up, the amount of oxygen it can hold in solution diminishes. Hence there is less oxygen to oxidize pollutants. Fish life in streams is also adversely affected. Unless effective controls are instituted, it is estimated that heat pollution will increase 100% between 1965 and 1975.

Other Sources of Pollution. *Land drainage wastes* include the silt, sediment, soils, mineral particles, agricultural pesticides, and fertilizers washed from the land by storms and floodwaters or drained off by rainwater. This may occur along an entire watershed. Sediment results from soil erosion, and this in turn is caused by denuding soil of its vegetative cover. Brush and forest fires may create this situation in some localities— giving the water of the nearby streams a "burnt" taste. More commonly land is denuded by bulldozers as the first step toward the erection of a housing development or the building of a new highway, which causes the same results.

Hard-surface runoff describes the waste material washed into streams by runoff of water from the hard-surfaced, chiefly urban areas—streets, highways, houses, industrial and other buildings, airports, etc. The urban runoff carries with it accumulated deposits, such as oils, organic matter, trash, soil, industrial dusts, other air pollutants, fertilizers, and pesticides used by weekend gardeners. The hard-surface runoff is nearly 100% of the rainfall, but a certain amount of this goes through sewer systems and water treatment plants.

Irrigation return flows are a major water pollution problem in 17 western states. As irrigation waters percolate through the soil, they dissolve significant amounts of minerals and other substances. Used over and over again, the concentration of mineral pollutants in these waters becomes damagingly high. Irrigation return flows often render streams unfit for further use, including irrigation, until their mineral content is diluted.

Agricultural pesticides and fertilizers have created perhaps the most important new land drainage problem involving water pollution. We shall discuss the pesticide and fertilizer problem later.

Recreation in and on the water—swimming, boating, water-skiing, etc.—can create measurable water pollution. Few recreational small crafts have proper waste disposal facilities, and they discharge galley and toilet wastes directly into the water. Motorboat and outboard motor exhaust wastes are becoming a serious problem in some areas. They leave in the waters significant concentrations of oil, lead, and combustion products, such as carbon monoxide, phenols, and benzpyrenes common to air pollution from automobile exhausts. Offshore drilling for oil has also contaminated once clear beaches, as at Santa Barbara, California in 1969.

Navigation is an old and still active source of water pollution in estuaries, harbors, and some coastal waters. With the opening of the St. Lawrence Seaway, which has opened the Great Lakes to 90% of the world's commercial vessels, the problem of water pollution in the Great Lakes has been greaty magnified. Many communities draw their drinking water from these lakes and there are many recreational beaches along them.

Few ships afloat today have any facilities for collection, treatment, or disposal of shipboard wastes. Ship pollution consists of bilge waters, sanitary sewage, garbage, spoiled cargo, oils, and anything else that can be thrown overboard. Theoretically bilge should be pumped outside a ten-mile harbor limit; but this regulation is not always honored. Stricter enforcement of sanitary regulations on the Great Lakes will be necessary as its cargo tonnage continues to increase.

How Can We Control Water Pollution? Unless the United States takes positive steps to control its increasing water pollution problem, it may find itself running out of safe, high-quality water for essential needs—personal, agricultural, industrial. The attack on the water-pollution problem must be threefold: (1) construction of more first-class water and sewage treatment facilities; (2) enforcement of laws against practices that create pollution; and (3) development of research procedures that will find ways to remove the new pollutants and better ways to get rid of the old contaminants.

The best modern sewage treatment plants provide a *primary* treatment, in which solids are given a chance to settle out; and a *secondary* treatment that depends on bacteriological action. This treatment removes only 75% to 90% of organic wastes, a smaller fraction of dissolved mineral solids, very little of the chemically new wastes. The U.S. Public Health Service is therefore encouraging *advanced waste treatment research,* through which it is hoped the conversion of waste water to fresh water may be genuinely achieved. In 1964 the Manufacturing Chemists Association undertook a research project to determine the behavior of organic chemicals in streams, lakes, and rivers. Among the new techniques for water purification under study, some of which may turn out to offer practical solutions to the water pollution problem, are absorption by carbon or other absorptive filter, distillation, foaming, freezing, ion exchange, solvent extraction, electrodialysis, and even electrolysis.

The individual can do relatively little, outside of obeying the laws against water pollution, to reduce this hazard of which he himself may fall a victim. He can as a *citizen,* however, raise a loud voice to encourage industry, voluntary agencies, and government agencies at all levels to do their jobs in controlling water pollution.

Measuring Water Quality. Realizing the need for continuing measures of water quality management through state, interstate, and other agencies, the U.S. Public Health Service in 1957 established a "National Water Quality Network." By 1962 more than one-third of the planned 300 sampling stations were in operation. Detailed analysis of samples is helpful in determining long-range water quality trends, in selecting sites for water use, and in developing comprehensive water resource programs. Another indicator of water pollution introduced by the U.S. Public Health Service is its annual "fish-kill" count, running into the millions (7.8 million in 1963). The U.S. Public Health Service has also undertaken a Pesticide Control Project to determine the presence of herbicides and insecticides in surface streams and ground waters so that their damage, if any, can be accurately assayed.

Water pollution control programs are now being developed for seven major river basins: Arkansas-Red, Colorado, Columbia, Great-Lakes-Illinois, Delaware, Chesapeake Bay, and Southeastern. As the nation grows, more and more developments in making pure water available will have to be undertaken. Industry will have to become more conscious of its responsibilities for water control and seek to provide clean, fresh water for economic as well as public health reasons. Water is now big business.

Food Contamination

The food a person eats is as much a part of his environment as the water he drinks or the air he breathes. Altogether air, water, and food provide the physical substance, the chemical elements, out of which living organisms, including man, are compounded. Just as population expansion and technological progress in civilization have created new problems of water and air pollution, they have also introduced new hazards of food contamination. True enough, the advances in microbiology and public health in the past century have happily eliminated some of the old hazards of unclean, impure food—for example, botulism and typhoid fever—but new risks have arisen.

The following statement from the *Report of the Committee on Environmental Health Problems to the Surgeon General* highlights the predicament of the 1970's:

The traditional food sanitation programs of [local] health departments generally speaking [cannot keep up] with the new responsibilities resulting from advances in food technology, changing eating habits, and population growth. So many new problems have arisen that many departments are no longer capable of providing adequate food protection. There is urgent need to reverse this trend toward obsolescence.

The food supply for metropolitan centers presents an increasing number and variety of public health problems, based on the potential hazards associated with technological changes, the continuing widespread occurrence of foodborne illnesses, rapidly changing economics and pattern of distribution, and the influence foods may have on man's response to environmental stresses. . . . Food protection is the keystone of environmental health.

The magnitude of the new problems faced by the official agencies responsible for food safety of the America public, that is, local and state health departments, the U.S. Public Health Service, and the Federal Food and Drug Administration (FDA) can be illuminated by the following fact: The American public spends $80 billion a year in retail stores for *food*. It spends another $35 billion for *meals* in restaurants, grills, hamburger stands, "drive-ins," etc. The American food industry devotes more than 1% of its income, a sum close to $1 billion a year, to research designed to develop *new* food products. In terms of budget alone the health agencies cannot keep up with the industry. New and unresolved problems are constantly arising as new foods are introduced. The food-protection service budgets of the Federal Food and Drug Administration and the U.S. Public Health Service operate in the low tens of millions of dollars.

The demand of the American public for foods of greater convenience, variety, and quality, and in ever-increasing quantity, is at the root of new problems in food safety. This human demand is certainly understandable. Man's relationship to his environment (including food supply) during his long evolutionary period was not unlike that of other animal species. The human race multiplied at a rate which was on the whole in excess of its food supply and accepted the marginal existence implicit in that multiplication. It is only today, and then only in a few countries like the United States, that people enjoy the possibility of having enough of the right kind of food to eat. Success in this direction has brought new kinds of problems of food contamination, and it has not eliminated all the old ones. It will be most illustrative to look at this in historical perspective.

Foods in America: An Historical Perspective. In general stores such as Abraham Lincoln kept when he was a young man fewer than a hundred food items were sold. These were mostly dried staples and produce from nearby farms. Perishable foods were consumed promptly or home-processed to preserve them a little longer. Milk was made into butter and cheese. Meat was salted down. The common preservative agents were salt, sugar, and vinegar. The causes of food-borne diseases and food spoilage were basically unknown.

Scientific advances in the second half of the nineteenth century led to remarkable progress in the production, manufacture, distribution, and service of food. Microbiology and epidemiology demonstrated the role of food (and milk) in spreading infectious diseases such as typhoid fever, tuberculosis, dysentery, and septic sore throat. Sanitation programs were set up, involving pasteurization of milk, inspection of dairy products, veterinary examination of food and dairy animals, inspection of restaurants, and education of food-handlers in hygienic practices. Adequate heat-processing of canned foods was insisted upon to destroy spore-forming bacteria which, without air, it was discovered, produced the highly virulent poison of botulism.

At about the turn of the twentieth century the traditional patterns of food marketing and consumption also began to change radically. Part of this was based on early urbanization; part on technological advances, such as the development of farm machinery, long-range railroad transportation, mechanical refrigeration in storage warehouses, and the commercial food industry. By 1900 food processing, chiefly canning, was moving rapidly from home kitchens to large factories and processing plants.

Then came shocking revelations of contamination and adulteration of commercially processed food. Housewives were terrified by public disclosure of filthy, fraudulent, and dangerous foods—foods doused with large amounts of dangerous chemical preservatives such as formaldehyde, salicylic acid, and boric acid; and candy colored with poisonous dyes. Such conditions led Congress to pass the original "Pure Food and Drug Law" of 1906. Appointed to enforce it was Dr. Harvey W. Wiley, the man whose 20-year fight against food contamination did most to show its need. Wiley conducted a dramatic "poison squad" experiment in 1903. In this sensational scientific experiment he fed a dozen young men measured amounts of chemical food preservatives and observed the harmful effects. Laws protecting food safety and purity have been strengthened many times since 1906.

Food production in the United States has advanced steadily in the twentieth century. Thanks to power-driven machinery, selection and hybridization of seed plants and animal sires, and agricultural chemicals, the American farmer now produces ten times as much food per acre as his Indian or African counterpart. But it is the agricultural chemicals, constantly being "improved," that have introduced new problems of food contamination. Agricultural chemicals include fertilizers, weed killers, feed supplements, fungicides, insecticides and pesticides. There are tens of thousands of them. Some are suspected of being carcinogenic (cancer-causing). Not all of them have been adequately tested. The pesticides in particular appear to offer the greatest risks, and a special amendment (1954) to the federal food and drug laws empowered the Food and Drug Administration to set safe limits or "tolerances" for residues of pesticides on fresh fruits and vegetables when shipped. We shall discuss the problem of pesticide contamination, which is an international problem, in great detail in the following chapter.

The technology of food processing, packaging, and distribution was changed radically after World War II. There came a still greater demand for complex, convenient, precooked foods, processed by increasingly complex machinery. Among the new foods were dried, precooked, and frozen products—which were not always sterile. New hazards were introduced—the risks of improper storage and the breakdown of refrigeration. Oldtime canning always included a step of heat sterilization. However, with use of some of the new packaging materials, foods are only partially sterilized—in the expectation that they will be preserved by unbroken refrigeration until consumed. This does not always happen.

Today, in contrast to Lincoln's day, you can buy 8000 different food items at America's supermarkets. Two dozen new ones are offered every day. The safety risks multiply, augmented by new modes of food service. Automatic vending machines now deliver both hot and cold foods and even complete meals. This business, presently around $300 million a year, is expected to increase. The American food industry in all its aspects probably does around $115 billion worth of business a year at retail prices. It is estimated that there are at least 450,000 establishments in the United States that manufacture, distribute, store, or sell food, in addition to 375,000 public eating places. The magnitude of the problems of inspection and surveillance is obvious!

And there is another mid-twentieth-century contaminant to which foodstuffs are liable: man-made radioactivity.

Three Basic Contaminants: Microbes, Chemicals, Radioactivity. The foodstuffs sold and served in America today run risk of contamination from three sources: (1) microbes, owing to faulty processing or handling; (2) chemicals, commonly known as "food additives," deliberately or indirectly added to food-stuffs; and (3) radioactivity, arising from controlled weapons testing, industrial, and accidental sources.

Not counting the occasional gastro-intestinal upsets that almost everyone experiences, it is estimated that a minimum of 1 million cases of definite food poisoning occur in the United States every year. The infective agents usually reported are the staphylococcal and salmonella or shigella organisms. In rare cases, such as the 1964 typhoid epidemic in Aberdeen, Scotland— traced to South American corned beef that had been prepared under less than the best sanitary precautions and had been kept in storage for many years—food infection and poisoning may be traced to other organisms.

There is another facet to this "poisoning" problem; namely, the long-range effect on health of chemicals directly or indirectly added to food. Studies of the results of cumulative effects of small amounts of food contaminants—chemical, microbial, and radiological—have just begun. The total risks are still undetermined.

Microbial Contamination of Food. Control of severe food-borne diseases, such as botulism and typhoid fever, in the past half-century has been so successful on the whole that it has left the impression that technical knowledge in this field is completely adequate. But current sanitation practices of the past decade and a half have failed to reduce a high incidence of food-borne infections. It is now believed that hitherto unsuspected fungi, bacteria, viruses, rickettsiae, and protozoa may be at least partly responsible for a number of these infections. For example, an outbreak of infectious hepatitis was traced to polluted shellfish, first in Sweden, then in the United States.

A local public health officer, William A. Dorsey, chief of the Richmond (Va.) Public Health Laboratories, pointed out in June, 1964, that there were significant changes in the way *Salmonella* food poisoning was attacking its victims. Formerly, the food poisoning occured as an epidemic and it was easy to trace the source of contamination. "Today," said Dr. Dorsey, "the poisoning is coming up as individual cases that are never concentrated in one particular area. In the Richmond area alone there are several hundred food plants putting out several thousand products. It's impossible to check them all. We're groping in the dark."

The situation described in Richmond is reflected nationwide. A survey of 63 frozen food plants conducted in 18 states in the mid-60's by the Food and Drug Administration revealed the same hazardous and unsanitary situation. After examining 3000 food samples, the Food and Drug Administration concluded: "Sanitary and operating practices in the plants were considerably below the levels desired."

The legal actions initiated by the Food and Drug Administration in recent years is *a priori* proof that strong steps, beyond a continuing program of persuasion and education, remain necessary to safeguard the food offered the American public from bacterial and chemical contamination. Approximately 3500 legal actions, that is, seizures, citations, prosecutions, and injunctions, are now instituted every year against food and drug manufacturers, wholesalers, retailers, and others who are apparently in violation of the laws. Approximately 7500 detentions of imported drugs and foodstuffs are recorded annually.

It is another interesting fact that industry often takes *voluntary* corrective actions as a result of Federal Food and Drug Administration inspections, which reveal batches of food to be adulterated or contaminated. In the first three years of the 1960's approximately 3500 members of the food industry voluntarily destroyed (or converted to feed, if allowable) nearly 60 million pounds of adulterated foods.

Chemical Additives; Radionuclides. Under the present operation of our scientific agriculture and highly technological food processing industry, it would be impossible to keep foreign chemicals—food additives—completely out of our foodstuffs and still feed the American people. It has been promulgated, for example, that if agricultural chemicals (principally fertilizers) were eliminated, the yield of American farms would drop by 10% to 90%. Among the food additives now commonly used in American foodstuffs are the following:

Nutrient supplements (e.g., vitamins, iodized salt); sugar substitutes (e.g., saccharin); preservatives (e.g., antioxidants, mold inhibitors, fungicides, sequestrants, citric acid, benzoic acid, salt, and vinegar); emulsifiers (e.g., lecithin, monoglycerides); stabilizers and thickeners (e.g., agar, gelatin); acids, alkalis, buffers, neutralizing agents (e.g., ammonium bicarbonate, calcium carbonate); flavoring agents (e.g., amyl acetate, methyl salicylate); bleaching agents, bread improvers (e.g., benzoyl peroxide, chlorine dioxide, chlorine); leavening agents; hardening agents; drying agents; chill-proofing agents; antifoaming agents; color additives (e.g., coal-tar colors); and livestock feed additives which leave a residue in milk, meat, eggs, and other human food.

A Food Additives Amendment became Federal law in 1958, and in 1960 the law was extended to bring all food colors under the same type of control. The Food and Drug Administration now receives animal feeding tests on proposed new food additives before they are marketed. If satisfied that the additive is safe, the Food and Drug Administration issues an order permitting its use and establishes its tolerance (the amount which may be used). This is a great improvement over previous practice, but it is not perfect.

As the Food and Drug Administration itself has said: "The danger [is] not theoretical—it [is] real, as shown by a number of instances of chemicals having been found injurious only after they had been in use for a considerable period of time, including a chemical used for flour aging and an ingredient of imitation vanilla extract. Both had to be removed from the market after years of presumed safety." The Food and Drug Administration has also pointed out that some of the coal-tar colors which it originally listed as "harmless" under provisions of the 1938 law were later found to produce injury when fed to animals in large amounts and had to be removed from the list of certified colors.

In all questions about the risks of food additives, one must bear in mind that fundamental axiom of pharmacology and clinical medicine: "The dose makes the poison." (*"Dosa venum facit."*)

Finally, we must briefly mention radionuclide contamination of milk and other foods by fallout from nuclear explosions, by-products of atomic reactors, and residues of radioactive waste. About five-sixths of the strontium 90 that gets into the human body comes through the food chain, especially dairy products (where strontium replaces calcium). A great deal of study remains to be done on radionuclide contamination through the food chain. We shall say no more about the subject here because we have included a detailed discussion on the radiation hazards faced by twentieth-century man in the following chapter. This too is an international subject of concern. In terms of the hazards it faces, the world is shrinking.

SUMMARY REVIEW QUESTIONS

1. What three essentials to life may be polluted or contaminated? What amount, on the average, of each of these three essentials are required daily by an adult?
2. What are some of the substances (name at least four) that may pollute the air we breathe? What might be some of the results of breathing this polluted air? In what areas is air pollution most likely to be a serious problem?
3. What are some of the methods by which the problem of air pollution can be abated? What is the relationship of the motor car to the problem of air pollution?
4. Are American water reserves adequate for the present? For the future? What is the key factor in providing water supplies for its many users? In addition to water necessary for daily human consumption, what other uses of water are essential to the American economy?
5. What are the principal water pollutants (name at least six) with which the United States must now contend? What are some of the sources (or reasons) of these old and new pollutants? How can water pollution be controlled? Whose responsibility is it?
6. What important steps have been taken in the United States since the middle of the nineteenth century to make food safer for human consumption? What new developments have taken place in the middle of the twentieth century to increase the risks of food contamination?
7. What are some of the principal "food additives" (name at least five) now used in the commercial processing of food sold to and consumed by the American public? What protection against dangerous food additives does the American public now have?
8. What in general would you say are the reasons for the new pollutions of air, water, and food which United States citizens of the middle twentieth century are facing?
9. Are the following statements sense or nonsense? Why? *Industry is the largest consumer of the American water supply. . . . All this talk about air, water, and food contamination is nonsense. . . . Ignorance and apathy are the real limitations upon the control of air pollution. . . . The causes of food-borne diseases and food spoilage are still basically unknown. . . . The dose makes the poison.*
10. What do the following terms mean to you: Salmonella, hard-surface runoff, pasteurization, smog, exhaust devices, organic wastes, "National Water Quality Network," agricultural chemicals, ciliary action, strontium 90?

Worth Looking Into: *A Study of Pollution—Air,* a staff report to the Committee on Public Works, U.S. Senate (88th Congress, 1st session). *A Study of Pollution—Water,* a staff report to the committee on Public Works, U.S. Senate. *What Consumers Should Know About Food Additives* (pamphlet), Federal Food and Drug Administration. *Environmental Health Problems,* report of a committee to the Surgeon General of the U.S. Public Health Service.

16

ENVIRONMENTAL HEALTH
AND WORLD HEALTH

THE PHYSICAL GEOGRAPHY OF THE GLOBE has remained basically fixed since long before the existence of man. Despite some minor evolutionary changes, the flora and fauna of the world have not altered within the memory of man. The fundamental physical and biological environments—background, framework, if you will—within which the human race has been set down on Earth have not changed. What has changed, easily within the memory of even young men, is the social environment of the globe. Much of this is the result of the improvement in the concepts and practices of environmental health that have occurred, at an increasingly rapid pace, within the last century. The gross outcome is what is today called "the population explosion."

The newly governing factor in today's world is its population, and the distribution of this population. Man is more a product and victim today of his social environment (with overtones of his ideological environment) than ever before in his history. Understanding of today's world, including its health problems, depends on appreciating the signficance of its population distribution—by continents, countries, and big cities (see accompanying table).

TEN LARGEST NATIONS

	Population in millions
1. China	697
2. India	441
3. U.S.S.R. (Soviet Union)	221
4. U. S. (United States)	200
5. Japan	96
6. Indonesia	96
7. Pakistan	96
8. Brazil	75
9. West Germany	57
10. United Kingdom	53
British Commonwealth of Nations (including India, Pakistan and the United Kingdom)	738

There are factors abroad in the world which will tend to push populations up—selectively by countries and continents. There are other factors which may starkly limit population growths. In this chapter we shall discuss both kinds of factors, for example, the question of the use of pesticides and insecticides, and activities of the World Health Organization.

Pesticides: Boon or Bane?

One of the major reasons for the present high population of the globe has been the discovery, control, and now hopefully eradication of insect-borne diseases. Until the turn of the twentieth century the population growth of every continent was dampened by death from insect-borne diseases.

The pressing questions about pesticides and insecticides—whether or not to use them, which ones to use if any, how to use them, what limitations to place upon their use—are still subject to debate, investigation, and research. They are unquestionably the leading environmental health questions on the stage of world health. Populations will undoubtedly rise or fall depending on how correctly these questions are answered. These new synthetic chemicals, of which the prototype is DDT, introduced in 1942, have stamped on insect-borne diseases in every country in the world. Before coming to the issue of the "great debate"—briefly, are pesticides going to do more harm than good?—it will be illuminating to present the history that leads up to it.

Insect-Borne Diseases

The opening of the Panama Canal in 1914 was a cogent triumph for Pasteur's germ theory of disease and a marked victory over insect-borne diseases. The isthmus of Panama had long had the reputation of being the "hellhole of the Pacific"; specifically, it was a hotbed of yellow fever. The French had attempted to build a canal across the isthmus between 1881 and 1888; but all the engineering genius of Ferdinand de Lesseps, who had previously built the Suez Canal, could not prevail against the country's sanitary conditions. It is estimated that the French lost through disease one-third of all their employees.

In 1902 President Theodore Roosevelt sent Colonel William C. Gorgas to Panama as chief sanitary officer. He knew what to do before the civil engineers could safely go to work—primarily, get rid of the mosquitoes. Behind this crucial knowledge, which made the building of the canal more a triumph of sanitary than civil engineering, stood the genius and heroism of the men who in the previous half a century had made epidemiology an eminently practical science.

The *proof* that communicable disease could be insect-borne, and the elaborate and peculiar ways in which this actually occurred, was a momentous step in the discovery of the common means of transmission of communicable disease. It had been vaguely and uncritically suspected for centuries. But it was the scientific work during the last quarter of the nineteenth century that made this crude suspicion a certainty and opened the way to practical public-health measures for the control of all insect-borne diseases.

The Itch Mite. Probably the first insect unquestionably indicted as a cause of disease was the itch mite, although in this case the tiny insect buried in the skin was itself the disease, called scabies or "the itch." It is claimed that an old woman proved this fact to the grave and learned physicians of the eighteenth century, who finally accepted her facts and proceeded to write scholarly books about it. Even in the nineteenth century it was folk wisdom that provided the hunch for the first definite, large-scale scientific proof that insects transmit the germs of disease.

The Tick. The American meat industry was menaced by attacks of "Texas fever" in northern cattle. The cowboys said it was caused by ticks; most scientists laughed at them. But not all. In 1889 the U.S. Department of Agriculture sent young Theobald Smith to investigage the cause of Texas fever. By ingenious and critical experiment he proved beyond a doubt that the cowboys were right. The ticks carried the microorganisms of the cattle infection. If the cattle were dipped to kill the ticks, Texas fever disappeared. Actually, as Smith had found out, baby ticks not blood-gorged adults transmitted the disease. In 1893 he published a classic paper on the subject. But since it dealt with an animal disease, it attracted relatively little public attention.

The Flea and the Rat. The following year there was an outbreak in Hong Kong of that most dreaded human disease, plague. Yersin, from Pasteur's laboratory, and Kitasato, a Japanese physician who was an assistant to the great Robert Koch, went to China to investigate it. They not only found the microorganism of the human disease, the plague bacillus; they also found it in rats and in the fleas that infested rats. This immediately suggested the chain of transmission of plague and the practical means of controlling epidemics. Get rid of the rats! Rat-proofing and deratization, especially of ships, have since become standard public-health procedures. The flea was now added to the list of vectors of disease, and the business of indicting other insects was in full swing.

The Tsetse Fly. Theobald Smith's paper on the insect transmission of cattle fever made a great impression on Dr. David Bruce, a disease-hunter in the employ of the British Army Medical Service. Bruce had already made a reputation for himself by discovering the microorganism of undulant fever in goats and goats' milk on the island of Malta. In 1895 Bruce went to South Africa to investigate *nagana*, a disease of horses. He had guessed that an insect might transmit the disease. He found that insect—the tsetse fly.

Later investigation by Bruce and others proved that African sleeping sickness, a disease of man, was also transmitted by the tsetse flies. And the tsetse flies, it was further proved, got it from the wild animals of the African jungles which were a reservoir of the microbe fatal to man.

Malaria Control. *The Mosquito.* The most dramatic tale in the quest for the insect vectors of disease is that of the mosquito. This insect was demonstrated by Ronald Ross and others to transmit malaria and by Walter Reed and others to carry yellow fever also.

Ross, like Bruce, was a member of the British Army Medical Service; he was also an accomplished mathematician and poet. Stationed in India, he desperately pursued proof of the opinion earlier vocied by Nott, King, and Manson that the mosquito did transmit malaria. On the hot evening of August 20, 1897, Ross peered through his microscope to discover one form of the malarial parasite in the minute, dissected stomach wall of a mosquito. He celebrated this discovery in verse. "I have found thy secret deeds,/Oh, million-murdering death," he wrote.

Within a year he had traced the parasites to the salivary gland of the mosquito. From this position they had free exit through the mosquito's stylet ("stinger"). These were the crucial facts in the proof that the *bite* of a mosquito infected with malarial parasites actually carried the disease to man.

A great deal of work remained to be done to find out exactly what kind of mosquitoes could convey the malarial parasites; they turned out to be females of the genus *Anopheles.*

Still more investigation was required into the life cycle of the mosquito and into the conditions under which these dangerous pests could be most effectively destroyed. The Italian scientist, Battista Grassi, shared the 1902 Nobel Prize with Ross for his discoveries in this direction. Mosquito control was thus shown to be the key to malaria control.

Contrary to some popular belief, mosquitoes do not travel far from their birthplace. Practically speaking, malaria control boils down to keeping mosquitoes from biting individuals who already have malarial parasites in their blood. The newer insecticides, of which DDT is a prime example, have revolutionized the techniques of mosquito control. They have not wiped out malaria yet—but they have made malaria eradication a reasonable and early possibility.

Yellow-Fever Control. The suspicion that the mosquito was associated with yellow fever had been advanced by Josiah Knott and most emphatically, in 1881, by Dr. Carlos Finlay, of Havana, Cuba. After the Spanish-American War, Cuba became for a time a United States responsibility. In 1900 Major Walter Reed, Dr. James Carroll, Dr. A. Agramonte, and Dr. Jesse W. Lazear were sent to Havana as a commission to study yellow fever, there rampant.

Lazear died of yellow fever early in the course of the investigation. A true martyr of science, he had permitted himself to be bitten by a mosquito suspected of carrying the disease. At Camp Lazear, named in his honor, Reed continued the essential experiments.

They required human volunteers who would permit themselves to be bitten by mosquitoes; others who would expose themselves to the contaminated bed clothing and other excretions of yellow-fever victims. Among those who offered themselves for the experiment were John R. Kissinger and John J. Moran. They refused any monetary compensation for running the risk of death. In an immortal phrase, Kissinger said that they had volunteered "solely in the interest of humanity and for the cause of science."

"Gentlemen," said Major Reed, rising and touching his cap, "I salute you."

With the help of his courageous volunteers, Reed indisputably proved that only persons bitten by mosquitoes who had previously bitten other persons with yellow fever could carry the disease. The offending mosquito, *Aëdes aegypti,* was a different brand from that which carried malaria. Mosquito control promptly controlled yellow fever in Havana, Panama, and wherever else it could be effectively applied. However, the disease remains endemic in Africa and is still found in monkeys in the South American jungles.

The New Insecticides

Insect control and destruction programs, based on available knowledge and materials, followed rapidly upon the momentous discoveries of the nature of the insect-borne diseases. The big break-through came during World War II with the introduction of DDT and other synthetic chemicals that came to be called insecticides and later pesticides. Scores of diseases have been conquered by them.

Epidemic typhus has plagued man for centuries. This "traditional" rickettsial disease, transmitted by the body louse, accompanies disasters. It has been known as war fever, famine fever, jail fever, ship fever, and camp fever. In World War II, specifically in 1943, typhus was again breaking out. When American troops arrived in Naples in December 1943, typhus was present. However, a vigorous campaign against it was immediately instituted, primarily with the insecticide, DDT. Freely blown into clothes with a dust gun, DDT quickly killed body lice and interrupted transmission of the disease. From this first blazing demonstration, DDT has gone on to control typhus wherever it lifts its head—even endemic (murine) typhus.

Insecticides have played a major role in the eradication of *Aëdes aegypti* and yellow fever from all of Central America and almost all of South America—probably also from Mexico—but the history is complicated because the eradication campaign has been going on for more than three decades and many things have changed. Earlier techniques called for sealing off and eliminating all possible breeding places. Later a perifocal, pinpoint method of applying DDT was developed, and this has provided a cheap and effective operational procedure.

Effective as campaigns against typhus and yellow fever have been, the greatest results of the use of insecticides have been against malaria. This disease has depopulated large areas, is accused of being responsible directly or indirectly for one-half of the world's mortality, and steals the "joy of living" from millions.

As noted, efforts to control malaria were made by other techniques (oil spraying) and other larvicides (e.g., Paris green) before DDT and other modern insecticides became available. It was hopeless to attack the anopheline mosquitoes in their enormous breeding areas, as in India, but another method proved effective. DDT is a contact poison which enters the mosquito through its feet. The mosquito was therefore eliminated by spraying indoor walls of homes with DDT—twice a year. When the mosquito, after eating, came to rest on the walls, it absorbed the poison. By this method the transmission of malaria was halted and the disease drained out of specific populations in less than three years. The effectiveness of the early campaigns encouraged the World Health Organization to undertake a malaria eradication campaign. DDT was generously used in the attack.

In 1968 World Health Organization revised its goals. It now believes that unless basic medical services in many countries become better developed in detection and treatment, total eradication of malaria is not attainable. Furthermore, the mosquito vectors have acquired resistance to many of the insecticides used in agriculture. However, by 1968, there were only 564 million people living under uncontrolled malarious conditions instead of the original 1420 million.

Another disease which has responded to DDT attack is onchoceriasis, often called river blindness. This disease is caused by a filarial nematode, which is transmitted by small black flies in Africa, South and Central America. Approximately 20 million people are infected. The microfilariae invade all the tissues of the skin, producing severe dermatitis with intense itching. It is worst in the eyes and may go on to produce total blindness. The vector flies of onchoceriasis breed in flowing water, mostly in small streams. Usually attached to stones, the larvae are highly susceptible to DDT. They can be killed by DDT applications as low as 0.1 p.p.m. (parts per million) applied for 15 minutes, although the chemical is usually applied at the rate of 0.05 p.p.m. for 30 minutes—which will not kill fish.

Another disabling disease of a large share of tropical mankind is bilharziasis, or schistosomiasis, commonly carried by snails in snail-infested waters. The infecting blood fluke (trematode) is spread in waters by urinary and fecal contamination. Its tiny larvae infect the snail. After a few weeks the snail liberates free-swimming cercariae, which penetrate the skin of people working, swimming, or wading in the stream. Like malaria, schistosomiasis causes a lifetime of disability. It is estimated that the disease is prevalent in 15 African and Middle Eastern countries. In Egypt possibly 26 million out of 107 million population are infected. The disease cannot be controlled by pesticides alone; other sanitary measures must also be employed.

"Pesticides Upset Balance of Nature." In 1962 there was a book published which rudely interrupted the success stories being piled up by the new insecticides and pesticides; and the "great debate" was on. The book was *Silent Spring* (Boston: Houghton Mifflin Co.); the author was Rachel Carson (d. 1964), a scientist, author, and brilliant observer of ecological cycles on the face of the globe. Miss Carson's book is a reasoned, well-documented, scientific, but impassioned plea against the indiscriminate use of pesticides, insecticides, herbicides, and other "agricultural chemicals" across the face of the globe. Her thesis is made clear in the following passage (quoted with permission):

The history of life on earth is a history of the interaction of living things and their surroundings. . . . It is only within the moment of time represented by the twentieth century that one species—man—has acquired significant power to alter the nature of his world, and it is only within the last twenty-five years that this power has achieved such a magnitude that it endangers the whole earth and its life. The most alarming of all man's assaults is the contamination of the air, earth, rivers, and seas with dangerous and even lethal materials. This pollution has rapidly become almost universal. . . .

It is widely known that radiation has done much to change the very nature of the world, the very nature of its life . . . [but] it is less widely known that many man-made chemicals act in much the same way as radiation; they lie long in the soil, and enter into living organisms, passing from one to another. Or they may travel mysteriously by underground streams, emerging to combine, through the alchemy of air and sunlight, into new forms, which kill vegetation, sicken cattle, and work unknown harm on those who drink from once pure wells. As Albert Schweitzer has said, "Man can hardly recognize the devils of his own creation."

The Statistical Evidence. The statistical evidence concerning pesticides gives some substance to Miss Carson's worry. Over 45,000 pesticide formulations are registered for sale with the U.S. Department of Agriculture! The new synthetics are rapidly replacing the older inorganic insecticides (arsenicals, copper, zinc sulfate, boron, sulfur). Each new pesticide brought on the market is usually more "powerful," that is to say, more toxic, than the one it is intended to supplant.

The quantities of pesticides, insecticides, and other "agricultural chemicals" now produced and used sounds almost fantastic. In the early 1960's this amounted to about 700 million pounds a year; and it was predicted that the output would be increased to 7 billion pounds a year by 1970. Most of these synthetic chemicals have been used by United States farmers. Primarily they have sprayed them one or more times a year on some 30 million acres of cultivated cropland. Some has gone for other purposes—application to pastures, highway right of ways, mesquite, and other nuisance plants. Many of these materials have a long residual toxicity in soil or water.

Most pesticides are removed only in part by ordinary water treatment. Water samples show them present in most major lakes and rivers. It can be assumed that they are washed in by normal land drainage processes. Some may be dropped or drift into the water. It is known that these water-borne pesticides are responsible for some large fishkills and that they wipe out certain chains of aquatic life. But the crucial question, hotly debated, remains unsettled: At what concentration will these pesticide residues become drinking water contaminants of serious toxicity? Opinions differ.

At the American Medical Association's 1964 Congress on Environmental Health Problems, Wayland Hayes, Jr., M.D., of the U.S. Public Health Service pointed out that pesticides kill about 200 people a year in the United States from accidental poisoning and that about 2000 cases of nonfatal pesticide poisoning occur. At the same meeting, Irma West, M.D., of Berkeley, California, declared vigorously: "There is no question that widespread, substantial contamination of the environment has arisen primarily from the massive use of the persistent chlorinated hydrocarbon pesticides. . . . Unforeseen, irrevocable, and undesirable side effects have risen on a sizable scale . . . because the chemicals involved were not checked out from all angles beforehand."

On the other hand another physician at the environmental health congress, Mitchell R. Zavon, M.D., of Cincinnati, Ohio, had a completely different opinion. He said: "The effect of pesticides on our general environment will probably require many years of research to evaluate. There is presently 'no evidence' . . . that the extremely small amounts of certain pesticides [e.g., dieldrin, lindane] which may be found in our food or in our general environment cause us any harm." He suggested that in some pesticide intoxications it may be the solvent which is the culprit.

The "great debate" on the hazard of pesticides appears in miniature in many scientific, technical, and popular journals. The following excerpts from an exchange of letters in *Science* (June 12, 1964, p. 1294) must stand as token for thousands more like it. A professor of biology writes:

"Thanks are due *Science* for the description of the Lower Mississippi fishkill by pesticides. . . . It is surprising that this was not first-page news all over the country. . . . In spite of repeated assurances that endrin and dieldrin were safe, obviously they are not safe. They have not been adequately tested. Have any of the new insecticides been adequately tested?"

A member of an Agricultural Experiment Station at a state university complains that the original *Science* report is "grossly unfair" because it condemns government regulation of pesticides as "weak and confused" and "piecemeal and inadequate" and "dissipated in political and bureaucratic bickering." The agriculturalist writes: "The use of pesticides is essential for the continued production of food and fiber crops, for the protection of human health through control of lice, flies, rats, and cockroaches. . . . Pesticides, when misused in high concentrations, can be dangerous. The public has a right to know. . . . However, in our worry about this problem let's not lose sight of the fact that we must have food and clothing from crops whose production would be impossible or much more expensive without pesticides."

The last word on pesticides (boon or bane?) will probably never be spoken. The latest words will depend on first-rate research. Some of the important research questions which must be taken up are: Do insecticides like DDT decompose in the soil or leach out? How are pesticides retained and released in various types of clays and other soils? What are the interactions between pesticides and soil microorganisms? Are pesticides retained by fish? Absorbed and accumulated by land and water plants? Some states have banned the use of DDT, and further research is going forward. Latest reports have asserted the risks of DDT and ask for substitutes for it.

Radiation Hazards

Mankind has been exposed to ionizing radiation ever since the very first stage of its evolutionary development. It worried no one, because no one knew about it. The first inkling of the existence of ionizing radiation and its production by what we now call atomic energy came in that "miracle decade" of modern science, 1895 to 1905. Then William Conrad Roentgen discovered X-rays, Henri Becquerel first observed natural radioactivity in the image of a key on a *wrapped-up* photographic plate inadvertently left in a drawer with a piece of uranium, and Pierre and Marie Curie isolated and discovered radium. Madame Curie correctly interpreted that its powerful radioactivity and gradual disintegration were being caused by an intra-atomic breakdown.

Atomic energy is produced when atoms break up. Among other things that happen under these circumstances is the emission of *gamma rays* from the site of the break-up. Gamma rays are electromagnetic waves, much like X-rays but of shorter wave length. Very powerful gamma rays and X-rays can penetrate several feet of lead. When atomic energy is kept under control, it is readily possible to protect against its hazards. When it is uncontrolled and reaches critically high levels, it may produce acute or delayed *radiation sickness,* which appears in many forms.

Human beings on Earth are being constantly bombarded by atomic energy from natural sources, such as cosmic rays and naturally occurring radium and other radioactive substances in the earth's crust. It is estimated that this amounts to about 3 *roentgens* (the standard measure of radiation) in 30 years.

Medical X-Ray Risks. Since 1900 the people of civilized countries have been exposed to a second major source of ionizing radiation—namely, medical and dental X-rays. The biological dangers of X-ray and radium were not appreciated at first by the early workers with these energy sources and a goodly number of physicians and scientists in the early 1900's died as "martyrs to radiation" used in examining and treating patients.

Medical necessity requires that X-ray pictures be taken to save life and limb and protect against ravages of disease. In fact more than 50 million diagnostic X-ray films or fluroscopic examina-

tions for medical purposes are now made annually in the United States. Dentists take twice as many, more than 100 million, X-ray pictures of teeth a year. The important thing is that all this X-raying be done with the highest possible safety standards.

It is now possible, however, to protect against a substantial part of the radiation hazards of medical and dental X-rays. This can be done, for example, by getting rid of all obsolete and badly working X-ray equipment, by using well-established protective devices such as lead shielding and new ones like aluminum filters and cone adaptors, by "faster" X-ray film, by periodic checking of all X-ray equipment, and by avoiding needless X-ray examinations and treatment. The National Tuberculosis Association and the U.S. Public Health Service have given up their past recommendations for mass or routine chest X-rays for screening populations for tuberculosis.

Particularly to be deplored and eliminated is the use of atomic energy by shoe clerks in shoe stores that employ fluoroscopes for fitting shoes. In some states, they have been banned.

Genetic-Mutation Risks. The individual risk from the medical use of X-rays must be evaluated against the potential seriousness of the conditions for which they are properly indicated. There is, however, another major danger from ionizing radiation—that of damaging the gonads (testes and ovaries) and creating harmful mutations of the genes that transmit hereditary characteristics. Geneticists strongly advise against provoking any gene mutations beyond those produced by natural background radiation.

While some geneticists would still argue the point, the present consensus is that the risk of any given individual having a child with inborn defects is not significantly increased above normal by submitting to the use of safely shielded X-rays for properly indicated medical or dental needs. The amount of theoretical harm done by correctly administered X-ray dosages is so small that it has never actually been detected or measured. Properly given dental X-rays involve such a limited area of the body that they contribute negligibly to whole body or gonadal radiation.

Nuclear Weapons—Atomic Fallout Risks.
The third source of radiation hazards to which the human race is now exposed came into existence in 1945 with the first atomic bomb. Since then there has been great scientific, popular, and political furor over the legitimacy of testing or using such weapons. The explosion of an atomic weapon above the surface of the earth causes atomic fallout, which creates dangers that by their very nature are beyond the control of exposed persons.

A particular problem is posed by the long-lived isotope strontium 90, chemically similar to calcium. Blown into the atmosphere and later descending to earth, this isotope could be absorbed by plants and passed on to man in meat, milk, and other foods. In the human body it would tend, like calcium, to lodge in the bones and might therefore damage the blood-forming organs and produce leukemia, especially in children. The reality of this theoretical risk is constantly being evaluated. For example, the U.S. Public Health Service has expanded to every state its program of measuring the kinds and amounts of radioactivity in the meals of selected school children. These regular diet studies permit more accurate estimates of the daily intake of radioactive substances by children and young adults.

The Federal Radiation Council, in a report issued in May 1963, stated:

Iodine 131 doses from weapons testing conducted through 1962 have not caused undue risk to health.

Health risks from the present and anticipated levels of strontium 90 and from fallout due to testing through 1962 are too small to justify measures to limit the intake by modification of the diet or altering the normal distribution and use of food.

In May 1964, John D. Harley, of the U.S. Atomic Energy Commission pointed out that natural radioactive isotopes (background radiation) give Americans a bigger dose of radiation every year than arrives through radioactive fallout, although the dose from fallout is a "significant fraction" of the natural dose.

Committee Reports on Radiation Hazards. In 1956 the U.S. National Academy of Sciences published a study on atomic-radiation hazards. The study committees sought, among other things, to decide what amount of radiation the male and female sex organs could safely take without undue risk of producing gene changes that might be harmful to future generations.

They arrived at the tentative conclusion that exposure to man-made radiation, including diagnostic and therapeutic X-rays, should not exceed 10 roentgens during the first 30 years of life, counting from the date of *conception.* They said, however: "This is a reasonable quota (for a population) not a harmless one. It should most emphatically not be assumed that any exposure less than 10 roentgens is, so to speak, all right. The idea is to stay as far under the quota as possible. As geneticists we say, 'Keep the dose as low as you can.'"

The National Academy of Sciences report also estimated that the amount of man-made radiation resulting from A-bomb and H-bomb tests continued indefinitely at the 1950 to 1955 rate would add $\frac{1}{2}$ a roentgen in 30 years of exposure to the other radiation hazards to which human beings are exposed.

The report further recommended that every effort should be made "to reduce the radiation exposure from X-rays to the lowest limit consistent with medical necessity."

"Proper safeguards always [should] be taken to minimize the radiation dose to the reproductive cells," the report emphasized.

In 1958 a United Nations Scientific Committee studying the effects of atomic radiation issued a report which in general confirmed the earlier American one. The United Nations committee pointed out that there are still vast areas of ignorance about atomic-radiation hazards since so many "conclusions" about its effects in man are based upon extrapolations of effects observed in rats and mice. The committee unanimously agreed that fallout from nuclear-weapons tests presents a hazard to mankind. "Even the smallest amounts of radiation," it stated, "are liable to cause deleterious genetic and perhaps also somatic (whole-body) effects."

However, on the key question of stopping nuclear-weapons tests or adopting other measures to control radiation dangers, the majority of the United Nations committee sidestepped. It held that these matters "involve national and international decisions which lie outside the scope of its work." The whole question is still debatable.

Cumulative Hazards of Ionizing Radiation. For a generation, ending in the middle 1960's, mankind can be said to have been living in the formative period of the nuclear age. Since World War II the problems of radiation have been magnified and dramatized. One of man's major problems for the seventies, and thereafter, is to control radiations from all sources, so that he can cope with the artificial environment created by the influence of the atomic industrial revolution. Even in the mid-sixties it was estimated that in the United States alone about half a million people were working on jobs in which radiation was an actual or potential danger.

In considering and planning against the hazards of radiological health, it must be admitted that there are major programs both in the United States and other nations specifically aimed at activities which could lead to exposure of large numbers of people. In these cases the health effects are weighed against considerations of national policy. Another major factor in the public health aspect of radiation is the difficulty in assessing the effects of ionizing radiation. The hazard to the individual is related to the cumulative total of radiation exposures continuously or intermittently received throughout life.

Many sources, old and new, as we have noted, contribute to the cumulative total of radiation which an individual receives through his lifetime. First, of course, there is the natural or "background" radiation, to which man has always been exposed. This includes cosmic rays from space and radiation from naturally radioactive materials present in all parts of the world. The average person in the latitude of the United States receives a total background dose of about 100 milliroentgens per year. Exposure to medical X-rays contributes roughly the same dosage level (when averaged out) as background radiation, especially in North America and Western Europe.

The greatest potential problem of radioactive contamination, if the problem goes uncontrolled, lies in the continuing development of atomic energy. A committee of the U.S. Public Health Service estimated that the accumulated volume of radioactive wastes will increase from about 1.5 million gallons in 1965 to 2 billion gallons in 1995!

The Division of Radiological Health of the U.S. Public Health Service has taken prime responsibility for protecting the American public against radiation dangers. The task, however, is an exceedingly complicated one in which other federal, state, and local government agencies must share. Since, except in rare accidents, acute radiation injury to individuals is rarely seen, the primarily objective of the Division of Radiological Health is the reduction of unnecessary radiation exposure, whatever its source and no matter how small the amount, in order to limit the possible long-term statistical effects upon large numbers of people.

How Much Radiation? A difficult question here has been whether there is such a thing as a safe threshold dose of radiation, below which adverse effects would not appear. Unfortunately, when calculated on a large scale, this does not seem to be the case. Accumulating evidence, particularly on the genetic effects of radiation, as noted, suggests that even small doses to the gonads prior to reproduction will be accompanied by an increase in genetic mutations, most of which will be deleterious.

Any dose chosen as "standard" must therefore be assumed to involve some risk of injury in exposed population groups. The setting of standards cannot therefore be an exclusively scientific task, since there is a need of balancing certain risks against acceptable standards. For use of United States government departments a radiation protection guide is established on the best judgment of the Federal Radiation Council (FRC). This council, incidentally, has estimated the harmful effects from the fallout of all nuclear tests through 1961 as astonishingly minor—

primarily affecting only about 110 people.

Once ionizing radiation is released into the environment, complex measures must be developed and applied to reduce its hazards. Though difficult, the task is not hopeless; and many hopeful experiments are under way. Some control of the radioactive iodine and strontium levels in milk, for example, can be achieved by altering the feeds of dairy cattle.

There can be no question but that in the last third of the twentieth-century mankind's *potential* risk from radiation hazards is bound to increase. However, with the ever-sharper attention and control measures, bulwarked by research directed to holding down or dissipating radiation effects, it is increasingly possible in a peaceful world for the operational hazards of ionizing radiation to be minimized. This is the goal for mankind to seek.

Atomic-Waste Disposal. The use of atomic energy for peaceful purposes also involves some radiation hazards, but up to 1960 these were not taken very seriously because so few (about a dozen) nuclear reactors were actually in operation. One risk is possible accident, but a far more pressing one is what to do with atomic wastes. We have no means of rendering atomic wastes harmless and they will continue to accumulate in the environment. You can't drop them into the ocean or scatter them to the winds. So far they have been buried in the ground, sometimes flushed down abandoned oil wells. The disposal of atomic wastes represents a real and only partially solved problem of environmental sanitation and public health.

Radiation Sickness. There appears to be a great public horror about the "mysterious" effects of radiation upon the human system. There is actually less mystery about this than popularly imagined.

The terms *radiation sickness, injury, or reaction* are used to describe the damage done to body tissues by exposure to radiation from X-rays, gamma rays, radium, radon, atomic energy, and other radioactive substances. The damage, of course, will depend both on the amount of exposure—the dose—and the individual's personal tolerance

for or resistance to radiation. The harmful effects may be acute or delayed.

Acute radiation sickness sometimes occurs in patients who are receiving X-ray treatment for conditions that cannot be expected to respond as adequately to other kinds of treatment, if available. The symptoms are loss of appetite, nausea, vomiting, and diarrhea. The treatment is symptomatic but the symptoms usually disappear in a day or two if no further exposure to X-ray radiation occurs.

Massive doses of radiation, as encountered in atomic explosions, can produce such severe reactions that death shortly ensues. The actual causes of death in these cases, however, can usually be attributed to severe *anemia,* since the blood-forming organs are exceptionally sensitive to radiation; to internal *bleeding,* since the capillary blood vessels are adversely affected; to secondary *infections,* since the white blood cells are knocked out; or to severe *burns,* with changes in the body-fluid balance, since any radiated energy is a form of heat.

In *delayed radiation sickness* the same mechanisms of body damage and possible death operate, but the severe symptoms develop more slowly and insidiously, sometimes over a course of many years. Early symptoms may include easy fatigue and lethargy and (in women) cessation of *menstruation.* Radiation injury in peace-time *can* be avoided by strict obedience to safety rules and regulations in establishments where possible radiation damage is a known hazard.

World Health Organization

Since the fourteenth century, when quarantine (40-day detention) was introduced at Italian seaports, it has been increasingly recognized that conditions affecting community health are not and cannot be contained within its political boundaries. Germs recognize no boundary lines, nor can ideas be kept in a bottle. Personal health and community health are interwoven with world health. What happens in Bangkok may have repercussions in Boston. Yellow fever in Guatemala can travel by plane to Georgia. Disease, like fire, is best fought at its source. The United States today has an inextricable stake in world health.

This responsibility is formally recognized in at least two ways: by United States membership in the World Health Organization—commonly abbreviated WHO—and by American participation in the World Medical Association, which is composed of over 50 national medical associations, including the American Medical Association. WMA now represents more than 700,000 physicians. The United States is the largest single national contributor to WHO.

WHO was organized in June 1946, in New York City, largely under United States leadership. It now includes over 130 member nations of the United Nations. Within the limitations of its small budget, WHO functions as an international public health agency. It is concerned with raising standards of medical education, fortifying national health services, assisting in campaigns for the control of communicable diseases, and codifying and classifying medical information of international importance. It runs up warning flags of epidemics and endemics anywhere. In protection of the health of its own citizens at home and abroad, and in many other ways, the U.S. has been amply repaid for its investment in WHO.

WHO is the latest in a hundred-year series of international conferences, conventions, and organizations devoted to safeguarding international health. The first international sanitary conference was held in 1851. By 1909 this seed had become the International Office of Public Health (*L'Office International d'Hygiene Publique*) with staff headquarters in Paris. Meantime, in 1902, the Pan American Sanitary Bureau was established at a conference in Washington, D.C. In 1923 the Health Organization of the League of Nations was established with central offices in Geneva, Switzerland. It outlasted the League itself and pointed the way for WHO.

WHO is governed by a World Health Assembly, to which three official delegates may be appointed by each member nation. It has six regional offices, which hold annual regional meetings of their own. Its genuine decentralization of offices, almost unique in international affairs, has considerably strengthened WHO by making it more responsive to the health needs of its member countries.

Principal World Health Problems. The programs to which WHO has assigned priorities for attention reflect the major health problems of the world at large. Its first three priorities were malaria, tuberculosis, and venereal disease. Other "priority" areas that WHO has spearheaded include maternal and child health programs, environmental sanitation, and campaigns against plague, cholera, yellow fever, smallpox, and typhus.

Some of WHO's most successful efforts have been in international disease reporting, in building corps of trained health workers in many countries, and in stimulating nations to the control of communicable diseases with modern techniques. For example, WHO sent six malaria experts to a demonstration area in Greece. With DDT, spraying equipment, and local cooperation, the farm production of this area increased by about 25% in one year! One of the knottiest problems WHO faces is nutrition, since this is related to the world food supply.

Its fundamental approach has been to help people of different nations to help themselves to healthier living. Under its impetus, for example, a midwife in Ceylon can be found conducting classes for mothers in a thatched health center built by the people of the little village where it stands. Continuing and intelligent health education is necessary to get people to adopt the health services by which they will profit.

In 1968 WHO celebrated its twentieth anniversary. Its accomplishments in the ten preceding years were considerable. It assisted 72 member states in establishing or improving health services; 16 of these projects were in Africa. Conferences on housing and urban development were held in Mexico, Madrid, Pittsburgh, and Stockholm. In 1968, 169 water supply projects were taking place in 83 countries. The membership of 131 nations at the 21st Assembly adopted a budget of $60,747,800 for

1969. It has established an international center at Delft, Netherlands for the purpose of coordinating research and acting as a clearinghouse of information.

"Little Dictionary of Infectious Diseases." In 1962 WHO issued a "Little Dictionary of Infectious Diseases" listing some of the more or less tropical ills it was fighting and telling how well it was doing against them. The following quotations are from the "Little Dictionary:"[1]

Bilharziasis. Disease caused by parasite that lives part of its life in freshwater snails. This disease hits young people and reduces working capacity. Irrigation often helps to spread. . . . Prevention is by sanitation, clearing water courses of aquatic plants and treating snail-breeding places with molluscicides. Synonym: snail fever, schistosomiasis.

Cholera. Intestinal disease caused by bacteria that contaminate water and food. The patient becomes dehydrated and can die in less than an hour. . . . With a vaccination jet-gun (useful in epidemics), injections can be given twenty times more rapidly than with usual syringe. Main areas of infection (1961): India and Pakistan. Prevention by clean water supplies.

Goiter. A disease caused by diet deficiencies. The remedy has been known for a century. Add iodine to kitchen salt. Still goiter affects 200 million people.

Leprosy. Ten million sufferers throughout the world, of whom only 20% receive treatment of any kind. Less infectious than tuberculosis. If detected in time, can be completely cured by sulfone drugs.

Malaria. Transmitted by mosquitoes. Fought with insecticides (to kill the mosquitoes) and drugs (to kill the parasites in the bloodstream of sufferers). 140 million cases estimated 1962. Difficulty: some mosquitos have developed resistance to certain insecticides.

Onchoceriasis (river blindness). Caused by minute worm transmitted to man by black flies. 200 to 300 million people are believed to be infected. Control measure: insecticides to reduce fly population.

Plague. Transmitted to man by fleas carried by rats. Natural reservoir of infection: wild rodents, including squirrels. Dread scourge of man for many centuries. In India alone an annual average of over 500,000

[1]"Little Dictionary of Infectious Diseases," *World Health,* The Magazine of the World Health Organization, 15: 4, 5–8 (July–August 1962).

deaths was reported between 1898–1908. [In 1967, 5619 cases were reported from South Vietnam, where the disease is endemic. However, great success in patient care. Prevention through rat control.]

Smallpox. Today, 150 years after the discovery of smallpox vaccine, this disease is an anachronism. It could be entirely eliminated if 80% of the world's population were vaccinated. Difficulties: fake certificates of vaccination, speed and volume of modern travel, lack of health workers. Countries most heavily infected: India, Pakistan, Central Africa. Revaccination necessary. [In 1967, about 120,000 cases were reported throughout the world.]

Trachoma. A virus disease that can lead to blindness. According to WHO, a sixth of the world's population (500 million people) is infected. In areas where practically the whole population has it, 1% of adults are totally blind and 4% are economically blind. Control through antibiotics.

Tuberculosis. 309 million persons were tuberculin-tested and 117 million vaccinated with BCG between 1941 and 1960 in 41 countries with a total population of 800 million. With modern drugs, particularly isoniazid, patients can be treated at home.

Typhus. Transmitted by lice. Killed hundreds of millions of people in the past. Control through DDT powder on body and clothes in order to destroy lice.

Yaws. A widespread, disfiguring, treponemal disease, causing deepseated infirmity if untreated. Can be cured by a single injection of long-acting penicillin (10 to 15 cents per treatment). 280 million people examined and 35 million treated between 1950 and 1960.

Yellow Fever. Transmitted to man by virus-carrying mosquito. Practically eliminated from the Americas. A few centers of infection remain in Africa. Not present in Asia. Forest reservoir of infection: mainly monkeys.

Zoonoses. Diseases transmitted from animal to man include psittacosis (parrot), Q-fever (goats, cattle), anthrax (cattle, horses), brucellosis (cattle, sheep, goats, etc.), and trichinosis (swine).

WHO alone cannot take credit for all the improvements in the world health that have occurred since World War II. But it has certainly taken some of the giant steps in that direction.

Other international organizations that contribute to world health include the Food and Agriculture Organization (FAO) of the United

Nations and UNICEF (United Nations International Children's Emergency Fund).

The United States State Department, under a program known as AID, supports and conducts many health programs throughout the world. In 1967, for example, the agency expended around $50 million on health projects.

A Healthier World. The world *is* getting healthier. Expectation of life at birth has increased appreciably, sometimes dramatically, throughout the world. In Puerto Rico it increased by 22 years in 15 calendar years (1941 to 1955)! In Ceylon it increased by 17 years! The lowest life expectancy is still in India (32 years at birth), the highest in the Netherlands (72.5), Sweden, Norway, Israel, England, New Zealnd, the United States, and Canada. In the Soviet Union the average length of life was 64 years in 1955—the figure at which the United States stood a decade earlier. Females outlive males in every country of the world except Guatemala, Ceylon, and India, where the males win by a fraction of a year.

Coupled with generally increased birth and marriage rates, the lowered death rates have added about 900 million people to the face of the earth since World War II. World population now stands over 3 billion! Asia claims more than half—over 1.75 billion. China, the largest nation, claims to have about 700 million people; India, next largest, 440 million. The United States, the wealthiest nation, has passed 200 million.

If the world's so-called population explosion continued at the rates of the early 1960's, it is estimated that the world population would reach 4 billion by 1980, 6 billion by 2000. This is unlikely, for the possible checks on population, as pointed out by Thomas Malthus back in 1798, will probably come into operation. The world cannot contain more people than it can feed.

The Space Age and Aerospace Medicine. We are living in what is called the "space age." If it must be dated by a specific event, it may be conceded to have begun on October 4, 1957, when the Russians launched the first artificial earth satellite, Sputnik I. We are also, however, living in the "atomic age" or "nuclear age,"

which may be dated back to December 2, 1942, when scientists working underneath the football stadium at the University of Chicago initiated and controlled the first self-sustaining, manmade, nuclear chain reaction. It is further asserted that we are now living in the "tranquillizer age" and the "aspirin age." Still we cannot claim that we have outlived the "electrical age," the "stream age" and the "iron age," all of much more ancient vintage.

The space age is interesting and characteristic in that it exhibits mankind's proclivity for exploring problems beyond his immediate ken long before he has resolved problems at home. We have put men on the moon before we have eliminated malaria, number one killer of mankind on earth. Practically speaking, the problem of surviving space travel affects the lives of only a few dozen earth dwellers, specially selected American astronauts and Russian cosmonauts. However, the intense research in aerospace medicine, the "human engineering," and particularly the development of new medical instrumentation and protective devices on their behalf may improve the health and welfare of millions of people who never get off the ground. Aerospace medicine, a step beyond global epidemiology, is a relatively new and fruitful medical and research specialty; but fascinating as it may be, it does not yet touch the lives of anywhere near so many people as such older and more mundane specialties as surgery and sanitary engineering.

Aerospace medicine is primarily concerned with the reactions of human beings under the special kinds of *stress* in space: for example, long and boring confinement in small capsules, wherein the normal cycles of day and night are lost; ability to withstand thrusts of pressure (acceleration) up to eighteen times the force of gravity (g); weightlessness; extreme heat; disorientation; tumbling; exposure to noise and vibration; and breathing an atmosphere ten times as loaded with carbon dioxide as the normal atmosphere on earth. Astronauts must also be protected against excess solar and radiant energy in space. The "ideal" build for the spaceman—stocky; short, sturdy neck; no heavy muscular development—is not necessarily the preferred physique for men who will spend their whole lives operating only against the perpetual pull of earth's gravity.

Man in His Social Environment: The Present Situation

It would be difficult to conclude this text more eloquently than in the words spoken by the great Canadian psychiatrist and humanitarian, first director of the World Health Organization, Dr. Brock Chisholm, at the 1962 International Conference on Health and Health Education in Philadelphia, as follows:

As is true for all other forms of life, man's environment has always been a very important, even determining factor in his physical, mental, and social development. His basic equipment of muscle, eye, ear, tactile sense, erect posture, opposable thumb, and his brain, plus a long gestation period, long period of defenselessness of his young, omnivorous digestive system, gregarious tendency, and other specific qualities, have determined or allowed the methods he has used of surviving and developing his social and cultural patterns.

Man's particular superiority over all other known forms of life seems to lie largely in the degree of development of his brain, his ability to think, to imagine, to plan for the future, and to base his decisions on a very wide range of information and experience. Man's ability to communicate, and thus to acquire experience from others, has been of immense importance to his rapid development, over the last few thousand years, of ability to manipulate or control his environment. His power of adjustment to wide variations of environment and of adaptation of the environment to his own requirements have increased very greatly even in this century.

At the present time it seems that man's most important and dangerous lag is in relation to the human part of his environment, in his social relationships. For the first time man is now capable of destroying mankind. His technical skills have now produced a new situation, totally unknown to any previous generation, in which this generation holds a veto power over continuing human evolution and even existence.

There is no precedent for this situation and no established patterns of adjustment to it or methods of dealing with it. Perhaps still worse, there is no tradition of concern in any culture for this kind of problem. The environment in which man now finds himself is, for the first time, dangerous to all mankind, and it appears that man's social organization and habitual behavior patterns are quite inadequate for dealing effectively with the new relationships involved in this new situation. Because our power to destroy life has become absolute, our ancient and universal method of survival, by competition to the death between survival groups, has become suicidal on a racial scale. . . .

If these observations are valid, as I believe they are, it is clear that a widespread reorientation is necessary, involving our own reeducation of ourselves into patterns of thinking and social behavior designed for survival in this new kind of world in which we, precariously, exist. No challenge of this degree of importance has ever before faced any human generation, but also no previous generation possessed the advantages we have of psychological and sociological understanding and of facility of communication.

Whether we will use those abilities effectively is still to be decided; that depends on our mental and social health. At the present time a large part of the responsibility for what will happen to the human race rests, inescapably, with the health professions. The very least that should be expected from the health professions is a demonstration of concern about man's ability to react appropriately and effectively to new and dangerous situations, with some appreciation of the factors in individual development which tend to facilitate or to obstruct progress toward a level of mental and social health necessary for human survival.

SUMMARY REVIEW QUESTIONS

1. What is the "population explosion"? What has brought it about? What is its principal significance? How, eventually, is it likely to be checked?
2. In terms of population, what are the three largest continents, the four largest nations, and the five largest cities in the world?
3. What are some of the most important insect-borne diseases (name at least four)? What roles in the conquest of insect-borne diseases did the following men play: William C. Gorgas, Theobald Smith, David Bruce, Ronald Ross, Walter Reed?
4. When, where, and how was DDT, the first of the well-known modern insecticides, first spectacularly used and thus established as an important means for the control of insect-borne diseases? How does DDT function in the control of malaria and yellow fever? What are some of the other tropical diseases against which DDT and other new insecticides offer a primary method of control?
5. What are pesticides? What are the risks arising from their indiscriminate use? How and where are they primarily used today? What are the arguments for the use of pesticides?
6. What are the present sources of ionizing radiation to which human beings in different countries are exposed? In what countries are the risks probably greatest—and why?
7. Exactly what are the risks of ionizing radiation in the United States? What measures are being taken to minimize these risks?
8. What is the World Health Organization (WHO)? How was it organized? What are its chief functions? What are some of the important world health problems it has tackled?
9. What are some of the infectious diseases (name four) which are still worldwide problems? In what ways, if any, has progress been made in controlling these diseases? How serious a problem on an international scale is blindness? Why?
10. What changes, if any, do you think must be made in the ideational environment of mankind to assure the survival of the human race?
11. Are the following statements sense or nonsense? Why? *This generation holds veto power over continuing human evolution and even its existence. . . . Pesticides are a boon. . . . The World Health Organization has failed in its basic purposes. . . . The population explosion of the twentieth century is one of the best things that has ever happened to the human race. . . . The risks of ionizing radiation are now completely under control. . . . Man can hardly recognize the devils of his own creation.*
12. What do the following terms mean to you: radiation sickness, ecology, WMA, genetic mutation, plague, *Anopheles,* zoonoses, trachoma, Thomas Malthus, social environment?

Recommended For Further Reading: *Silent Spring* by Rachel Carson. *An Essay on the Principle of Population* by Thomas Malthus (1798). *Plague on Us* by Geddes Smith. *Doctors to the World* by Murray Morgan. *The Next Million Years* by Sir Charles Galton Darwin.

GLOSSARY AND SELECTIVE DICTIONARY
OF COMMON MEDICAL TERMS

abdomen. Body cavity bounded above by the diaphragm and below by the pelvis. It contains the stomach, intestines, and other internal organs.

abnormal. Outside the range of the normal, irregular.

abortion. The detachment and expulsion from the uterus of the embryo or fetus before it has become capable of living. It can occur spontaneously or be artificially induced.

abrasion. Rubbing or scraping off of skin or mucous membrane.

abstinence. The act of completely giving up something, such as liquor, sexual intercourse, narcotics.

accommodation. Power of the eyes to focus.

Achilles tendon. The tendon that binds the muscles in the calf of the leg to the heel bone.

acid. A chemical substance that, in solution, releases hydrogen ions. Acids taste sour, turn blue litmus paper red, unite with bases to form salts, and in general have chemical properties opposed to those of *alkalis* (or bases).

acidosis. A higher than normal acid content of the blood. It occurs, for example, in an advanced condition of diabetes.

acne. A skin disorder caused by an inflammation of the sebaceous glands of the skin.

ACTH. A hormone manufactured in the pituitary gland which stimulates the adrenal gland to release the hormone cortisone.

acute illness. Severe, usually critical, often dangerous illness.

addiction. The state of being completely in the grip of some habit. Drug addiction is characterized by an overwhelming compulsion, desire, or need to continue use of a drug, and producing psychological and physical dependencies on it.

Addison's disease. "Bronze skin" disease, named after Thomas Addison (1803–1860), a British physician. It results from underactivity of the adrenal glands.

adhesions. The sticking together of body tissues not normally joined. Distressing adhesions sometimes follow surgery.

adrenals. Endrocrine glands, above the kidneys, that secrete adrenalin and other hormones.

aerosol. A solution atomized into a fine mist, either a drug for inhalation or a substance for spraying in a room.

afterbirth. Placenta and membranes expelled from the womb a few minutes after the birth of a child.

aggression. A forceful, attacking action or feeling usually directed toward another person, and generally having a great emotional content.

airsickness. A form of motion sickness resulting from unaccustomed rapid motion.

alarm reaction. The first reaction to stress placed upon a person or any part of his mind or body.

albinism. Congenital absence of pigment in the skin, hair, and eyes; hence usually white in color.

alcoholism. An illness resulting from the prolonged and repeated use of alcoholic beverages frequently as a compensation for deep-seated personality problems.

alkali. The opposite of an acid; chemically a basic substance that turns red litmus paper blue.

allergy. An oversensitivity and overreaction to something in the internal or external environment. Examples of allergic reactions (or diseases) are hay fever and "strawberry rash."

alopecia. A condition in which the hair falls out; baldness.

altitude sickness. A condition that sometimes occurs at high altitudes, as on mountain tops or in airplanes, caused by lack of oxygen in the blood and brain.

alveolus. Air sac of the lungs; also socket of the teeth.

amblyopia. Dim or poor vision.

ameba. A microscopic, one-celled animal.

amino acid. Any one of some 30 or more chemical compounds, all containing nitrogen, that are the building blocks of body protein.

amnesia. Loss of memory; especially inability to remember past experiences.

amniotic sac. So-called "bag of waters"; an "elastic bottle" in which a growing infant floats during its life in the mother's womb.

amphetamine. A drug used to stimulate the central nervous system, increase blood pressure, reduce both appetite and nasal congestion. A common ingredient in "pep pills."

analgesia. The relief of pain without loss of consciousness.

anemia. A blood disease, of which there are many types; most commonly result from the failure of the blood-forming system in the bone marrow to manufacture enough or the right kind of red blood cells.

anesthesia. Loss of feeling or sensation.

aneurysm. The bulging out of the wall of an artery —or vein.

angina. A spasmodic or suffocating pain, or the disease that causes it. *Angina pectoris* is pain in the chest, a form of heart disease.

anopheles. The kind of mosquito that carries malaria.

antibiotics. A group of drugs that kill or stop the growth of harmful microorganisms in the body. Most antibiotics (such as penicillin) are derived from cultures of molds or bacteria.

antibody. A substance produced in and by the body that protects against specific disease infections.

antidote. Anything that counteracts a poison.

antigen. Anything, usually a chemical substance, that prompts the body to manufacture antibodies.

antihistamine. A drug that counteracts the effect of histamine in the body; commonly used in treating allergy.

antitoxin. A substance in the blood that particularly fights a specific toxin (poison); for example, diphtheria antitoxin.

anxiety. A state of uneasiness, or apprehension arising in the unconscious mind, related to a fear which is nonspecific (i.e., a vague danger).

aphrodisiac. Anything that stimulates sexual desire or appetite.

apoplexy. A stroke resulting from a damaged blood vessel in the brain.

appendicitis. Inflammation of the useless, worm-shaped appendix, a small pocket or projection, one to six inches long, that protrudes from a part of the large bowel.

arteriosclerosis. The thickening and hardening of the arteries.

artery. Any of the blood vessels leading away from the heart.

arthritis. Literally, inflammation of a joint. It is one of the number of diseases and disorders called rheumatism.

asthma. A wheezing type of breathing and shortness of breath often resulting from an allergy.

astigmatism. A structural defect of the shape of the cornea or crystalline lens of the eye which distorts vision.

ataraxics. Class of tranquillizing drugs, used to calm the mind without depression of mental faculties.

atherosclerosis. A serious form of hardening of the arteries which arises from deposits of fat on the inner lining of the blood vessels.

"athlete's foot." Slang for ringworm of the feet.

atrophy. Wasting away of flesh, tissue, cell, or organ. For example, tonsils atrophy with increasing age.

anorexia. Extreme loss of appetite for food.

autonomic. Self-governing, as the autonomic nervous system.

autopsy. Examination of a body after death (post mortem) to determine exact cause of death.

avitaminosis. Mild or severe disease state caused by lack of vitamins.

axon. A nerve cell process which conducts nerve impulses away from the central cell body.

bacillus. A microbe, a germ; specifically a rod-shaped bacterium.

bacteria. Germs or microbes, more exactly, one-celled plants; they can be seen only under a microscope. "Pathogenic" bacteria cause disease, but not all bacteria are pathogenic.

barbiturates. A class of narcotic drugs; chemical compounds of many varieties and names, commonly used as sleeping pills, sedatives, and hypnotics.

basal metabolism. The minimum amount of energy required by the body at rest to keep up its normal functions such as food digestion, blood circulation, and maintenance of body temperature.

"bends." An occupational disease of "sand-hogs," deep sea divers, or others who work in an atmosphere of compressed air. Unless slowly decompressed, nitrogen bubbles form in the victim's blood stream, producing terrific pain.

benign. Harmless, not malignant; usually refers to tumors, new growths of body tissue.

beriberi. A deficiency disease due to lack of vitamin B (thiamine); characterized by inflammatory changes in the nerves.

bile. A complex body fluid that dissolves fat. It is manufactured in the liver, stored in the gall bladder. Bile backing up into the blood stream produces *jaundice,* a yellowing of the skin.

biopsy. The removal and microscopic examination of living tissue from the body. It is important in the diagnosis of cancer.

bisexual. Having both male and female sexual interests or characteristics.

"bleeder's disease." *See* **hemophilia.**

blood count. A laboratory test useful in the diagnosis of disease. A small sample of blood is dropped on a square-ruled glass slide, which is examined under a microscope in order to count the number of red blood cells, white blood cells, and other blood elements per square millimeter.

blood pressure. The force exerted by the blood beating against the artery walls.

blood test. Any laboratory test performed with a blood sample.

blood vessels. Elastic tubes of various sizes that carry blood throughout the body to and from the heart.

Blue Cross. Hospital insurance; specifically, the symbol for prepaid, voluntary group plans which pay hospital bills. It may protect not only the subscriber but also his dependents.

Blue Shield. Medical insurance; specifically, the symbol for certain voluntary, prepaid health insurance plans which pay surgical and medical bills.

botulism. An extremely dangerous type of food poisoning arising from food comtaminated with *botulinum,* which is sometimes found in improperly canned or preserved foods.

brain stem. All of the brain except the cerebrum and cerebellum. It includes the motor and sensory nerve tracts, and the nuclei of the cranial nerves.

bronchi. The two main branches of the wind-pipe going into the lungs.

bursitis. Inflammation of a *bursa,* the small sac of heavy fluid found in various joints, such as the knee and elbow.

Caesarean section. Delivery of an infant through an incision in the mother's abdominal wall and the uterus.

caffeine. A stimulating drug present in coffee, tea, cocoa, and some cola drinks. It stimulates the heart, nervous system, and kidneys.

calorie. A unit of heat. The large calorie is the amount of heat needed to raise one kilogram of water one degree Centigrade. Commonly used as the measure of energy (heat) yielded by different foods.

cancer. A group of diseases characterized by abnormal and uncontrolled growth of body cells.

canker sore. A small ulcer, chiefly of the mouth and lips.

cannabis. The dried flowering tops of hemp plants, *Cannabis sativa,* known as marihauna, hashish and bhang.

capillaries. The smallest of the blood vessels in the circulatory system.

carbohydrate. An organic chemical compound; one of the chief classes of foodstuffs, represented by starches, sugars, dextrins, and other energy foods.

carbon dioxide. A gas (CO_2). It is normally formed in the human body through oxidation of foodstuffs. It is also the gas used to give the "fizz" to carbonated beverages.

carbon monoxide. A highly poisonous gas (CO) formed by incomplete burning (combustion) of carbon. It is a regular byproduct of automobile exhaust gases.

carcinoma. A malignant new growth (cancer) arising in epithelial cells (skin or glands). The condition may respond to treatment or may spread (metastasize).

cardiac. Relating to the heart.

cardiovascular system. The entire system of heart and blood vessels.

caries, dental. Tooth decay.

castration. Commonly refers to removal of a male's sexual organs (usually testicles, but sometimes penis also). Castration of the female means removal of both ovaries.

cataract. Clouding of the crystalline lens of the eye; it usually occurs in later life.

cementum. The bony material covering the root of a tooth, located underneath the tooth enamel.

cerebellum. The part of the brain behind and below the cerebrum.

cerebral palsy. Primarily a lack of muscular control caused by brain damage before, during, or soon after birth.

cerebrum. The large, main, upper "thinking" part of the brain, divided into two hemispheres.

cervix. A neck or narrow part; most commonly, the neck (or forward part) of the uterus.

chancre. The first open sign of syphilis. It is a small, painless sore or ulcer that appears at the site where the infecting spirochete of syphilis entered the body.

chancroid. Soft chancre; an uncommon venereal disease.

chemotherapy. The treatment of disease with chemical substances (drugs).

chiropodist. Podiatrist; an individual who diagnoses and treats disorders of the feet.

cholesterol. A fatlike substance found in all animal fats and oils, and in many other tissues of the human body.

chromosomes. Colored bodies, thread or rod-like in shape, which can be seen under a microscope when a "mother cell" is dividing into two "daughter cells." Genes, which control heredity, are located at specific positions along the chromosome threads.

chronic illness. A persistent, prolonged, and recurring illness.

chyme. The semifluid, homogeneous, creamy material produced in the stomach by gastric digestion of food.

ciliary muscles. Small muscles of the eye that help control its focus.

circumcision. The cutting away of the foreskin or some part of it.

cirrhosis. Hardening of a bodily organ as the result of inflammation or other disease process. Cirrhosis of the liver means destruction of its important functioning cells. This condition is usually brought on by chronic alcoholism.

claustrophobia. The abnormal fear of being shut up in a closed space.

cleft palate. An opening or fissure in the roof of the mouth; usually accompanied by harelip. Both of these conditions are first discovered at birth. No cause is known.

climacteric. "Change of life." The syndrome of endocrine, somatic, and psychological changes taking place at the ending of the reproductive period in the female (menopause), or accompanying the normal lessening of sexual activity in the male.

coagulate. To clot, as blood; to curdle, as milk solids becoming cheese.

cocaine. A narcotic drug obtained from coca leaves; addictive. Cocaine salts are sometimes used as local anesthetics.

cochlea. Snail-shaped bony structure of the inner ear, about the size of a pea. It carries end-organ receptors of the hearing process.

codeine. A narcotic drug derived from opium and related to morphine.

coitus. Sexual intercourse.

colitis. Inflammation of the bowels.

communicable disease. A disease which is capable of being transmitted from one person to another; sometimes through a chain of carriers (vectors). For example, malaria is carried by the mosquito.

compulsion. The act of being irresistibly driven to perform some action, often irrational.

conception. The fertilization of the ovum by the sperm; the beginning of pregnancy.

congenital. Conveyed from mother to child during intrauterine life, such as congenital syphilis; not inherited in the genes.

conjunctivitis. Inflammation of the conjunctiva, the tissue lining the outer surface of the eyeball and the inner surface of the eyelid.

contact lenses. Small lenses, made of glass or plastic, that fit directly over the cornea of the eye and under the eyelid.

contraception. Birth control; the prevention of conception by any means.

convulsion. A "fit" or seizure; usually uncontrollable by the afflicted person. Convulsions are a symptom of brain irritation; hence they occur as a result of such conditions as brain inflammation, brain tumor, skull fracture, or epilepsy.

cornea. Transparent outer surface of eyeball.

coronary. Usually refers to the "crown" of small blood vessels (arteries) that supply the nourishment of the heart itself.

coronary occlusion. Anything that stops the flow of blood through the coronary arteries of the heart. This is the form of heart disease usually called a "heart attack."

coronary thrombosis. A blood clot in the coronary arteries causing coronary occlusion.

cortisone. A hormone normally produced in the cortex of the adrenal glands. It is now manufactured as a drug and is useful in treating many diseases; for example, arthritis and some eye and skin ailments.

cretin. A dwarfed, misshapen, mentally retarded individual whose condition was caused by a prenatal lack of thyroxin, owing to lack of iodine in his mother's diet.

cryptorchidism. Undescended testes; the failure of the testes to descend normally into scrotal sac.

cutaneous. Relating to the skin.

cyanosis. Blue skin resulting from lack of oxygen in the blood.

cyst. A membranous sac enclosing a thin or heavy fluid. Cysts in the ovary are quite common.

cystitis. Inflammation of the bladder.

DDT. A powerful, common, cheap, and potentially hazardous pesticide. Its full name is dichloro-diphenyl-trichloro-ethane.

deficiency disease. Disease caused by lack of foodstuffs (or medication) containing elements, such as vitamins and minerals, essential to life and health.

degenerative diseases. A class of diseases (in contrast to infectious or psychogenic diseases) which are characterized by deterioration of tissues. Examples are rheumatism, heart attack, and cancer.

dehydration. A condition occurring when excessive or abnormal amounts of water are removed from the body, as by profuse sweating or frequent urination.

delirium. A state of restlessness, excitement, and wild talk, that sometimes follows a high fever, head injury, or disease.

delirium tremens (D.T.'s). An acute mental disturbance characterized by delirium with trembling and great excitement, accompanied by anxiety, sweating, some hallucinations. It is one of the symptoms of alcoholic psychosis, also seen in addiction to opium.

delusion. A false belief or irrational idea that is clung to despite logical proof to the contrary. Delusions of persecution or grandeur sometimes occur in mental illness.

dementia. Loss of mind; mental deterioration.

depilatory. Substance or method for removing unwanted hair from the surface of the skin.

depression. "The blues," a melancholy and downcast mood. If extreme or prolonged, it can be considered as a form of mental illness.

dermatitis. Inflammation of the skin from any cause.

dermis. Inner layers of the skin.

diabetes mellitus. A metabolic disorder in which the body is unable to burn its intake of sugar, starches, and other carbohydrates because of faulty activity of the pancreas.

diagnosis. The doctor's (or clinics') best judgment as to what is specifically wrong with a patient. This is the core of the art of medicine. Rational treatment depends on correct diagnosis.

diaphragm. The sheet of muscle that separates the chest cavity from the abdominal cavity. Moving up and down, it supplies most of the muscle power for breathing. A *vaginal diaphragm* is a fitted rubber or plastic cap that covers the mouth of the womb to prevent entrance of semen during sexual intercourse. It is one of the means of achieving birth control.

diarrhea. Frequent or excessive bowel movements.

diastole. The resting stage of the heart between beats (systole). Diastolic blood pressure is the pressure recorded at this in-between time.

digestion. The conversion of food into materials to be assimilated by the body cells.

digestive system (alimentary system). Comprises a 24 to 36 foot long flexible tube, beginning at the mouth and ending in the anus. It transforms food taken into the mouth into nutrient substances that can be assimilated by the cells of the body.

dipsomania. Severe addiction to alcohol.

disorientation. The loss of proper bearings; a state of mental confusion as to time, place, or identity.

diuretic. Anything that promotes excretion of urine.

DNA (deoxyribonucleic acid). One of the exceptionally long spiral molecules that are in fact the *genes* on the chromosomal chains. They determine the genetic constitution of living matter. DNA forms the genetic pattern; RNA, sometimes called "messenger RNA" carries it to the new cells where it will be adapted.

dorsal. The backside of any organism, as contrasted with the ventral (front or belly) side.

ductless gland. Endocrine gland which pours its secretions (hormones) directly into the blood stream without passing through any specific duct.

dysentery. A bowel disorder, characterized by pain in the abdomen, diarrhea, cramps, and sometimes bloody stools.

dysmenorrhea. Difficult and painful menstruation.

dyspnea. Difficult breathing; shortness of breath.

ecology. The study of organisms (including man) as they relate to each other in a stable or changing environment.

-ectomy. A word ending that means that something has been cut out or removed; for example, *tonsillectomy*, or removal of tonsils.

ectopic. Out of place.

ectopic pregnancy. A pregnancy in which the fertilized ovum attaches itself and begins to grow somewhere in a uterine tube instead of the womb.

eczema. A skin disease of uncertain origin. The skin is rough and red and has patches of rashes.

edema. Swelling of body tissues as a result of being waterlogged with fluid.

ego. That portion of the unconscious mind which possesses consciousness, maintains its identity, and recognizes and tests reality.

electrocardiogram. Often abbreviated EKG or ECG, it is a wavy, graphic, "picture" on a tape that records the electrical action of the heart muscle. EKG's are used in diagnosing, treating, and managing heart diseases.

electroencephalogram (EEG). A graphic picture of the electrical impulses of the brain on a moving tape; "brain waves."

electrolysis. A method or removing unwanted hair.

emasculation. Castration of the male; removal of testes or testes and penis.

embolus. Anything carried along in the blood stream that causes sudden blockage of a vein or artery. Often the embolus results from a thrombus (a clot of blood broken off from the spot where it was formed).

embryo. Unborn, developing infant-to-be during first few months of intrauterine growth.

embryology. The science and study of life before birth; notably conception and intrauterine life.

empathy. Recognizing and entering in to the feelings of another person or set of circumstances. Empathy thus goes beyond sympathy, which is feeling for, but not acting out of feelings and impulses.

emphysema. A lung disease, most common in older people, in which the air sacs of the lungs have been stretched too thin and broken down.

empyema. A collection of pus within a body cavity, usually the chest.

encephalitis. An inflammation of the brain.

endemic disease. Disease confined to a particular group of people or locality.

endocrine glands. The ductless glands whose secretions (hormones) regulate and control most bodily functions. The seven important endocrine glands, from the head downward are: pituitary, thyroid, parathyroid, thymus (?), adrenals, islet cells of the pancreas, and gonads (testes or ovaries).

endogamy. Marriage within the tribe, caste, or social group.

endometrium. Inner lining of the uterus. Part of it is shed during menstruation.

enuresis. Bed-wetting; involuntary discharge of urine.

enzymes. Organic substances, mostly proteins, capable of entering into and bringing about chemical reactions in living organisms. Enzymes act as chemical catalysts.

epidemiology. The study of disease as it spreads and involves large groups of people.

epidermis. Outer layers of the skin.

epidermophytosis. Fungus infection of skin, notably "athlete's foot."

epilepsy. A disease characterized by seizures ("fits") with impairment or loss of consciousness.

epithelial. A type of body cells that make up the skin, mucous membranes lining body organs, and glands.

erythema. Reddening of the skin from various attacks upon it.

erythrocyte. Red blood cell.

etiology. The causes of disease.

eugenics. The effort to improve the human race by attention to mating and breeding.

euphoria. A sense of extreme well-being; sometimes exaggerated and unwarranted.

eustachian tube. Auditory tube; narrow passageway from the middle ear to the back of the throat (pharynx). It was named after the Italian anatomist, Bartolommeo Eustachia (1520–1574) who first described it.

exhibitionism. The display of one's body for the purpose, conscious or unconscious, of indirectly satisfying sexual urges.

exogamy. Marriage outside of the same kinship group or clan.

extrovert. A personality type whose interest is turned outward toward external values. The extrovert is frequently trying to escape his own inner thoughts and emotional conflicts. He is restless.

fainting. Temporary loss of consciousness as a result of diminished supply of blood to the brain.

fallopian tubes. Tubes from the ovaries to the womb; oviducts. Named after Gabriello Fallopius (1523–1562), Italian anatomist who first described them.

fantasy. A psychological mechanism by which a harsh reality is converted into an imaginary experience to satisfy the individual's subjective demands.

fatigue. "That tired feeling," "loss of pep," can be one of the most important symptoms of disease. Fatigue may be physical, resulting from physical labor, or emotional, the result of conflicts in the unconscious mind.

feeblemindedness. Old name for mental retardation of varying degrees.

fertility. The ability to sire, conceive, or bear offspring.

fetishist. A person who gets sexual gratification from an object (such as a lock of hair) regarded with unreasoning devotion.

fetus. The developing infant-to-be in the uterus after the first eight weeks of pregnancy; before eight weeks, called an embryo.

fibroid. Generally describes a type of harmless or benign tumor or new growth inside the uterus.

fibrositis. A form of muscular rheumatism.

filariasis. The name for several tropical diseases, caused by threadlike worms, which block the lymph channels. This causes enormous swellings of arms, legs, and scrotum.

flatus. Gas or air on the stomach or in the intestines; sometimes expelled from the mouth as a belch or from the anus as "passing wind."

fluoridation. Addition of fluorides to (public) water supply to aid in preventing tooth decay.

fluoroscope. A machine used to examine, not photograph, the interior of the body by means of roentgen rays shining on a fluorescent screen.

follicle (of hair). The hair roots from which the hair grows. (*See also* **graafian follicle.**)

foot-candle. A standard unit in measurement of intensity of illumination from a source of light; the amount of light projected at one foot from the flame of a standard candle.

fracture. Broken bone.

frigidity. A woman's lack of normal interest in, sometimes an aversion to, sexual intercourse.

frustration. A condition of increased emotional tension resulting from failure to achieve sought gratifications.

functional. A word used to describe many disease conditions in which no visible or laboratory evidence can be found to explain the patient's complaints. The opposite state is "organic," in which something definitely wrong with the body can be found.

fungicide. Anything that kills a fungus.

fungus. A low form of plant life; most commonly a microscopically small vegetable organism. Some fungi (plural of fungus) can cause annoying and sometimes dangerous infections. Most fungus infections are on the skin. Athlete's foot is typical.

galactosemia. A hereditary disorder of carbohydrate metabolism in early infancy; characterized by vomiting, diarrhea, jaundice, poor weight gain, and malnutrition.

gallstones. Concretions of elements that make up bile; for example, cholesterol. These have backed up and accumulated in the gallbladder.

gamma globulin. A fraction of the blood plasma which carries antibodies.

ganglion. A knotlike mass of nerve-cell bodies located outside the central nervous system. May also refer to a form of cystic tumor on a tendon, as in the wrist.

gangrene. Death of body tissue over an area large enough to be visible; caused by damage to the circulation of blood.

gastric. Relating to the stomach; as, for example, gastric juice.

gene. The biological unit of heredity; self-reproducing and located in a definite position on a particular chromosome. Genes are *molecules* of the nucleic acids, DNA or RNA.

genetics. The study of heredity as determined by the genes.

genitalia. The reproductive apparatus (organs).

genotype. The genetic make-up of an organism; its fundamental hereditary constitution, as determined by its genes.

geriatrics. That branch of medicine that is concerned with the diseases and disabilities of older people.

german measles. *Rubella;* a mild virus disease. Hazardous in early months of pregnancy, it may cause malformation of fetus.

germicide. Anything that kills germs.

germs. Disease-producing microorganisms. The concept of the germ theory of diseases was established in the late 19th century by Pasteur and Koch.

gingivitis. Inflammation of the gums.

glands. Body organs that manufacture some fluid that they secrete from their cells. Thus we have glands, like the sweat glands and mammary glands (breasts), that secrete their "product" through definitely defined ducts, and also ductless glands, such as the endocrine glands (pituitary, thyroid, etc.) that secrete their hormones directly into the blood stream.

glaucoma. A serious disease of the eye, marked by hardness of the eyeball, causing vision impairment or blindness.

globulin. A fraction of blood serum, that can be separated out of it.

glucose. Sugar in the form in which it usually appears in the blood stream (blood sugar).

gluteal. Related to the buttocks, which are made up of the large *gluteus maximus* muscles.

glycogen. Animal starch formed by and stored in the liver, where it is reformed into glucose (blood sugar).

goiter. Enlargement of the thyroid glands in the neck.

gonads. Essential sexual glands; testes in the male, ovaries in the female.

gonorrhea. The most common and most curable veneral disease; caused by the *gonoccocus* micro-organism; effectively treated with penicillin and other antibiotics.

gout. A metabolic disease in which the body fails to get rid of uric acid. The typical picture of gout is that of a middle-aged man with an exquisitely sensitive and swollen big toe.

graafian follicle. "Pocket" in the ovary in which an individual ovum matures (one each month) and from which it is released when ripened.

group therapy. A group discussion or other activity with a therapeutic purpose, generally consisting of a therapist and several clients or patients.

gynecologist. Specialist in diseases of women.

habituation. The condition resulting from the repeated use of a drug, with a compulsion to continue its use. There may be psychic but *not physical* dependence on the drug, which is the distinction between habituation and addiction.

halitosis. Bad breath.

hallucination. Hearing, seeing, or feeling things that do not actually exist; a mental mirage.

hardening of the arteries. A condition marked by thickening, hardening, and loss of elasticity in the walls of the arteries. Deposits of sodium salts and hardening take place chiefly in the middle layer of the arteries.

harelip. A notch in the upper lip, giving it the appearance of a rabbit's (hare's) lip. This congenital malformation is usually accompanied by cleft palate.

hay fever. A catarrhal inflammation of the nose and eyes, caused by allergy to various plant pollens, especially ragweed.

heartburn. A burning sensation in the food tube (esophagus), which passes near the heart on the way to the stomach. Heartburn has nothing to do with the heart.

hemiplegia. Paralysis of one side of the body.

hemoglobin. The red coloring matter of the blood which carries the oxygen.

hemophilia ("bleeder's disease"). A hereditary disease in which the blood lacks the elements necessary for clotting.

hemorrhage. Bleeding.

hemorrhoids (piles). Swollen or distended varicose veins situated just outside, inside, or across the walls of the anus.

hepatitis. Inflammation of the liver. *Infectious hepatitis* is caused by a virus. *Serum hepatitis* is transmitted by way of blood, as in use of inadequately sterilized needles.

heredity. The genetic transmission of a quality or trait from parent to child; for example, the tendency for red-haired parents to have red-haired children (and grandchildren).

hermaphrodites. Individuals of doubtful or obscure sex, since they usually have sex organs of both sexes.

hernia. The protrusion of a loop or part of some internal organ of the body through an abnormal hole or slit. In *inguinal hernia* a loop of bowel protrudes into the scrotum.

heroin. A narcotic drug; probably the most dangerous.

herpes. A virus infection, in which blisters develop on the skin and mucous membranes.

heteroxesual love. Love for a person of the opposite sex.

Hippocratic oath. The physician's oath, dating back to the great Greek physician, Hippocrates (460–377? B.C.). It promises among other ethical promises, that the physician will guard his life and art (medicine) in "purity and holiness."

histamine. A chemical substance occurring in all animal and vegetable tissues. When the human body becomes oversensitive to its quantity of histamine, an allergy may result.

hives. *See* **urticara.**

Hodgkin's disease. A malignant disease first described by the British physician, Hodgkin, in 1852. It brings about the swelling of the lymph glands in many parts of the body.

homeostatis. The tendency of the internal environment of the body to return to normal whenever it is disturbed or assaulted.

homicide. Murder; sometimes justifiable.

homosexuality. The sexual attraction toward those of the same sex. Lesbianism is female homosexuality.

hormones. Chemical substances, produced in the body by the endocrine glands and having specific effects on the activities of certain other organs and of each other.

hydrophobia. Literally means fear of water. It is a common name for the virus disease, *rabies,* as it appears in human beings.

hydrotherapy. Any treatment with water; commonly hot-and-cold baths.

hymen (maidenhead). A thin, perforated, mucous membrane that stretches across the opening of the vagina. The hymen is usually broken by first sexual intercourse, but it may be broken in other ways.

hyper-. A prefix meaning too much, above normal.

hyperkinetic. Abnormally increased body movements.

hyperopia. Farsightedness.

hypertension. Consistent elevation of the pressure of blood above a normal range. Generally called "high blood pressure."

hyperthyroidism. Excessive secretion from the thyroid gland, usually causing goiter.

hypnosis. An artificially induced passive state (trance) in which there is responsiveness to suggestions and commands if these do not conflict seriously with the subject's own conscious or unconscious wishes.

hypo-. A prefix to medical terms which indicates too little, not enough, or below normal. Also used with reference to a hypodermic syringe for giving injections under the skin.

hypochondriac. One who has a morbid anxiety about his health; a person who "enjoys" poor health.

hypodermic. Under the skin; the same as subcutaneous. Also refers to a hypodermic syringe for giving injections ("shots") under the skin.

hypokinetic. Abnormally decreased movements.

hypotension. Low blood pressure.

hysterectomy. Surgical removal of the uterus.

hysteria. A psychoneurosis, the emotional conflicts of which are often converted into physical symptoms. Some characteristics are: lack of control over acts and emotions, morbid self-consciousness, anxiety, and simulating various physical disorders (hysterical blindness, deafness, paralysis, etc.).

iatrogenic. Caused by the doctor. Originally applied to disorders caused by autosuggestion based on physician's remarks at examination of the patient.

id. The prime mover of the unconscious mind, out of which develop the ego and superego.

idealization. Unconscious habit of looking up to other people, usually parents.

illusion. A false or misinterpreted sensory impression; that is, seeing, hearing, or otherwise sensing something that is not really there.

immunity. The power of an individual to resist an infection to which he might be susceptible. Immunity can be *active* or *passive.*

immunization. Vaccination (the two words now mean practically the same thing); providing immunity against some specific diseases by injections (or "shots"). Infants are routinely immunized against such diseases as whooping cough, tetanus, diphtheria, polio, mumps, and measles.

impacted. Usually refers to wisdom teeth so firmly imbedded in the jaw that they do not normally erupt above the gum line.

impetigo. A highly contagious infection of the skin, principally found among newborn babies and young children.

impotence. Inability of the male to have an erection of the penis so that he can have sexual intercourse.

incest. Sexual intercourse between individuals whose relationship is too close to permit a legal marriage.

incontinence. Inability to hold back urine or bowel movements.

incubation period. The time between contact with a source of infection and the outbreak of symptoms.

infection. The entry, presence, and multiplication of disease-producing microorganisms in the body, and the reaction of the tissues to their presence and to the toxins generated by them.

influenza. A virus-caused disease that may attack the respiratory, nervous, or gastrointestinal system.

infrared. The range of electromagnetic waves beyond red in the visible spectrum of light. Infrared rays provide intensive heat for careful, dry heat treatment.

injection. A "shot"; anything forced into the body through a hollow needle with a syringe and plunger behind it.

ink-blot test. *See* **Rorschach test.**

insemination. Fertilization of an ovum by a sperm; conception.

insomnia. The inability to sleep.

instinct. A native or hereditary factor in behaviour which leads to a goal natural to a species.

insulin. A hormone formed by the islet cells of the pancreas and secreted into the blood, where it regulates the metabolism of sugar. Used in treating diabetes.

intern. A medical school graduate who is working (and often living) in a hospital to get at least a year of practical training before being licensed to practice medicine.

intravenous. Inside a vein.

introvert. An individual whose interest is focused within himself.

I. Q. Intelligence quotient; the numerical result of a test which attempts to measure intelligence.

irradiation. Treatment with any form of radiant energy: heat, light (sunlight), x-ray, radium emanations, or radioisotopes.

islet cells. Part of the pancreas, they secrete insulin necessary for carbohydrate digestion.

isometric exercise. The practice of performing muscular contractions to maximum ability for brief periods of time (seconds) to increase muscle strength.

isoniazid. A group of drugs, given by mouth, which are highly effective in the treatment of tuberculosis.

isotonic exercise. Ordinary exercise in which the body or limbs move as a result of making contractions and extensions of the muscles.

-itis. A suffix denoting inflammation and usually disease of a body part, for example; tonsill*itis*.

jaundice. A disease symptom that causes the skin and the whites of the eyes to turn yellow.

keratin. The hard protein substance, containing sulfur, that is the chief component of hard body tissues, such as hair, nails, horns (in animals), and the outer layer of the skin.

ketosis. "Vinegar breath"; a disturbance of normal acid-base relationships in the body. It is sometimes a complication of diabetes.

kinesiology. The study and science that deals with human motion and locomotion.

kinesthesia. The combination of sense perceptions and judgment by which a human being "feels" muscle tension and thus judges in himself and in others muscular motion, weight, and position.

kleptomania. An uncontrollable compulsion to steal; a form of mental illness.

laceration. A tear; any wound or injury in which skin, muscle, or other tissue is torn.

lactation. The act and time of giving milk from the breasts.

lactic acid. A thick, almost colorless, liquid that sours milk, disinfects wounds, and accumulates in the muscles as they become fatigued.

lanolin. Wool fat; used in some cosmetics.

laryngitis. Inflammation of the larynx; sore throat.

laughing gas. The popular name for nitrous oxide, sometimes used for inhalation anesthesia.

leprosy. An ancient, serious and chronic disease caused by infection with a specific microorganism (*Hansen's bacillus*). One form of leprosy particularly affects the skin; another, the nerves.

lesbianism. Homosexuality between women.

lesion. An injury to any part of the body from any cause that results in damage to the part.

leukemia. A serious disease of the blood-forming organs, which then produce too many white blood cells. Leukemia is sometimes called cancer of the blood.

leukocyte. White blood cell.

libido. The psychic energy of the unconscious mind; sometimes refers to sexual desire and drive.

ligament. A tough band of tissues that connects bones or supports body organs.

liver extract. Processed from the livers of meat animals, it is used in the treatment of pernicious anemia.

lobotomy. A cutting into a lobe of the brain to sever fibers as a treatment for certain types of mental illness. Now rarely used.

lockjaw. Tetanus; an acute, infectious disease. Its major symptom is the tightening of the jaw muscles, called trismus.

lues. Another name for syphilis; the adjective is "luetic."

lymph. The fluid, outside the blood vessels, in which the cells and tissues of the body are constantly bathed.

lymphatic system. The channels and small vessels that collect tissue fluid (lymph) and transport it back to the veins so that it re-enters the circulating blood stream.

maidenhead. *See* **hymen.**

malaise. A generally sick feeling, often accompanied by nausea and vomiting.

malaria. A mosquito (*anopheles*)-borne disease, characterized by intermittent attacks of chills, fever, and sweating.

malignant. Refers primarily to cancer. A truly cancerous growth or tumor is called malignant. The phrase "malignant hypertension," a rapidly increasing high blood pressure, is also used.

malnourishment. Failure to receive adequate nourishment for any reason. The usual cause is a diet inadequate in vitamins, minerals, and other nutritional substances.

malocclusion. Failure of teeth in upper and lower jaws to come together properly.

malpighian cells. Second (from the top) layer of skin whose growing cells contain skin pigment (melanin) that largely determines human skin color.

malpractice. Failure of a physician to treat a patient with the skill and attention that could reasonably be expected of him.

mammary. Relating to breasts.

mania. Frenzy or madness, a sign of mental illness. It may be characterized by violence of behavior, overtalkativeness, wild ideas, or undue excitement.

manic-depressive psychosis. A mental illness characterized by mood swings in the direction of excitement (manic phase) or extreme fatigue and despondency (depressive phase). It may be cyclic or periodic.

Mantoux text. A skin test for tuberculosis.

marihuana. A drug produced from the tops and leaves of the female *cannabis* plant; it is considered a hallucinogen, not a narcotic, but it produces a psychological dependency.

masochism. The psychological tendency to take pleasure in receiving pain; in its extreme form, a sexual perversion.

mastication. The act of chewing food.

mastoiditis. Inflammation in the mastoid bone, on the side of the head near the ear.

matriarchy. A pattern of social organization in which the mother is the dominant figure, descent is traced in the female line, and all children belong to the mother's family line.

M. D. Doctor of Medicine.

megalomania. Irrational belief in one's own greatness; delusions of grandeur.

melancholia. The deeply melancholy state of mind and body in which fear, anxiety, pessimism, indecision, and unwillingness to act dominate the mental outlook.

melanin. A dark pigment found in the skin, hair, and other body parts.

menarche. Onset of menstruation.

Mendelian laws. Patterns of heredity, in terms of dominant and recessive characteristics, first evolved by the Austrian abbot, Gregor Mendel (1822–1884).

meningitis. Inflammation of the meninges, the membranes that envelop the brain and spinal cord.

menopause. "Change of life"; the time when menstruation stops, marking the end of the childbearing period.

menorrhagia. Profuse menstrual bleeding.

menstruation. The periodic discharge of blood from the vagina, usually about every 28 days. This blood and other tissue come from the inner lining of the uterus. The function of this lining is to receive a fertilized ovum. If none appears, the lining is again shed, with some bleeding.

mental illness. The exaggeration of personal behavior to the point where it strikes other people as queer, odd, abnormal, or dangerous. The bulk of so-called mental illness is really emotional maladjustment. The most common of the severe mental illnesses is schizophrenia.

mental mechanisms. The defenses adopted by the ego for the relief of painful conflicts in the unconscious mind. These defenses include: regression, projection, rationalization, and fantasy.

mental retardation. A condition characterized by faulty development of intelligence, which damages an individual's ability to learn and to adapt to the demands of society.

meprobomate. A chemical substance used as a tranquilizer.

metabolism. All of the physical and chemical processes that take place in the living body; the building up (anabolism) and breaking down (catabolism) processes that release energy for the use of the body.

metastasis. The spread of disease within the body, usually by way of the blood stream or lymph channels. Metastasis is particularly used to describe the migration of cancer cells from the site of their original growth to other parts of the body.

metatarsal. Any one of the five more or less parallel bones of each foot that reach from the ankle joint to the toes. They form the metatarsal arches of the feet.

metazoa. Comparatively large wormlike organisms that cause disease; for example, tapeworm, hookworm.

microbe. A tiny living organism, a microorganism, that can be seen only under a microscope. The smallest of these organisms are viruses and can be seen only with an electron microscope. Microbes are also germs; but only relatively few of them cause illness in man.

microbiology. The science which is concerned with the study of microorganisms; synonymous with bacteriology.

microorganism. A minute living organism, visible through a microscope. (*See* **microbe**.)

migraine. A type of headache usually confined to one side of the head, and often preceded by warning signals, such as flashes of light before the eyes.

miscarriage. A spontaneous abortion; premature expulsion of contents of the pregnant uterus.

mitosis. The common method of cell division into two "daughter cells" from one "mother cell."

mongolism. A condition of severe mental and physical retardation, characterized by an oblique slant of the eyes and a short flat-bridged nose.

monogamy. Marriage with one person at a time.

mononuclueosis, infectious. An acute, infectious disease characterized by fever and swelling of the lymph nodes in the neck. It is sometimes called the "kissing disease" or the "student's disease."

mons veneris ("mount of Venus"). The pad of rounded fatty tissue just above the female sex organs.

morbidity. Sickness.

moron. A person of low intelligence, whose mental age is between eight and twelve years.

morphine. A narcotic drug derived from opium.

motion sickness. Dizziness, headache, nausea, and vomiting produced by unaccustomed motions of vehicles of transportation. The seat of the illness is in the semicircular canals of the ears, where the sense of balance resides.

motor nerves. The nerves leading from the central nervous system out to the nerve endings in different parts of the body. These parts are put into action by the nerve impulse.

mucus. The thick, slippery fluid excreted by the mucous membranes of the body; for example, by the lips.

multiple sclerosis. A crippling disease of the central nervous system and nerve pathways; usually attacking young adults. The insulating tissue that covers the nerve fibers (the myelin sheath) degenerates in patches and is replaced by scar tissue. Hence messages from the brain to the muscles and organs are "short-circuited."

muscle tone. Describes the state of a muscle when it is partially and firmly contracted and is on the alert to contract more.

muscular dystrophy. A progressive disease whose principal characteristic is the wasting away of the striped, voluntary muscles of the body. It begins in early childhood.

myocardium. Heart muscle.

myopia. Nearsightedness.

myxedema. An endocrine disorder caused by thyroid deficiency. It is a disease of middle life; far more common in women than in men. Puffy face and hands, low body temperature, are some of its symptoms.

narcissism. Self-love. Narcissus, in Greek mythology, fell in love with his own image as reflected in a pool.

narcolepsy. A condition in which there is uncontrollable desire to fall asleep at any time of the day or night.

narcotics. Any drugs that produce sleep and stupor and at the same time relieve pain. Most narcotics are derivatives of opium, for example, morphine and heroin.

nausea. Tendency to vomit; sick at the stomach.

necropsy. Autopsy; postmortem examination of a body.

necrosis. Death or destruction of body tissue (or cells) while still in place and surrounded by living tissue. Gangrene and bedsores are examples.

neisserian infection. Another name for gonorrhea.

neoplasm. Any new growth or tumor. Malignant neoplasm means cancer.

nephritis. Inflammation of the kidneys.

nervous breakdown. A popular term for any kind of mental illness which is serious and prolonged.

neuralgia. Pain in a nerve, arising from a specific nerve and running along its course in the body. Examples: migraine headache, toothache.

neurasthenia. Nervous weakness or exhaustion; a mild form of mental illness characterized by extreme fatigue and loss of energy.

neuritis. Inflammation of a nerve. The body areas served by these nerves are usually tender and painful.

neurologist. A medical specialist concerned primarily with disorders of the nervous system.

neuron. A nerve cell.

neurosis. (Also called psychoneurosis.) A disturbance in an individual's psychic constitution. It is a milder form of mental illness, less severe than a psychosis. The disease is produced by conflicts in the unconscious mind, often too severe to be relieved without psychiatric treatment.

niacin. Nicotinic acid; the pellagra-preventive factor of the vitamin B complex.

nicotine. The principal active substance (alkaloid) in tobacco. Pure nicotine, even in small doses, is a dangerous poison.

nucleic acids. Acids formed in the nucleus of a cell. The two important ones are DNA (deoxynucleic acid) and RNA (ribonucleic acid), which provide the genes (molecules) that govern heredity.

nucleus (of cell). The cell's core, center, and reproductive system. It contains the thread-like chromosomes that separate into two chains when one cell breaks down into two cells.

nullipara. A woman who has never borne a child.

nutrient. Nourishing; any substance that supplies food to the body.

nutrition. The essential body process of assimilating food. Failure of nutrition may result from a faulty, limited diet or from the body's failure to absorb food.

nymphomania. Extreme, abnormal sexual desire in the female; comparable to satyriasis in the male.

obesity. Fat and overweight.

obstetrics. The medical speciality that deals with the events of pregnancy and childbirth.

occlusion. The condition of being closed. The closure of the small arteries of the heart brings on coronary occlusion. In dentistry, occlusion describes the fit of the teeth of the upper and lower jaws when the mouth is closed.

occupational diseases. Those arising out of the course of one's work or occupation, unless adequate safety or preventive measures are taken. Examples: lead poisoning in painters, black lung in coal miners.

occupational therapy. Part of the process of total rehabilitation. It means providing the patient (in or out of a hospital) with interesting opportunities to exercise those muscles and talents that can be strengthened and lead toward a life as normal as possible. Included in occupational therapy projects are such things as weaving, painting, carpentry, dance, and many other hobby-crafts.

oculist. Eye specialist; an older term for ophthalmologist.

Oedipus complex. A construct in Freudian psychoanalysis. The name derives from Oedipus Rex who, in Greek mythology, was destined by the gods to kill his father and marry his mother. The Freudian theory contends that there is a normal stage in the psychological development of a male child, usually around the ages of five to seven when he wants to replace his father in the affections of his mother.

olfactory. Related to the sense of smell.

ophthalmia. Inflammation of the eyes; conjunctivitis. The gonococcus germ often threatens the sight of the newborn if the mother herself has gonorrhea. To prevent damage to the eyes of the newborn (*gonococcal ophthalmia*) the physician is required by law to instill in all newborn babies' eyes some drug or antibiotic which will kill the gonococcus.

ophthamologist. Eye specialist; physician; also called oculist.

opiate. Any painkiller or narcotic, particularly one derived from the opium poppy.

opium. The crude product of the resins derived from the flowering tops of the female poppy plant (*papaver somniferum*).

optician. A technician who grinds the lenses of eye glasses and adjusts their frames.

optometrist. A person licensed to give limited eye care; to examine the eyes for the purpose of prescribing eye glasses and recommending specific eye exercises.

organism. Any living thing, from a polio virus to a whale.

orgasm. The climax; the moment of the highest pitch of sexual excitation.

orthodontics. A speciality of dentistry which deals with straightening and realigning the teeth to achieve proper occlusion of the upper and lower teeth.

orthopedics. The medical specialty that deals primarily with the results of disease or accident to the bones, joints, and muscles.

osmosis. The passage of fluid solutions through membranes that ostensibly separate them. For example, the nutrient-carrying blood plasma seeps through capillary blood vessels to bring needed nourishment.

osteopath. Abbreviated to D. O. for Doctor of Osteopathy; a medical practitioner who has been trained in and accepts the teachings of osteopathy. Some D. O.'s are also M. D.'s.

otitis. Inflammation of the inner, middle, or outer ear.

otologist. Ear specialist.

otosclerosis. A form of progressive deafness caused by formation of spongy bone around the tiny inner bones of the ear.

oviducts. The tubes, one on each side of the body, through which the ova descend from the ovary to the womb. (Also called uterine tubes or fallopian tubes.)

ovulation. The time when a mature ovum is released from the ovary; approximately the midpoint of the menstrual cycle.

ovum. Egg; the human ovum is the female reproductive cell, a sphere approximately $\frac{1}{20}$ of an inch in diameter.

palliative. A drug or treatment which relieves or alleviates pain but has little or no affect on its underlying cause.

palpation. Examination by hand; feeling with the fingers or whole hand for signs of disease.

palpitation. Rapid heartbeat of which a person is acutely aware.

palsy. Paralysis.

pancreas gland. A large, long internal organ, located behind the lower part of the stomach. It is an important part both of the digestive system and endocrine system. Scattered through it are islet cells which secrete insulin necessary for proper digestion of sugars and starches (carbohydrates).

"Pap test." Laboratory examination for detection of possible uterine cancer. Named after originator, Dr. George Papanicolaou.

"paramedical" specialties. A growing list of minor specialties, whose work complements that performed by the physician. Thus, for example, we have physical and occupational therapists, x-ray technicians, and more recently "physician's aides."

paranoia. A chronic form of mental illness in which the patient suffers from delusions of persecution or illusions of grandeur.

paraplegia. Paralysis of both legs and lower part of the body. It results from accident to or disease of the spinal cord.

parasite. A plant (for example, a fungus) or an animal (protozoa) that lives and feeds on another plant or animal, presumably to the detriment of its host. A virus is a type of parasite in a cell.

parathyroid glands. Endocrine glands, four small ones, attached to each of the two thyroid glands in the neck.

paresthesia. Abnormal feeling, heightened sensibility, such as burning, pricking, or crawling sensation on the skin.

parietal. Refers to walls of any body cavity, usually the skull.

Parkinson's disease. A degenerative disease in which some unknown process takes place at the clusters of nerve cells at the base of the brain. The disease is named after the English physician, James Parkinson (1755–1824) who first described it.

parotid glands. The saliva-producing glands in the back of the mouth, near the ears.

pasteurization. A method of "sterilizing" milk, wine, and other fluids without boiling or destroying their intrinsic flavors. Named after the French chemist, Louis Pasteur (1822–1895).

pathogenic. Anything that causes disease, whether a microorganism or any other material.

pathological. A diseased condition.

pediatrics. The medical specialty relating to the care of children.

pediculosis. Lousiness; infestation with lice.

pellagra. A vitamin deficiency disease, once common in the South. The vitamin lacking in this condition is niacin, a part of the vitamin B complex. The symptoms of pellagra include sore tongue and mouth, skin eruptions, digestive disturbances (diarrhea), mental depression, backache, and general weakness.

penicillin. An antibiotic derived from the mold, *Penicillium notatum*. Effective against a wide range of microbes, including those that cause syphilis, gonorrhea, pneumonia, and sore throat.

perfectionist. An individual who, to avoid criticism, sets his goals so high that he cannot be reasonbly criticized for failure to reach such impossible goals.

periodontal disease. Inflammation, infection, or other disorder of the periodontal membranes; commonly called *pyorrhea*.

periodontal membrane. Soft tissue surrounding teeth.

periosteum. The elastic lining around the bones; consisting of two layers of fibrous tissue.

periphereal nervous system. The nerves that reach the outer surfaces of the body and return sensations, felt on their end-organs (sensory nerves), to the central nervous system which immediately dispatches "orders" to the part by way of the motor nerves.

peristalsis. The wavelike motion, brought about by alternating contraction and relaxation of the smooth muscle tissues of the gastrointestinal tract. This motion carries food and gastic juices along from the stomach to the rectum.

peritoneum. The strong membrane that lines the abdomen.

peritonitis. Inflammation in or of the peritoneum.

pertussis. Whooping cough.

pesticides. A wide range of chemical substances, starting in the 1940's with DDT, which are applied to dwellings or field crops to kill undesirable insect pests; for example, the *anopheles* mosquito which carries malaria.

peyote. A hallucinating drug obtained from Mexican cactus.

phagocyte. A white blood cell that engulfs and destroys microbes that infect the body.

phallus. The male organ; the penis and representations of it, as found in phallic worship rites.

pharmacist. Druggist, apothecary, licensed to fill physicians' prescriptions.

pharmacology. The science that deals with drugs; in particular the formulation and testing of new drugs.

pharmacopoeia. An authoritative and official treatise or book that describes drugs and tells in exact detail how to make and use them. Many countries have an official pharmacopoeia.

pharyngitis. Sore throat.

phenotype. The individual organism resulting from the reactions between its genotype (the purely hereditary factors) and its environment.

phlebitis. Inflammation of the walls of a vein.

phlegm. Thick mucus, coughed up or spit out of the mouth.

phobia. Abnormal, morbid fear; for example, claustrophobia; fear of enclosed places.

physical therapy. The treatment of disease by physical methods. Among these are the use of heat, cold, water (hydrotherapy), ultraviolet light, massage, and exercise.

physiology. The science and study of the functions or actions of living organisms in their gross or minute structures.

piles. *See* **hemorrhoids.**

pink eye. *See* **conjunctivitis.**

pituitary gland. An endocrine gland located at the base of the brain; sometimes called the "master gland."

placebo. A sugar pill or other "make-believe" medicine, given merely to satisfy the patient's desire for drug treatment; or used as a control in a scientific medical experiment.

placenta. The pancake-shaped tissue attached to the wall of the uterus during pregnancy. Through it the fetus is nourished from its mother's blood. The placenta is normally expelled from the uterus five to ten minutes after birth.

plasma (blood). The fluid part of the blood in which the various blood cells are suspended.

plastic surgery. The reconstruction of facial and other skin and soft tissues to relieve disfigurements, deformities, and other visible blemishes.

plexus. A knot or tangle of tissues, usually applied to nerves or veins. The *solar plexus* is a large network of nerves located on the outside of the stomach.

pneumonia. A serious, infectious disease of one or more lobes of the lungs; caused by invasion of the pneumococcus germ.

podiatrist. Chiropodist; nonmedical specialist in the care of the feet.

poliomyelitis. Polio; acute virus disease characterized by fever, sore throat, headache, and vomiting, frequently with stiffness of the neck and back. It may be minor or major, with possible crippling or fatal effects. Since vaccines for the prevention of polio were introduced in the United States in the mid-fifties, the incidence of the disease has fallen to fewer than 100 cases a year.

polyandry. The union of one woman to several husbands at the same time.

polygamy. Multiple or plural marriage; sometimes construed as the exclusive right of one man to several wives at the same time.

polygyny. The right of one man to several women, concubines as well as wives, concurrently.

polyps. New growths of body tissue; overgrowths of the mucous membranes that line many body cavities.

postmortem. After death. Usually refers to a postmortem examination of the body; an autopsy.

postnasal drip. A collection of mucus at the back of the nose from where it drips down to the throat.

postnatal. Following childbirth.

premature. Too soon, before expected; usually applied to an infant born before the full nine months of pregnancy.

prenatal. Before birth.

presbyopia. Old-sightedness; a type of farsightedness that comes with advancing years.

procaine. A local or topical anesthetic.

proctology. The medical specialty dealing with diseases and disorders of the rectum and anus.

progesterone. A female sex hormone.

prognosis. The physician's opinion, based on past experience, of the probable outcome of a specific disease or injury.

projection. The mental mechanism in which people project the blame for their own shortcomings on other people or things.

prophylaxis. The prevention of disease; frequently refers to the means of preventing venereal disease through the use of a condom.

proprietary. Any drug that can be sold without a doctor's prescription, including "patent medicines."

prostate gland. A gland in the male located just below the bladder and encircling the urethra. Enlargement of the prostate (usually in older men) causes difficulties in urination.

prosthesis. Any artificial replacement or substitute for a part of the body that has been lost or is missing. For example; a false tooth, a glass eye, a wooden leg, a plastic arm, or an artificial heart.

protein. The "meat" of a body; the prime component of the flesh of any living organism from the one-celled ameba to the blue whale. Some form of protein, or its "building blocks," the amino acids, are essential to a life-sustaining diet.

protoplasm. Living matter.

protozoa. One-celled "animals" of a variety of shapes and sizes; usually larger than bacteria. Typical example is the plasmodium which causes malaria.

pruritis. Itching.

pseudocyesis. False pregnancy. A woman believes herself to be pregnant and displays some of the early signs of pregnancy, for example, morning sickness and enlarged abdomen.

psittacosis. "Parrot fever"; transmitted to man by parrots, parakeets, and domestic fowl. It is a virus disease, causing an atypical pneumonia.

psoriasis. A chronic recurring skin disorder of unknown cause.

psyche. Mind; taken from the Greek word for soul, it is now used to describe the processes that arise in the conscious and unconscious mind.

psychiatry. The medical specialty dealing with mental illness and the restoration and maintenance of mental health.

"psycho." Slang expression for an individual currently or in the past afflicted with mental illness.

psychoanalysis. It has three meanings: (1) a method of treatment for some of the milder forms of mental illness (notably neuroses); (2) a method of research throwing light on mental illness and the nature of man's mind, both conscious and unconscious; and (3) a theory on how the human mind operates.

psychogenic. Caused by mental or emotional factors.

psychologist. An individual trained in the science of psychology; that is, the scientific study of the mind and the whole range of human and animal behavior. A well-trained clinical psychologist who treats emotional disorders usually has a Ph.D. degree.

psychoneurosis. *See* **neurosis.**

psychosis. The term now used to describe the more severe forms of mental illness; notably, schizophrenia, manic-depressive psychosis, and alcoholic psychosis.

psychosomatic. An illness or disorder in which the mental component seems to have a great or direct bearing; for example, hysterical paralysis and stomach ulcers.

psychotherapy. A planned and organized pattern of action, chiefly conversation between doctor and patient, designed to cure or alleviate mental illness. It is designed to give a patient greater insight into the nature of his illness.

ptomaine poisoning. Old fashioned and incorrect name for serious food poisoning. Ptomaines are a class of substances formed in the decay of flesh.

puberty. The years during which sexual maturity occurs. In the female it is marked by the onset of menstruation.

public health. Attention to the health of the community at large. The health officer and his staff take the steps necessary to achieve a healthy environment; for example, sanitation, epidemic control, and recording of vital statistics. Public health departments are tax-supported and have police power over situations within their realm of protective and preventive services.

pudenda. External sex organs, male or female.

puerperal. Related to childbirth and the days immediately following.

pulmonary. Related to the lungs.

pulmonary embolism. The blocking or closure of the pulmonary artery by a blood clot (an embolus); a frequent cause of sudden death.

purgative. A strong laxative.

pus. The fluid that accumulates around an inflammation. It contains dead cells and many white blood cells.

pyelitis. Infection of the kidney, usually its inner core.

pyorrhea. Literally, a flow of pus. The term is usually used to describe infection of the gums and the membranes that cover the roots of the teeth below the gum line.

quackery. False pretense to medical skills and achievements; charlatan is another name for a quack doctor.

quarantine. Means legal and, if necessary, forceable restriction of people from entering and especially from leaving countries or premises where communicable or contagious disease exists (or may be presumed to exist). The American astronauts who first set foot upon the moon were held in quarantine for two weeks after splashdown, to avoid the possiblity that they were carriers of unknown and potentially dangerous microorganisms from the moon.

quinine. Bark of the cinchona tree; a specific drug for treating all forms of malaria.

rabies. Called *hydrophobia* when it occurs in man; a virus disease, fatal if not treated with rabies vaccine. The disease is transmitted by the bite of rabid animals.

radiation. Emission of radiant energy, electromagnetic waves; as evident in x-ray beams, radium emanations, and atomic explosions.

radiation sickness. Injury or bodily damage occurring as the result of overdoses of radiant energy. Many survivors of Hiroshima suffered from delayed radiation sickness.

radiology. Sometimes called roentgenology; the medical specialty that deals with the use of radiant energy (for instance, x-rays) for the diagnosis and treatment of disease.

radioisotope. Any isotope of a chemical element or its compounds that has been made radioactive by treatment in an atomic energy pile. For example, radiocobalt is now used in the treatment of cancer.

rash. An abnormal, reddish coloration, or blotch on some part of the skin. The causes are many, including irritation, infection, and allergy.

rationalization. A common mechanism of the unconscious mind, through which an individual finds acceptable reasons for doing or thinking things that his superego does not approve.

rauwolfia. A drug derived from the Indian snakeroot plant(*Rauwolfia serpentina*) which grows in southeast Asia. In purified forms, which became available in the 1950's, it has proved an exceptionally valuable drug for the treatment of high blood pressure and an effective tranquilizer for use in treatment of mild to severe mental illness.

receptor. A nerve ending in a sense organ that responds to particular stimuli; thus the eye is stimulated by light, the ear by sound.

red blood cells. The cells that give blood its color. These cells contain iron in the form of hemoglobin. They transport oxygen to all cells of the body (via the blood stream) and bring back for exclusion (via the lungs) the waste product of cell metabolism, carbon dioxide.

reflexes. Involuntary acts performed in response to some stimulus from the nervous system. For example, the eyes blink when a light is flashed upon them.

refraction. (1) The deviation of light rays when they pass from one transparent medium to another (as from air to glass lenses). (2) The testing of eyesight for errors of refraction of the crystalline lens of the eye and prescribing lenses to correct these errors.

regression. The unconsciously motivated psychological mechanism in which a person reverts to earlier, childish types of behavior.

rehabilitation (medical). The restoration of a disabled person toward self-sufficiency or gainful employment at his highest possible skill as rapidly as possible.

renal. Related to the kidneys.

repression. A fundamental mental mechanism by which disagreeable, unpleasant, or painful thoughts and feelings are submerged into the unconscious mind.

reserpine. A drug, related to *rauwolfia,* for the treatment of heart disease and high blood pressure.

resident. A graduate physician, licensed to practice, who remains in the hospital framework to further his education in a medical specialty.

respiratory system. Includes the lungs and other parts of the body that have to do with the mechanism of breathing.

resuscitation. Artificial respiration; various kinds of maneuvers to restore breathing when it has been stopped by such events as drowning or electric shock.

rheumatic fever. An infectious disease that is most damaging when it scars the heart muscle or valves of the heart and thus produces rheumatic heart disease.

rheumatism. The popular term for *arthritis.* It describes a multitude of aches and pains in muscles, bones, and joints.

Rh factor. A substance included in red blood cells; important for typing blood for transfusions and in obstetrics. It is an hereditary characteristic.

rhinitis. Inflammation, usually with some swelling, of the inner lining of the nose.

rhythm method. A "safe-period" system of contraception based on knowledge of the fertility cycle.

rickets. A deficiency disease; specifically the lack of vitamin D in infancy and childhood. Lack of vitamin D causes brittleness and softness of the bones.

rickettsia. A class of microbes, larger than viruses but usually smaller than bacteria. It is named for Howard Taylor Ricketts (1871–1910), an American scientist. Among the diseases caused by rickettsia are typhus fever and Q fever.

RNA (ribonucleic acid). An exceptionally long spiral molecule that carries the genetic pattern from its model, DNA, to the cells newly being formed. *See* **DNA.**

roentgen. The roentgen or *r* is a measure of the amount of radiation exposure that will produce a certain amount of ionization in a specific volume of air. This unit is named after the German physicist, Wilhelm Conrad Roentgen (1845–1923), who first discovered x-rays (also called roentgen rays).

Rohrschach. A test in which the subject is shown a standard series of ink blots and asked to describe what he sees; used to determine aspects of personality.

rubella. *See* **German measles.**

rubeola. Measles.

rupture. The popular term for hernia. *See* **hernia.**

sacroiliac. The lower part of the back; the joints between the sacrum and ilium (hipbone) and the ligaments that join them. A common site of backache.

sadism. Deliberate cruelty, usually for the satisfaction of open or disguised sexual impulses.

salicylates. A large class of drugs that have the same general effects as aspirin, which is one of them.

salmonella. A genus of bacteria frequently responsible for food poisoning.

sarcoma. Cancer arising from connective tissues, such as the bones.

satyriasis. Abnormal and excessive sexual desire in the male. In the female this condition is called nymphomania.

scabies. "The itch"; a skin disorder caused by the boring of the itch mite beneath the surface of the skin.

schistosomiasis. A tropical disease caused by infestation of a particular kind of parasite (*schistosome*). These parasites are dependent on snails for one part of their life cycle.

schizophrenia. A term for dementia praecox (early madness) which is interpreted as a "split" in the mental functions. In general terms, it implies withdrawal from the real world into a fantastic (but sometimes logically fantastic) world of one's own. Schizophrenia is the most serious form of psychosis.

sclerosis. Hardening. It is used in such terms as arteriosclerosis; hardening of the arteries.

scurvy. A vitamin C deficiency disease.

sebaceous glands. Small glands near the surface of the skin and adjacent to hair follicles. These glands secrete sebum, an oily substance, which helps keep skin soft.

seborrhea. Excessive secretion of oily substance, sebum, from the sebaceous glands of the skin; an important factor in the development of adolescent *acne.*

"second sight." Better vision for reading and seeing in the later years of life. This improved vision is a result of the thickening of the lens of the eye.

However, this is usually a forerunner of cataracts of the eyes.

sedative. Any drug that reduces activity and allays excitement or overt anxiety.

semen. The white, slightly sticky, fluid produced by the male sex organs and ejaculated from them; the vehicle for sperm.

sensory nerves. A system of nerve endings that pick up sensations (for example, heat or bad smells) and convey them back to the central nervous system.

sepsis. Poisoning by microbes or their by-products in the living organism. It is the root of the words *asepsis* and *antiseptic.*

septicemia. Blood poisoning.

serology. The branch of science that deals with the study of antigens and antibodies in blood serum. Blood tests like the Wassermann and other similar tests for syphilis, are actually serologic tests.

shingles. A virus disease, caused perhaps by the same virus that brings on chicken pox. The first symptoms are a crop of small blisters on the skin.

shock. In medicine it usually means the rapid and sometimes fatal fall in blood pressure following injury (for example, a blow on the head), operation, or administration of anesthesia. The term shock is also used to designate *electric shock* given in some cases of mental illness. *Psychic shock* refers to emotional reaction to a sudden, shocking event.

"shots." Popular term for injections.

sign. Any objective evidence of a disease condition. Signs, in contrast to *symptoms,* can be seen, heard, felt, or even smelled by the examiner.

silicosis. An occupational disease of the lung caused by long-time inhalation of stone or sand dust.

sinusitis. Inflammation of a sinus; generally refers to the sinuses of the nose.

sleeping pills. Usually barbiturate drugs. Overdoses can be fatal.

sleeping sickness. Occurs as the result of some damage or disorder in the brain. Most commonly refers to African sleeping sickness, transmitted from domestic and wild animals to man through the bite of the *tsetse fly* and similar insects.

smog. A fog made heavier, darker, and irritating to the eyes by the smoke emitted from a city's smoke stacks and also by exhaust fumes from motor vehicles.

socialized medicine. A system of medical practice in which all physicians are employed by the state and all people in the state have the right to medical help without direct payment of a fee for service.

soma. Taken from the Greek word meaning "body" and used in contrast to *psyche,* or mind.

somnambulist. Sleep-walker.

spastic. Marked by muscle spasms; involuntary, repeated contractions of any set of muscles. A spastic child or adult is usually one whose rigid, stiff muscles or awkward muscular movements reflect some brain damage.

specimen. A sample for further study or medical laboratory examination; frequently refers to small sample of urine.

sperm. The fully developed male sex cell formed in the testes and capable of fertilizing the female ovum.

spirochete. A cork-screw shaped microorganism; such as the pale spirochete (*Treponema pallida*) that causes syphilis.

staphyloccus. Often abbreviated to "staph," this is the general name for a particular group of round, ball-shaped bacteria that grow in bunches like a cluster of grapes.

sterility. Barrenness; inability to bear or sire children. May be relative, not absolute.

sterilization. (1) The process of making surgical instruments and dressings completely free of germs by autoclaving under steam. (2) It also means making an individual incapable of further reproduction, often by simple surgical procedure.

stethoscope. An instrument that enables the physician to hear better what is taking place inside the body, by conducting sound.

stimulant. A drug that excites or stimulates some organ or part of the body to greater function or activity. Amphetamines and caffeine, for example, stimulate the central nervous system.

strabismus. Squint; cross-eye or wall-eye.

streptoccocus. Often abbreviated to "strep," this is the name for a class of dangerous microbes associated with several serious illnesses; for example, sore throat and rheumatic fever.

streptomycin. An antibiotic isolated from a soil mold.

stress. Pressure, physical or mental, usually persistent, that leads to the development of the stress syndrome.

stroke. Any sudden, severe attack of illness; usually an apopletic stroke, or apoplexy. This condition is caused by the breaking or clogging of a blood vessel in the brain.

"student's disease." *See* **infectious mononucleosis.**

subcutaneous. Under the skin.

sublimation. The directing, channelizing, and converting of basic drives and instincts into personally satisfying, socially acceptable, and useful activities.

sulfa drugs. A great number of powerful germ-fighting drugs, all of which (such as sulfanilamide) contain in some combination the chemical group called a sulfonamide radical which includes sulfur.

superego. Roughly, the conscience, in particular, the unconscious censor of an individual's thought, feeling, and action. It partially controls the ego.

suture. (1) Threadlike material, such as catgut, wire, silk, or cotton thread, for sewing up a wound. (2) Suture also describes the lines where the bones of the skull join together.

symptom. Subjective evidence of disease; something the patient feels but the doctor cannot see; for example, a headache.

synapse. The "spark" by which nerve impulses jump from one neuron to another.

syndrome. A set of signs and symptoms which, taken together, often point to the diagnosis of a specific illness.

syphilis. A contagious venereal disease, caused by a microorganism (*Treponema pallidum*), almost always transmitted by sexual intercourse. It leads to many structural and skin lesions if unchecked; but is curable with massive doses of antibiotics.

syphilophobia. Exaggerated and abnormal fear of syphilis.

systole. The short period of time when the heart muscle contracts to force blood through the arteries. This is the moment when blood pressure is at its highest in all the arteries in the body. Readings of blood pressure at these moments are also at their highest. When the heart is not in systole (working) it is in *diastole* (at rest).

taboo. Forbidden.

tachycardia. Rapid heart beat; usually over 100 beats per minute.

tampon. A plug of cotton or other absorbent material introduced into a body cavity to stop bleeding or soak up secretions. Tampons are safely and comfortably inserted into the vagina to absorb menstrual flow.

tendons. The glistening white connective tissues in which muscle fibers end and which attach the muscles to bones or other body organs. The *Achilles tendon* runs from the calf muscle of the leg to the heelbone.

testes. The male sex organs suspended in the sac of the scrotum at the groin outside the abdominal cavity.

testosterone. Male sex hormone.

tetanus. *See* **lockjaw.**

tetany. A disease state, marked by muscular twitching, tremors, spasms, and cramps. It can be traced to a fall in the amount of calcium in the blood stream. *Not* the same as tetanus.

thalamus. A part of the brain, situated at its base; the main relay station for sensory nerve impulses to the higher centers of the cerebrum.

thalidomide. A drug once commonly used in Europe as a tranquilizer or sedative. It was later discovered to produce fetal damage (deformed infants) if taken by a pregnant woman.

therapy. A technical word for treatment by any means.

thiamine. Part of the vitamin B complex.

thorax. The chest cavity, reaching from the neck to the abdomen.

thrombosis. Means the clogging of a blood vessel as a result of the formation of a blood clot within the vessel itself. When a thrombus breaks off from the site where it was formed and enters the blood stream, it is called an *embolus*.

thymus gland. An accessory gland, in the chest, whose function is not really known. It is sometimes considered an endocrine gland, but it wastes away during childhood.

thyroid glands. The two endocrine glands in the neck that secrete the hormone, thyroxin. When they are enlarged, they produce the condition called goiter.

thyroxin. The hormone secreted by the thyroid gland. It partially controls body metabolism.

tic. A twitching of muscles, especially of the face, constantly repeated.

"tired blood." Anemia.

tissue. A collection of body cells of the same kind in sufficient quantity to form a definable part of the anatomy; for example, skin tissue.

tolbutamide. Oral drug for treatment of mild forms of diabetes.

tolerance. The ability of the human body or other living organisms, notably microbes, to resist successfully the anticipated effects of drugs, poisons, or other stress.

tonometer. Instrument for determining the pressure inside the eyeball; useful in detecting early glaucoma.

tonsillectomy. Surgical removal of tonsils by snare, knife or electrocoagulation; the most common surgical operation.

torticollis. Wry-neck; head twisted on shoulders.

toxemia. Poisoning by way of the blood stream, usually from toxins (poisons) released by microbes. Toxemia also occurs in pregnancy, for reasons still uncertain.

toxicology. The scientific study of poisons and their antidotes.

toxin. A poison.

trachoma. A serious eye disease; a form of conjunctivitis.

traction. Pulling, drawing, or stretching action. It often refers to methods for setting broken bones.

tranquilizer. A drug which acts on the emotional state to calm without affecting clarity of consciousness.

trauma. An injury or wound to living tissue. *Birth trauma* means injury in the process of being born. In psychiatry, this may imply that being born is in itself a traumatic experience. *Psychic trauma* is an emotional shock that makes a lasting impression on the conscious or unconscious mind.

tremor. Involuntary shaking, trembling, or quivering of any part of the body or of the body as a whole.

"trench mouth." Vincent's infection; inflammation of the gums with ulcerations that may also extend to the tonsils.

trichinosis. A disease caused by infestation with a hairlike parasite, *Trichinella spiralis.* The infestation is transmitted from pigs to man by the eating of insufficiently cooked pork or pork products.

trypanosome. A protozoan (comparatively large) microorganism which infects the blood stream to cause a disease such as sleeping sickness.

tsetse fly. The insect carrier of African sleeping sickness.

tubercle. A nodule or small rounded mass sometimes found on the skin, bones, or in the lungs; especially the characteristic little nodule found in the lungs in the presence of tuberculosis.

tuberculosis. An infectious disease caused by the presence of the tubercle bacillus in the lungs (and sometimes other parts of the body).

tumor. New growth in the body of useless cells, benign or malignant (cancerous).

typanic membrane. Ear drum.

typhoid fever. A serious communicable disease caused by infection with a specific microbe (*Salmonella typhosa*). The disease, sometimes called an intestinal fever, is spread through the excretion of the microbe in feces (bowel movements).

typhus. Describes a large class of diseases (fevers) caused by microbes called *rickettsia.* They are all transmitted from man to man or from animal to man by insects (ticks).

ulcer, peptic. Open lesions in the stomach or duodenum.

ultraviolet rays. They are the electromagnetic radiations that occur beyond the violet end of the visible spectrum (rainbow) of light.

unconscious mind. The hidden, buried, and temporarily forgotten part of the human mind. Here occur the conflicts between its three parts (or constructs); the id (instincts), the ego (self) and the superego (conscience). This theoretical construct of the unconscious mind is central to *psychoanalysis.*

undulant fever. Also called Malta fever and brucellosis; perhaps the most common animal disease transmitted to man.

urea. The nitrogen-containing chemical substance which is the chief end-product of the decomposition of protein foodstuffs in the human or animal body. It is present in blood, lymph, and especially urine.

uremia. Poisoning by accumulation in the blood stream of waste products like *urea* that should normally be passed off into the urine by the kidneys.

urinalysis. Examination of patient's urine as an aid in detecting and diagnosing disease.

urticaria. Hives; an allergic reaction of the skin characterized by elevated white, pink, or red patches, which often itch.

uterus. Womb: the chief female sex organ.

vaccination. Immunization against specific diseases by inoculation, injection, or ingestion (oral vaccines) of any product of biologic origin designed to prevent or alleviate those diseases. Originally vaccination meant only inoculation with cowpox to prevent smallpox.

vaccine. Any biological material administered to protect against microbial invasion or damage. The vaccines are usually attenuated forms of the microbes against which they protect. They may confer brief or long-lasting immunity against the specific microbes which cause such diseases. There are about a dozen successful vaccines now available (polio, smallpox, diphtheria, yellow fever, measles, mumps, whooping cough, lockjaw, cholera, typhoid, paratyphoid fever, and rabies).

vagina. The birth canal and female organ of sexual intercourse.

valve. Usually refers to the structures of the heart and veins which keep blood from flowing the wrong way.

varicose veins. Dilated or swollen veins. The veins of the legs are by far the most commonly affected.

vascular. Relating to the blood vessels.

"V. D." Venereal disease.

vector. Anything that carries and thus tends to spread a specific disease. For example, malaria is carried by the *Anopheles* mosquito.

vein. Any blood vessel leading to the heart.

venereal disease. Diseases spread primarily by sexual intercourse; notably syphilis, gonorrhea, and chancroid.

ventral. Bellyside or frontside; the opposite of *dorsal* or backside.

vertebrae. The odd shaped bones that, piled one on top of the other, make up the spinal column or backbone. The adult human has 26 vertebrae.

vertigo. Dizziness; the sensation that the environment is revolving around you.

vessel. In medicine it means blood vessel; vein or artery.

veterinary medicine. The diagnosis, treatment, and prevention of disease in animals.

virus. A tiny parasite living, growing, and reproducing its kind inside a host cell. Viruses are the smallest of microbes. When viruses damage or destroy the host cells they invade, they produce virus diseases; for example, polio, smallpox, and rabies.

viscera. Internal organs of the abdomen and chest.

vitamins. Organic chemical substances, widely distributed in natural foodstuffs, that are essential to normal metabolic function in man, lower animals, and birds. Vitamins, also called accessory food factors, are needed only in small amounts, but lack of this necessary amount results in a vitamin deficiency disease (avitaminosis). Examples are scurvy, rickets, beriberi, and pellagra.

voyeurism. Sexual satisfaction through merely seeing sexual organs or watching sex acts.

Wassermann test. A blood test for detecting the presence and severity of syphilitic infections.

WHO. World Health Organization.

x-rays. Electromagnetic waves of very short wavelength. They have the property of (1) penetrating solids to produce an image on sensitized film or screen, and (2) in large doses, inducing certain chemical changes in living tissue that are beneficial in the treatment of malignant diseases. Wilhelm Conrad Roentgen, their discover in 1895, named them "x-rays," although in his honor they are now frequently called roentgen rays.

yaws. A tropical disease caused by a spirochete (*Treponema pertenue*).

yellow fever. An acute virus disease carried by mosquitoes and marked by fever, albuminuria, and jaundice (which gives a yellow color to the skin of the victim).

zoonoses. Animal diseases that can be transmitted to man.

zygote. A fertilized ovum in its earliest stages.

ACKNOWLEDGMENTS

Every book is the product of many minds and hands. I wish in this place to express sincerest thanks and make most grateful acknowledgment for assistance to the many individuals and organizations who have contributed in one way or another, mainly through critical reviews of material or by permission to quote them, to the completion of this book and its previous editions.

For critical reviews of material that appears in this book either in original or revised form, I want to thank:

Maurice Irvine, Ph.D., professor of English at Sarah Lawrence College, Bronxville, N. Y.*

Louis J. Peterson, Ph.D., San Jose State College, San Jose, Calif.

Ella Harris, M.D.; Sherwin Kaufman, M.D.: Rudolf Ekstein, Ph.D.; Marie Coleman; Richard G. Thurston, Ph.D.; Ralph Sikes, M.D.; Norman Goldsmith, M.D.*; David B. Kimmelman, M.D.; Ruth Frankel, Ph.D.; Clarence Frankel, D.D.S.; Perry Sandell* (American Dental Association); William J. Plunkert and Terence J. Boyle (National Council on Alcoholism); Laurence Wyatt and Henry Van Zyle Hyde, M.D. (Division of International Health, U.S. Public Health Service.

For introductions and forewords to this and previous editions of *Healthier Living:*

William Hammond, M.D., Editor of the *New York State Journal of Medicine.*

John E. Sawhill, M.D., formerly University Physician, New York University.

Howard R. Craig, M.D., Director Emeritus of the New York Academy of Medicine.

For original artwork: Robert A. Jones; Louise Bush, Ph.D.

*Deceased.

For permission to use and quote specific material in the text, credit goes to the following organizations and individuals:

The American Association for Health, Physical Education and Recreation, for permission to quote from its committee report entitled "The Role of Exercise in Physical Fitness."

American Journal of Public Health, for extracts from "Evaluation of Development in Contraceptive Technology," by Howard C. Taylor, Jr., M.D., published in the January 1966 supplement.

The American Medical Association, for permission to reprint quotations from the *Journal of the American Medical Association* and the *A.M.A. Archives of Neurology and Psychiatry;* and also the A.M.A. Communications Division, News Department, for specific information on physicians and hospitals and news releases on a variety of subjects.

Harper and Brothers, for a selection from *The Mind in the Making* by James Harvey Robinson. Copyright 1921 by Harper and Brothers; copyright 1949 by Bankers Trust Company.

Houghton Mifflin Company, for permission to quote from *Silent Spring* by Rachel Carson.

J. P. Lippincott Company, for an extract from *Sex, Marriage and Family* by Thurman B. Rice.

Metropolitan Life Insurance Company for permission to use its height-weight tables, reprinted herein under caption "What Should You Weigh?"

National Council of Churches of Christ in the United States of America, for extracts from *Christian Marriage,* copyright, 1952, National Council of Churches; also from *Social Ideals of the Churches,* published by the Federal Council of Churches.

National Research Council, Food and Nutrition Board, for permission to reprint the "Table of Recommended Daily Dietary Allowances, Revised 1968.

Random House, for an extract from *Mind and Body: Psychosomatic Medicine* by H. Flanders Dunbar, copyright 1947.

Saturday Review, for permission to quote observations by Dr. Sarah Gibson Blanding from the issue of May 31, 1958. Permission also from Dr. Blanding, president of Vassar College.

W. B. Saunders Company, for extracts from *Sexual Behavior in the Human Male* by Alfred C. Kinsey, et al. (permission also from Dr. Kinsey and Dr. Paul C. Gebhard), and also from *Introduction to Medical Biometry and Statistics,* third edition, by Raymond Pearl.

Union of American Hebrew Congregations, for excerpts from *Judaism and Marriage* by Rabbi Felix Levy; and from *Wife of Thy Youth,* by Rabbi Stanley R. Brav.

The publisher and I wish to express our gratitude to the respondents to our surveys, whose helpful comments and suggestions have materially aided in shaping this book.

Justus J. Schifferes, PH.D.

INDEX